JOINT MOTION AND FUNCTION ASSESSMENT

A Research-Based
Practical Guide

JOINT MOTION AND FUNCTION ASSESSMENT

A Research-Based Practical Guide

Hazel M. Clarkson, M.A., B.P.T.
Formerly Assistant Professor, Department of Physical Therapy,
Faculty of Rehabilitation Medicine, University of Alberta,
Edmonton, Alberta, Canada

Photography by **Jacques Hurabielle**, Ph.D., and **Sandra Bruinsma**
Illustrations by **Heather K. Doy**, B.A., B.F.A.,
Joy D. Marlowe, M.A., C.M.I., and **Kimberly Battista**

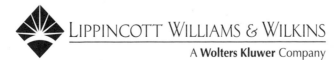

LIPPINCOTT WILLIAMS & WILKINS
A **Wolters Kluwer** Company

Philadelphia · Baltimore · New York · London
Buenos Aires · Hong Kong · Sydney · Tokyo

Editor: Pamela Lappies
Managing Editors: Linda Napora and Andrea M. Klingler
Marketing Manager: Mary Martin
Production Services: Maryland Composition
Printer: Courier Kendallville

Library of Congress Cataloging-in-Publication Data

Clarkson, Hazel M.
  Joint motion and function assessment : a research-based practical guide / Hazel M. Clarkson ; photography by Jacques Hurabielle and Sandra Bruinsma ; illustrations by Heather K. Doy, Joy D. Marlowe, and Kimberly Battista.
      p. ; cm.
  Includes bibliographical references and index.
  ISBN 0-7817-4061-4 (alk. paper)
  1. Musculoskeletal system—Diseases—Diagnosis. 2. Joints—Range of motion—Measurement. 3. Muscle strength—Measurement. I. Title.
  [DNLM: 1. Range of Motion, Articular. 2. Joints—physiology. 3. Movement. 4. Muscles—physiology. 5. Physical Examination—methods. WE 300 C613j 2005]
RC925.7.C52 2005
616.7'075—dc22

                                                                    2005016552

To my wonderful and supportive family:
my husband, Capt. Hans Longerich;
my parents, Dr. and Mrs. Graham; June Clarkson;
and all other members of my family
who are very close to my heart:
Wendy Carter, Ron Clarkson, Bruce Clarkson,
Simonne Longerich, Walter Longerich, and
Ryan, Scott, Christine, and Curt Carter,
who all kept enthusiastically asking:
"Is the book not done yet?"

Preface

Valid and reliable assessment and measurement of joint range of motion (ROM) and the ability to relate the findings to function are important clinical skills in the practice of physical and occupational therapy. This book was created in response to the need for an in-depth joint ROM textbook—one that balances academic and practical requirements for optimal clinical application of joint ROM assessment and measurement. My previous textbook, *Musculoskeletal Assessment: Joint Range of Motion and Manual Muscle Strength*, published in 2000, includes the assessment and measurement of joint ROM and the evaluation of muscle strength using manual muscle testing. The joint ROM section of that textbook served as a starting point for the development of *Joint Motion and Function Assessment: A Research-Based Practical Guide*, which provides a more in-depth research-based look at the assessment and measurement of joint ROM.

Organization

This book is divided into three sections. **Section I** includes Chapters 1 and 2 and discusses principles and methods, and the comparison of joint ROM assessment and treatment methods. Chapter 1 discusses the factors pertinent to evaluation of joint ROM, including the evaluation of muscle length. The methods used to assess ROM are based on the principles of assessment, articular function, and movement. A firm foundation of the principles, methods, and associated terminology presented in this chapter is necessary for the specific techniques presented in subsequent chapters.

Although the guidelines for diagnosis and treatment protocols are beyond the scope of this text, Chapter 2 links the procedures used to assess deficiencies in active range of motion (AROM), passive range of motion (PROM), and muscle length with the procedures (used when appropriate) to treat these deficiencies. Through descriptions and illustrations, the reader is provided with an overview of the similarities and differences between clinical assessments presented in Chapters 3 through 9 and similar treatments. Understanding the links between assessment and treatment facilitates the learning of these skills and is essential to integrate patient assessment and treatment in the clinical setting.

Section II, Chapters 3 through 9, focuses on the specific techniques of ROM evaluation of the extremities, temporomandibular joints, and spine. Each chapter is devoted to a specific joint complex and all are organized in the same format.

Through illustration, description, and practice the reader is provided with the knowledge and practical instruction required to gain proficiency in the clinical skills of assessment and measurement of AROM, PROM, and muscle length. These skills and knowledge are essential for the reader to accurately assess a patient's present status and plan treatment, and to assess the patient's progress, the effectiveness of the treatment program, and the patient's ability to perform ADLs.

In the final section of each chapter, the specific function of the joint complex is described and the functional ROM at the joint is documented. Emphasis is placed on the ranges required for performance of daily activities. Through knowledge of the ROM required in daily activities, the therapist is able to elicit meaningful information from the joint ROM assessment findings. The therapist links the assessment findings with the patient's ability to perform daily activities and, in conjunction with other physical assessment measures, plans an appropriate treatment plan to restore or maintain function.

Section III includes the appendices. Appendix A contains a Sample Numerical Recording Form for Joint ROM measurement used to record ROM findings. Appendix B, an adjunct to Chapter 9, provides more in-depth summaries of the validity and reliability research of selected instruments used to measure AROM of the temporomandibular joint and spine. Reading the summaries, the reader should be able to better appreciate the context within which the summaries in Chapter 9 are made. However, reading the research literature firsthand is ideal. After reviewing the validity and reliability data, the need for a planned research approach to identify the most valid tools and reliable methods to evaluate joint ROM becomes evident.

Appendix C provides a summary of "preferred" and "alternate" patient positioning for the assessment and measurement of joint ROM and selected tests of muscle length. With this summary, the reader is provided with the knowledge essential to performing an organized and efficient evaluation of joint ROM and avoiding unnecessary patient position changes and fatigue.

Appendix D is a summary of the joint ROM requirements of normal gait.

The Practical Test Forms in Appendix E include the criteria, presented in a chart/checklist format, for the clinical skills of assessment and measurement of joint ROM and muscle length. During the practice of joint ROM assessment and measurement skills, the Practical Test Forms are helpful in evaluating proficiency.

Appendix F is the Answer Guide for the chapter Questions and Exercises, to be used to assist the reader in successfully completing the learning process.

Appendices A, E, and F should be used in conjunction with Chapters 3 through 9.

Features

Joint Motion and Function Assessment: A Research-Based Practical Guide includes many helpful features, which have been added to enhance the reader's understanding and ability to apply knowledge and skills clinically. They include:

- Chapter Rationales and Objectives
- In-depth descriptions of articulations and movements at each joint complex
- An introduction to arthrokinematics
- Reviews of validity and reliability research and summaries of data for the different tools and methods that can be used to measure joint ROM at different joints
- Description and illustration of the application of inclinometers (i.e., the standard inclinometer, OB "Myrin" Goniometer, and the CROM) to measure joint ROM
- Illustrations of the anatomical structures that must be palpated to perform reliable measures of joint ROM; alignment of the universal goniometer and position of the therapist's hands in relation to the deep anatomical structures with the patient in the positions used to measure joint ROM; and anatomical structures that normally limit joint motion and the motion(s) limited identified
- Description of the most common methods of recording ROM, including the SFTR method, with examples illustrating the recording of joint ROM using numerical and pictorial ROM recording forms
- Joint ROM requirements for activities of daily living (ADLs) are presented in table format for easy reference
- Summary of patient positioning to encourage the organization of a streamlined approach to assessing and measuring joint ROM and muscle length
- Questions and Exercises and the accompanying Answer Guide to facilitate learning of the theoretical and practical components of joint ROM assessment and measurement

- Practical Testing Evaluation Forms that include the criteria for the assessment and measurement of joint ROM and muscle length, presented in a chart/checklist format

Reliability and Validity

Reliability and validity are important clinical issues when evaluating joint ROM. The most immediate means of improving reliability in clinical practice techniques is to ensure clinicians are well trained and practiced in the techniques. To this end, emphasis is placed on the need for standardized and consistent application of joint ROM assessment and measurement techniques. Becoming proficient in the clinical skills of joint ROM assessment and measurement requires knowledge, attention to detail, and practice of the physical skills.

Throughout the book, extensive use is made of illustrations and photographs. These are intended to help the reader visualize and develop an intuitive sense regarding the ROM evaluation techniques and to facilitate the learning and practice of reliable joint ROM evaluation. *Joint Motion and Function: A Research-Based Practical Guide* also provides an understanding of similar treatments and sets high standards of clinical evaluation of joint ROM.

It is my intent to provide physical and occupational therapists with a research-based practical approach to reliably assess and measure ROM and identify when these clinical findings affect a patient's health and/or function. Learning a clinical skill requires both classroom and clinical environments; therefore, the presentation style used in this book will serve as a useful adjunct to self-directed learning in these environments.

Joint Motion and Function Assessment: A Research-Based Practical Guide serves as a guide to the evaluation of joint ROM, including muscle length and functional ROM. The content was written with the assumption that the reader possesses prerequisite knowledge of musculoskeletal system anatomy. This textbook is primarily intended for students in physical and occupational therapy programs, regardless of the academic level of entry to the professions, since the study of the evaluation of joint ROM remains the same. Because of the presentation style, this textbook will also serve as a useful clinical reference for the practicing therapist.

Hazel M. Clarkson

Acknowledgments

I wish to thank those who assisted with the successful completion of this book. The visuals created for this textbook would not have been possible without the contributions of several talented individuals. For the production of photographs, a special thanks to Dr. Jacques Hurabielle. Thanks also to Sandra Bruinsma and Kelly Redinger for assisting with additional photographs for the text. Troy Lorenson and Ron Clarkson, with never ending patience, served as excellent models. My thanks to Sandra Hanington, Service Manager Medical Services, Worker's Compensation Board of Alberta, for providing the inclinometers for the measurement of spinal ROM. For the artwork, three talented artists, Kim Battista, Heather Doy, and Joy Marlowe created unique illustrations to facilitate learning and enable the reader to "visualize" the deep anatomy when applying clinical techniques.

Ian Trenholm, Liza Burgess, and Alison Webster were most helpful in collecting the literature while also managing their busy physical therapy studies. Ron Clarkson also assisted with further literature searches.

Critiques of one's work is essential to promote excellence. I thank all colleagues who provided reviews, suggestions, and encouragement. To Wendy Brook, Physical Therapist at the Glenrose Rehabilitation Hospital, many thanks for generously sharing time, expertise, and enthusiasm in reviewing my early manuscripts. Thanks also to Ruth Moellenbeck, Occupational Therapist and President of Moellenbeck Consulting, and to Rita Koenig, Staff Physical Therapist at Capital Health Home Care and the Cross Cancer Institute, for sharing their perspectives, expertise, and opinions. I am so glad to be able to thank George Beneck, Rachel Diamant, Suzy Dougherty, Ruth Freeman, Nancy Gann, Mary Hudak, Joy Karges, and Kelly Sass for their reviews of the text.

I thank Florence Kendall for inviting me to participate in the Retreat on the Standardization of Certain Musculoskeletal Tests, along with Dr. Shirley Sahrmann, Dr. Jules Rothstein, and other colleagues. This session was enlightening and reinforced my belief in the importance for the physical therapy profession to promote standardization and practice excellence in the fundamentals (e.g., evaluation of joint ROM and muscle strength).

Thanks to my former colleagues at the University of Alberta who support my work. I am also grateful to the physical therapy and occupational therapy students with whom I worked at the University of Alberta and from whom I learned so much regarding teaching and learning.

A special thank you to the reference librarians at the John W. Scott Health Sciences Library, University of Alberta, for their continuing ever-accommodating assistance.

My thanks are also extended to the team at Lippincott Williams & Wilkins for being so helpful. This book would not have been possible without them. A special thanks to Linda Napora, Managing Editor, who has been so consistently helpful over the many years we have worked together. I have indeed been fortunate to have a highly respected publisher.

I thank my husband, Hans Longerich, for his patience and support during the production of this book, and for serving as a model, photography assistant, and artwork reviewer. Also, thanks to my family for the encouragement and support they have given over the years.

Reviewers

Ruth Freeman, MEd
Program Manager, PTA
Daytona Beach Community College
1200 International Speedway Blvd.
Daytona Beach, FL 32120

Nancy Gann, PT, DPT, MS, OCS
Associate Professor
University of Texas Health Science Center
3223 Howard #63
San Antonio, TX 78212

Joy Karges, PT, EdD, MS, CLT
Assistant Professor and Academic Coordinator of Clinical
    Education
University of South Dakota
USDSMHS Physical Therapy
414 E. Clark St.
Medical Arts Building, 25 S. Plum St.
Vermillion, SD 57069

Suzy Dougherty, MPT
Department of Physical Therapy
Texas State University–San Marcos
601 University Dr.
San Marcos, TX 78666

Kelley Sass, MPT
Associate and Assistant Academic Coordinator of Clinical
    Education
The University of Iowa
1-241 Medical Education Building
Iowa City, IA 52242-1190

Rachel Diamant, MS, OTR/L, BCP
Associate Professor
Arizona School of Health Sciences
5850 E. Still Circle
Mesa, AZ 85206

George Beneck, MS, PT, OCS
Lecturer
University of California at Long Beach
1250 Bellflower Blvd.
Long Beach, CA 90840

Mary Hudak, PT, MSPT
Duquesne University
106 Health Science Center
Pittsburgh, PA 15282

Contents

SECTION I

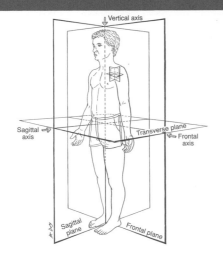

Vertical axis

Sagittal
axis

Transverse plane

Frontal
axis

Sagittal
plane

Frontal plane

Principles
and Methods

1

Chapter Rationale

Assessment and measurement of joint range of motion (ROM) are essential clinical skills in the practice of occupational and physical therapy. The methods used to assess ROM are based on the principles of assessment, articular function, and movement. A fundamental requisite to the study of evaluation of joint ROM is the knowledge of evaluation principles and methodology. This chapter discusses the factors pertinent to evaluation of ROM. A firm foundation of the principles, methods, and the terminology presented in this chapter is necessary for application of the specific techniques presented in subsequent chapters.

Chapter Objectives

Upon completion of Chapter 1: Principles and Methods, for assessing and measuring joint ROM, the reader should be able to:

- demonstrate, define, and describe (i.e., identify the axis/plane of movement) the movements at the joints in the human body.

- explain how the therapist applies osteokinematics and arthrokinematics when assessing joint ROM.

- identify when the assessment of active ROM (AROM) and passive ROM (PROM) is contraindicated or when special care should be taken.

- identify the information gained from the assessment of AROM and PROM.

- demonstrate how to assess and measure AROM using the universal goniometer.

- demonstrate how to assess and measure PROM using the universal goniometer.

- demonstrate how to assess and measure muscle length using the universal goniometer.

- identify how reliability of ROM measurement is best achieved using the universal goniometer.

- explain how the OB "Myrin" goniometer, a compass inclinometer, is designed and applied to measure joint ROM.

- identify the advantages and disadvantages of using the OB "Myrin" goniometer to measure joint ROM.

Communication

When conducting a physical assessment, introduce yourself to the patient and explain the rationale for performing the physical assessment and the component parts of the assessment process as these are carried out. Use lay terms, provide concise and easily understood explanations, speak slowly, and encourage the patient to ask questions at any time. It is essential for the patient to understand the need to expose specific regions of the body and assume different body positions for the examination, and the need to communicate any change in his or her signs and symptoms during and after the assessment procedures. Inform the patient that he or she might experience a temporary increase in symptoms following an assessment, but the symptoms should subside within a short period.

Visual Observation

Visual observation is an integral part of assessment of joint ROM. The body part being assessed should be adequately exposed for visual inspection. Throughout the initial assessment of the patient, the therapist gathers visual information that contributes to determining the patient's problems and formulating an appropriate assessment plan. Information that is gained visually includes such factors as facial expression, symmetrical or compensatory motion in functional activities, body posture, muscle contours, body proportions, and color, condition, and creases of the skin.

Palpation

Palpation is the examination of the body surface by touch. Palpation is performed to assess bony and soft tissue contours, soft tissue consistency, and skin temperature and texture. The therapist uses visual observation and palpation to "visualize" the deep anatomy (1).

Palpation is an essential skill to assess and treat patients. The therapist must be able to locate the bony landmarks to align a goniometer, tape measure, or inclinometer correctly when assessing joint ROM. To stabilize one joint surface and move the opposing joint surface to isolate movement at a joint when assessing joint ROM or mobilizing a joint, palpation is used to locate the bony segments that make up the joint. Bony landmarks are used as reference points to assess limb or trunk circumference. A therapist must be proficient in palpation to determine the presence or absence of muscle contraction when assessing strength or conducting re-education exercises. Palpation is also used to identify bony or soft tissue irregularities and to localize structures that require direct treatment.

Proficiency at palpation is gained through practice and experience. It is necessary to practice palpation on as many subjects as possible to become familiar with individual variations in human anatomy.

Palpation Technique

- The patient is made comfortable and kept warm, and the body or body part is well supported to relax the muscles. This allows palpation of deep or inert (noncontractile) structures such as ligaments and bursae.
- The therapist visually observes the area to be palpated and notes any deformity or abnormality.
- The therapist palpates with the pads of the index and middle fingers and occasionally uses the thumb pad. Fingernails should be kept short.
- The therapist's fingers are in direct contact with the skin. Palpation should not be attempted through clothing.
- To instill a feeling of security, the therapist should use a sensitive but firm touch. Prodding is uncomfortable and may elicit tension in the muscles.
- To palpate muscles and tendons, the patient isometrically contracts the muscle against resistance, followed by relaxation of the muscle. The muscle is palpated during contraction and relaxation.
- To palpate tendons, the tips of the index and middle fingers are placed across the long axis of the tendon and gently rolled forward and backward across the tendon.

Therapist Posture

When performing assessment techniques, apply biomechanical principles of posture and lifting. The therapist's posture and support of the patient's limb are described.

Posture

Stand with your head and trunk upright, feet shoulder width apart and knees slightly flexed. With one foot ahead of the other, the stance is in the line of the direction of movement. Maintaining a broad base of support attains balance and allows effective weight-shifting from one leg to the other. When performing movements that are parallel to the side of the plinth, stand beside the plinth with the leg furthest from the plinth ahead of the other leg (Fig. 1-1). When performing movements that are perpendicular to the side of the plinth, face the plinth with one foot slightly in front of the other (Fig. 1-2). When performing diagonal movements, the therapist's stance is in line with the diagonal movement and one foot is slightly ahead of the other.

Protect your lumbar spine by assuming a neutral lordotic posture (the exact posture varying based on comfort and practicality) and avoiding extreme spinal flexion or extension (2). Gain additional protection by keeping as close to the patient as possible, avoiding spinal rotation by moving the feet to turn, and using your leg muscles to perform the work by flexing and extending the joints of the lower extremity. Adjust the height of the plinth so that you can assume a neutral lordotic posture, keep close to the patient, and avoid fatigue.

Supporting the Patient's Limb

To move a limb or limb segment easily, support the part at the level of its center of gravity, located approximately at the junction of the upper and middle third of the segment (3). Ensure all joints are adequately supported when lifting or moving a limb or limb segment.

Use a relaxed hand grasp, with the hand conforming to the contour of the part, to support or lift a body part (Fig.

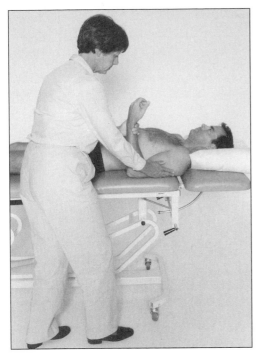

Figure 1-1 Therapist's stance when performing movements parallel to the side of the plinth.

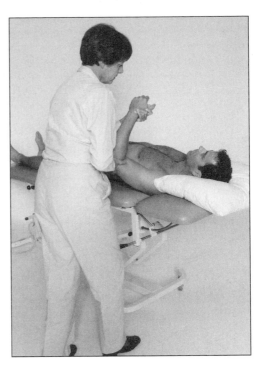

Figure 1-2 Therapist's stance when performing movements perpendicular to the side of the plinth.

1-3) (3). Give additional support by cradling the part with the forearm.

JOINT RANGE OF MOTION

Movement Description: Osteokinematics

Kinematics is the term given to the study of movement (4). *Osteokinematics* is the study of the movement of the bone in space (4). The movement of the bone is assessed, mea-

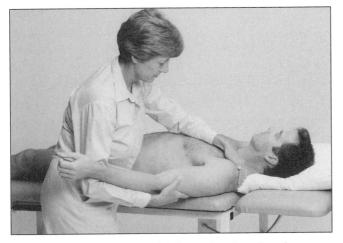

Figure 1-3 The limb supported at the center of gravity using a relaxed hand grasp.

sured, and recorded to represent the joint ROM. ROM of the joint is the amount of movement that occurs at a joint to produce movement of a bone in space. To perform AROM, the patient contracts muscle to voluntarily move the body part through the ROM without assistance. To perform PROM, the therapist or another external force moves the body part through the ROM.

To assess the ROM at a joint, the therapist must have a sound knowledge of anatomy. This includes a knowledge of joint articulations, motions, and normal limiting factors. These factors are discussed separately.

Joint Articulations and Classification

An anatomical joint or articulation is formed when two bony articular surfaces, lined by hyaline cartilage, meet (5) and movement is allowed to occur at the junction. The movements that occur at a joint are partly determined by the shape of the articular surfaces. Anatomical articulations are classified as described and illustrated in Table 1-1 (Figs. 1-4–1-10).

In addition to classifying a joint according to the anatomical relationship of the articular surfaces, a joint may also be classified as a syndesmosis or a physiological or functional joint. A *syndesmosis* is a joint in which the bones are joined together by ligaments (Fig. 1-11) (7). Movement is possible around one axis. A *physiological* (5) or *functional* (8) joint consists of two surfaces, muscle and bone (scapulothoracic joint) or bursa and bone (subdeltoid joint), moving one with respect to the other (Fig. 1-12).

TABLE 1-1   Classification of Anatomical Articulations[6]

Ball-and-socket (spheroidal)

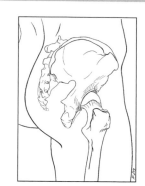

Figure 1-4 Ball-and-socket articulation (hip joint). A ball-shaped surface articulates with a cup-shaped surface; movement is possible around innumerable axes.

Hinge (ginglymus)

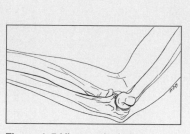

Figure 1-5 Hinge articulation (humeroulnar joint). Two articular surfaces that restrict movement largely to one axis; usually have strong collateral ligaments.

Plane

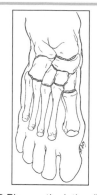

Figure 1-6 Plane articulation (intertarsal joints). This articulation is formed by the apposition of two relatively flat surfaces; gliding movements occur at these joints.

Ellipsoidal

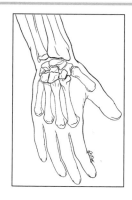

Figure 1-7 Ellipsoidal articulation (radio-carpal joint). This articulation is formed by an oval convex surface in apposition with an elliptical concave surface; movement is possible around two axes.

Saddle (sellar)

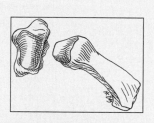

Figure 1-8 Saddle articulation (first carpometacarpal joint). Each joint surface has a convexity at right angles to a concave surface; movement is possible around two axes.

Bicondylar

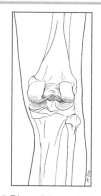

Figure 1-9 Bicondylar articulations (femorotibial joint). Most movement occurs around one axis; some degree of rotation is also possible around an axis set at 90° to the first; formed by one surface having two convex condyles, the corresponding surface having two concave reciprocal surfaces.

Pivot (trochoid)

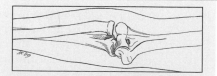

Figure 1-10 Pivot articulation (superior radioulnar joint). Formed by a central bony pivot surrounded by an osteo-ligamentous ring; movement is restricted to rotation.

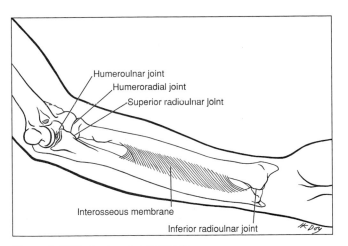

Figure 1-11 Radioulnar syndesmosis.

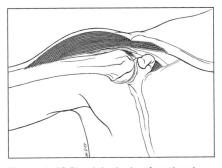

Figure 1-12 Physiological or functional joint (subdeltoid joint).

Movements: Planes and Axes

Joint movements are more easily described and understood using a coordinate system that has its central point located just anterior to the second sacral vertebra, with the subject standing in the anatomical position. The *anatomical position* is illustrated in Figures 1-13 through 1-15. The "start" positions for assessing ranges of movement described in this text are understood to be the anatomical position of the joint, unless otherwise indicated.

The coordinate system consists of three imaginary cardinal planes and axes (Fig. 1-16). This same coordinate system can be transposed so that its central point is located at the center of any joint in the body. Movement in, or parallel to, the cardinal planes occurs around the axis that lies perpendicular to the plane of movement. Table 1-2 describes the planes and axes of the body. Many functional movements occur in diagonal planes located between the cardinal planes.

Movement Terminology

Visual depiction of the following movement terminology is provided in subsequent chapters.

Angular Movements

Angular motions refer to movements that produce an increase or a decrease in the angle between the adjacent

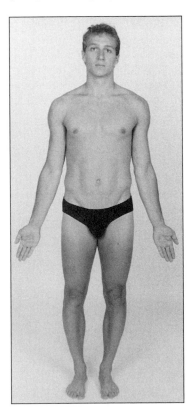

Figure 1-13 Anatomical position—anterior view. The individual is standing erect with the arms by the sides, toes, palms of the hand and eyes facing forward and fingers extended.

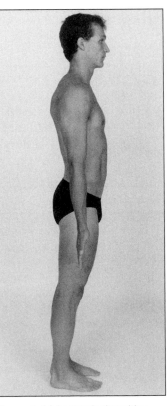

Figure 1-14 Anatomical position—lateral view.

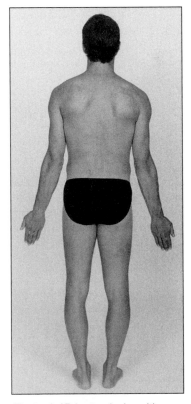

Figure 1-15 Anatomical position—posterior view.

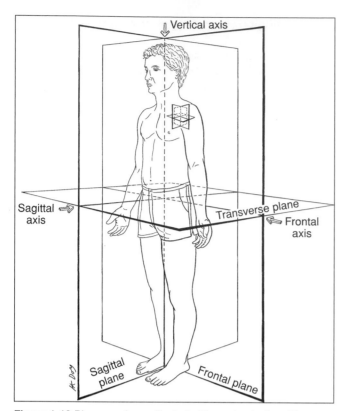

Figure 1-16 Planes and axes illustrated in anatomical position.

bones and include flexion, extension, abduction, and adduction (68).

Flexion: bending of a part so the anterior surfaces come closer together. *Special considerations*: Flexion of the thumb—the thumb moves across the palm of the hand. Knee and toe flexion—the posterior or plantar surfaces of the body parts, respectively, come closer together. Ankle flexion—when the dorsal surface of the foot is brought closer to the anterior aspect of the leg, the

movement is termed *dorsiflexion*. Lateral flexion of the neck and trunk—bending movements that occur in a lateral direction either to the right or left side.

Extension: the straightening of a part and movement is in the opposite direction to flexion movements. *Special consideration*: Ankle extension—when the plantar aspect of the foot is extended toward the posterior aspect of the leg, the movement is termed *plantarflexion*.

Hyperextension: movement that goes beyond the normal anatomical joint position of extension

Abduction: movement away from the midline of the body or body part. The midline of the hand passes through the third digit, and the midline of the foot passes through the second digit. *Special considerations*: Abduction of the scapula is referred to as *protraction* and is movement of the vertebral border of the scapula away from the vertebral column. Abduction of the thumb—the thumb moves in an anterior direction in a plane perpendicular to the palm of the hand. Abduction of the wrist is referred to as *wrist radial deviation*. Eversion of the foot—the sole of the foot is turned outward; it is not a pure abduction movement because it includes abduction and pronation of the forefoot.

Adduction: movement toward the midline of the body or body part. *Special considerations*: Adduction of the scapula, referred to as *retraction*, is movement of the vertebral border of the scapula toward the vertebral column. Adduction of the thumb—the thumb moves back to anatomical position from a position of abduction. Adduction of the wrist is referred to as *wrist ulnar deviation*. Inversion of the foot—the sole of the foot is turned inward; it is not a pure adduction movement because it includes adduction and supination of the forefoot.

Shoulder elevation: movement of the arm above shoulder level (i.e., 90°) to a vertical position alongside the

TABLE 1-2   Planes and Axes of the Body

Plane	Description of Plane	Axis of Rotation	Description of Axis	Most Common Movement
Frontal (coronal)	Divides body into anterior and posterior sections	Sagittal	Runs anterior/posterior	Abduction, adduction
Sagittal	Divides body into right and left sections	Frontal (transverse)	Runs medial/lateral	Flexion, extension
Transverse (horizontal)	Divides body into upper and lower sections	Longitudinal (vertical)	Runs superior/inferior	Internal rotation, external rotation

head (i.e., 180°). The vertical position may be arrived at by moving the arm through either the sagittal plane (i.e., shoulder flexion) or the frontal plane (i.e. shoulder abduction), and the movement is referred to as *shoulder elevation through flexion* or *shoulder elevation through abduction*, respectively. In the clinical setting, these movements may be referred to as *shoulder flexion* and *shoulder abduction*. The plane of the scapula lies 30° to 45° anterior to the frontal plane (9), and this is the plane of reference for diagonal movements of shoulder elevation. *Scaption* (10) is the term given to this midplane elevation (see Fig. 3-77).

Rotation Movements

These movements generally occur around a longitudinal or vertical axis.

Internal (medial, inward) rotation: turning of the anterior surface of a part toward the midline of the body. *Special consideration*: Internal rotation of the forearm is referred to as pronation.

External (lateral, outward) rotation: turning of the anterior surface of a part away from the midline of the body. *Special considerations*: External rotation of the forearm is referred to as supination.

Neck or trunk rotation: turning around a vertical axis to either the right or left side.

Scapular rotation: described in terms of the direction of movement of either the inferior angle of the scapula or the glenoid cavity of the scapula (Fig. 1-17).

Medial (downward) rotation of the scapula—movement of the inferior angle of the scapula toward the midline and movement of the glenoid cavity in a caudal or downward direction.

Lateral (upward) rotation of the scapula—movement of the inferior angle of the scapula away from the midline and movement of the glenoid cavity in a cranial or upward direction.

Circumduction: a combination of the movements of flexion, extension, abduction, and adduction.

Opposition of the thumb and little finger: the tips of the thumb and little finger come together.

Reposition of the thumb and little finger: the thumb and little finger return to anatomical position from a position of opposition.

Horizontal abduction (extension): occurs at the shoulder and hip joints. With the shoulder joint in 90° of either abduction or flexion, or the hip joint in 90° flexion, the arm or the thigh, respectively, is moved in a direction either away from the midline of the body or in a posterior direction.

Horizontal adduction (flexion): occurs at the shoulder and hip joints. With the shoulder joint in 90° of either abduction or flexion, or the hip joint in 90° flexion, the arm or the thigh, respectively, is moved in a direction either toward the midline of the body or in an anterior direction.

Tilt: describes movement of either the scapula or the pelvis.

Anterior tilt of the scapula—"the coracoid process moves in an anterior and caudal direction while the inferior angle moves in a posterior and cranial direction" (11, p 303).

Posterior tilt of the scapula—the coracoid process moves in a posterior and cranial direction while the inferior angle of the scapula moves in an anterior and caudal direction.

Anterior pelvic tilt—the anterior superior iliac spines of the pelvis move in an anterior and caudal direction.

Posterior pelvic tilt—the anterior superior iliac spines of the pelvis move in a posterior and cranial direction.

Lateral pelvic tilt—movement of the ipsilateral iliac crest in the frontal plane either in a cranial direction (elevation or hiking of the pelvis) or in a caudal direction (pelvic drop).

Shoulder girdle elevation: movement of the scapula and lateral end of the clavicle in a cranial direction.

Shoulder girdle depression: movement of the scapula and lateral end of the clavicle in a caudal direction.

Hypermobility: an excessive amount of movement; joint ROM that is greater than the normal ROM expected at the joint.

Hypomobility: a reduced amount of movement; joint ROM that is less than the normal ROM expected at the joint.

Passive insufficiency of a muscle occurs when the length of a muscle prevents full ROM at the joint or joints that the muscle crosses over (Fig. 1-18) (12).

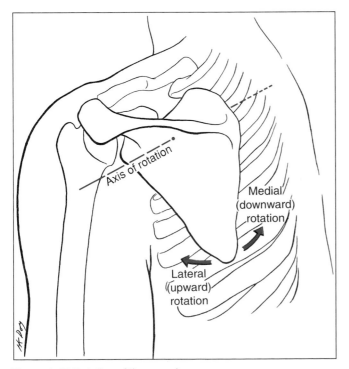

Figure 1-17 Rotation of the scapula.

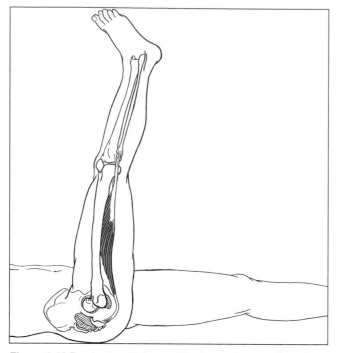

Figure 1-18 Passive insufficiency of the hamstring muscles. Hip flexion ROM is limited by the length of the hamstring muscles when the knee joint is held in extension.

Arthrokinematics

The study of movement occurring within the joints, between the articular surfaces of the bones, is called *arthrokinematics* (4). Arthrokinematic motion can be observed and determined indirectly through observation of bone movement when assessing active and passive joint ROM and with the knowledge of the shape of the articular surfaces.

Joints are classified on the basis of the general form of the joint (see Table 1-1). Regardless of the classification of a joint, the shape of all articular surfaces of synovial joints is, to varying degrees, either concave or convex, even for articulations classified as plane (4). All joint surfaces are either convex or concave in all directions, as in the hip joint (see Fig. 1-4) (i.e., the head of the femur is convex and the acetabulum is concave), or sellar (i.e., saddle-shaped). The saddle-shaped surface has a convexity at right angles to a concave surface, as in the first carpometacarpal joint (i.e., formed by the surface of the trapezium and base of the first metacarpal) (see Fig. 1-8). At all joints convex articular surfaces mate with corresponding concave surfaces.

When movement occurs at a joint, two types of articular motion—glide (i.e., slide) and roll—are present (4). Both glide and roll occur together in varying proportions to allow normal joint motion. *Glide* is a translatory motion that occurs when a point on one joint surface contacts new points on the opposing surface. Glide at a joint is analogous to a car tire sliding over an icy surface

when the brakes are applied. *Roll* occurs when new points on one joint surface contact new equidistant points on an opposing joint surface. Roll is analogous to a car tire rolling over the ground.

According to Kaltenborn (13), decreased motion at a joint is due to decreased glide and roll, with glide being the more significant motion that is restricted. In the presence of decreased joint ROM due to decreased joint glide, an appropriate treatment plan to restore normal motion is determined based on the therapist's knowledge of the normal direction of glide at the joint for the limited joint movement. The therapist determines the normal glide that occurs at a joint for a specific movement by knowing the direction of movement of the bone during the AROM or PROM and the shape of the moving articular surface, and applying the concave–convex rule. The direction of bone movement is observed during the assessment of the ROM, and the shape of the articular surface is described at the beginning of each chapter. The concave–convex rule (13) states:

1. When a convex joint surface moves on a fixed concave surface, the convex joint surface glides in the opposite direction to the movement of the shaft of the bone (Fig. 1-19A). For example, during glenohumeral joint abduction ROM, the shaft of the humerus moves in a superior direction and the convex humeral articular surface moves in an inferior direction on the fixed concave surface of the scapular glenoid fossa. Therefore, restricted inferior glide of the convex humeral head would result in decreased glenohumeral joint abduction ROM.

2. When a concave joint surface moves on a fixed convex surface, the concave joint surface glides in the same direction as the movement of the shaft of the bone (see Fig. 1-19B). For example, during knee extension ROM, the shaft of the tibia moves in an anterior direction and the concave tibial articular surface moves in an anterior direction on the fixed convex femoral articular surface. Therefore, restricted anterior glide of the concave tibial articular surface would result in decreased knee extension ROM.

Arthrokinematics, specifically the glide that accompanies the bone movement for normal ROM of the extremity joints, is identified in subsequent chapters. The normal joint glide is introduced to facilitate integration of osteokinematic findings (i.e., bone movement) with arthrokinematics (i.e., the corresponding motion between the joint surfaces) when assessing and measuring ROM of the extremity joints. The techniques used to assess and restore joint glide are beyond the scope of this text.

Spin (4), the third type of movement that occurs between articular surfaces, is a rotary motion that occurs around an axis. During normal joint ROM, spin may occur alone or accompany roll and glide. Spin occurs alone during flexion and extension at the shoulder and hip joints, and pronation and supination at the humeroradial joint (Fig. 1-20). Spin occurs in conjunction with roll and glide during flexion and extension at the knee joint.

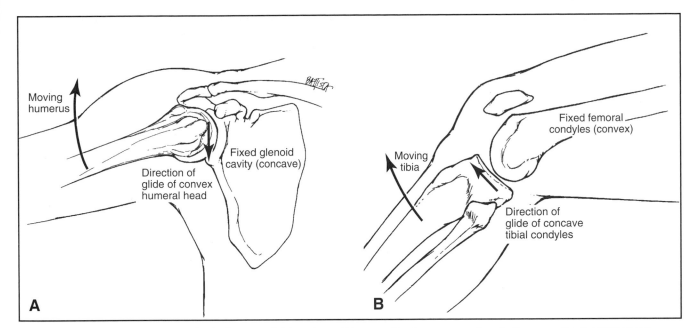

Figure 1-19 The concave–convex rule. **A.** A convex joint surface glides on a fixed concave surface in the opposite direction to the movement of the shaft of the bone. **B.** A concave joint surface glides on a fixed convex surface in the same direction to the movement of the shaft of the bone.

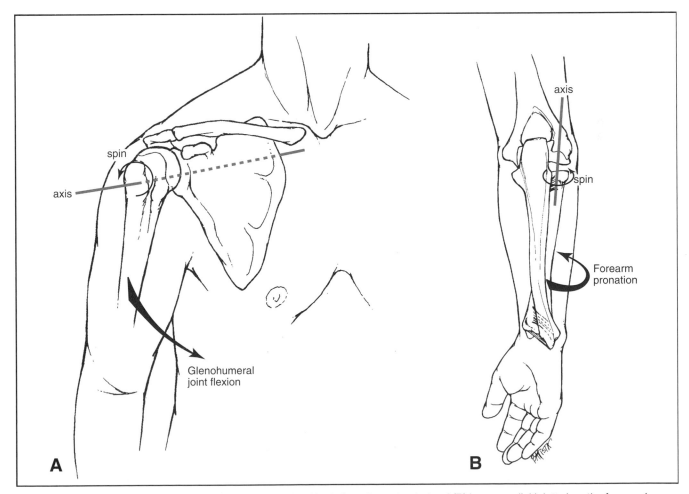

Figure 1-20 Spin at the **(A)** glenohumeral joint when the shoulder is flexed or extended and **(B)** humeroradial joint when the forearm is supinated or pronated.

ASSESSMENT AND MEASUREMENT OF JOINT RANGE OF MOTION

Contraindications and Precautions

AROM or PROM must not be assessed or measured if contraindications to this assessment exist. In special instances, the assessment techniques have to be performed with a modified approach.

Both AROM and PROM assessment techniques are contraindicated where muscle contraction (AROM) or motion (AROM and PROM) of the part could disrupt the healing process or result in injury or deterioration of the condition. Examples of this are:

1. If motion to the part will cause further damage or interrupt the healing process immediately after injury or surgery.

2. If the therapist suspects a subluxation or dislocation or fracture.

3. If myositis ossificans or ectopic ossification is suspected or present, AROM and PROM should not be undertaken without first ensuring the patient is assessed by a professional who has expertise in the management of these conditions (14).

After ensuring no contraindications to AROM or PROM exist, the therapist must take extra care when assessing AROM and PROM if movement to the part might aggravate the condition. Examples of this are:

1. In painful conditions.

2. In the presence of an inflammatory process in a joint or the region around a joint.

3. In patients taking medication for pain or muscle relaxants, because the patient may not be able to respond appropriately and movement may be performed too vigorously.

4. In the presence of marked osteoporosis or in conditions where bone fragility is a factor, perform PROM with extreme care or not at all.

5. In assessing a hypermobile joint.

6. In patients with hemophilia.

7. In the region of a hematoma, especially at the elbow, hip, or knee.

8. In assessing joints if bony ankylosis is suspected.

9. After an injury where there has been a disruption of soft tissue (i.e., tendon, muscle, ligament).

10. In the region of a recently healed fracture.

11. After prolonged immobilization of a part.

After ensuring no contraindications to AROM or PROM exist, the therapist must take extra care when performing AROM assessment where strenuous and resisted movement could aggravate or worsen the patient's condition. Examples of this are:

1. Following recent surgery of the abdomen, intervertebral disc, or eye (15); in patients with herniation of the abdominal wall; or in patients with a history of cardiovascular problems (e.g., aneurysm, fixed-rate pacemaker, arrhythmias, thrombophlebitis, recent embolus, marked obesity, hypertension, cardiopulmonary disease, angina pectoris, myocardial infarctions, and cerebrovascular disorders). These patients should be instructed to avoid the Valsalva maneuver during the assessment procedure.

Kisner and Colby (16) describe the sequence of events in the Valsalva maneuver, which consists of an expiratory effort against a closed glottis during a strenuous and prolonged effort. A deep breath is taken at the beginning of the effort and held by closing the glottis. The abdominal muscles contract, causing an increase in the intra-abdominal and intrathoracic pressures, and blood is forced from the heart, causing a temporary and abrupt rise in the arterial blood pressure. The Valsalva maneuver can be avoided by instructing the patient not to hold his or her breath during the assessment of AROM. Should this be difficult, the patient may be instructed to breathe out (17) or talk during the test (16).

2. If fatigue may be detrimental to or exacerbate the patient's condition (e.g., extreme debility, malnutrition, malignancy, multiple sclerosis, chronic obstructive pulmonary disease, or cardiovascular disease), strenuous testing should not be carried out. Signs of fatigue include complaints or observation of tiredness, pain, muscular spasm, a slow response to contraction, tremor, and a decreased ability to perform AROM.

Assessment of Active ROM

An overview or scan of the AROM available at the joints of the upper or lower limb can be attained using tests that include movement at several joints simultaneously (see Figs. 3-13, 3-14, and 6-11–6-14). For a detailed assessment of the AROM, the patient performs all of the active movements that normally occur at the affected joint(s) and at the joints immediately proximal and distal to the affected joint(s). The therapist observes as the patient performs each active movement one at a time and, if possible, bilaterally and symmetrically (Fig. 1-21). Assessment of the AROM provides the therapist with information about the patient's willingness to move, coordination, level of consciousness, attention span, joint ROM, movements that cause or increase pain, muscle strength, and ability to follow instructions and perform functional activities. AROM may be decreased due to the patient's restricted joint mobility, muscle weakness, pain, inability to follow instructions, or unwillingness to move.

In the presence of muscle weakness, the effect of gravity on the part being moved may affect the AROM. When the part is moved in a vertical plane against the force of gravity rather than in a horizontal plane when gravity is not a factor, the AROM may be less. Therefore, the thera-

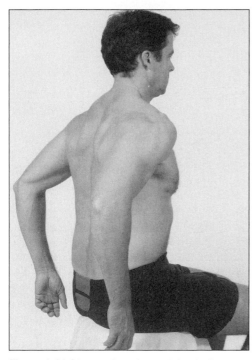

Figure 1-21 Observation of the AROM indicates the patient's willingness to move, coordination, level of consciousness, attention span, joint ROM, movements that cause or increase pain, muscle strength, and ability to follow instructions and perform functional activities.

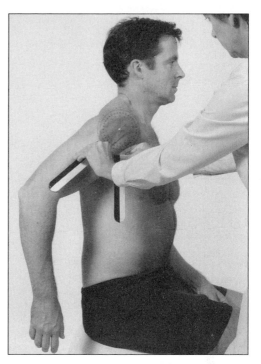

Figure 1-22 Using an instrument (e.g., universal goniometer) to measure the AROM.

pist must consider the patient's position and the effect of gravity on the movement to correctly interpret the AROM assessment findings. Although the detailed assessment of muscle strength is beyond the scope of this textbook, when manually assessing muscle strength, a grade is assigned to indicate the strength of a muscle or muscle group. The grade indicates the strength of a voluntary muscle contraction and the AROM possible relative to the existing PROM available at the joint. Therefore, the muscle grade assigned to indicate muscle strength provides a general indication of the AROM from which the therapist can also evaluate the patient's functional capability.

Active movement is used to perform functional activities. In the presence of decreased AROM, it may be difficult or impossible to perform these activities. For an objective measure of the patient's ability to perform functional activity, the therapist measures the AROM. Assessment of AROM is followed by an assessment of PROM and muscle strength.

Measurement of AROM

The measurement procedures for the universal goniometer (Fig. 1-22) and the OB "Myrin" goniometer (see Figs. 4-26 through 4-29) are described in the section on measurement of ROM (see p. 15). The measurement of AROM may use the same or different positions to those used for PROM; for example, functional positions or activities may be used to measure AROM. When the patient actively

moves through the range, emphasize the exactness of the movement to the patient so that substitute motion at other joints is avoided.

Assessment of PROM

PROM is assessed to determine the amount of movement possible at the joint. PROM is usually slightly greater than AROM owing to the slight elastic stretch of tissues and in some instances due to the decreased bulk of relaxed muscles. However, the PROM can be much greater than the AROM in the presence of muscle weakness. Taking the body segments through a PROM allows the therapist to estimate the ROM at each joint, determine the quality of the movement throughout the ROM and the end feel, note the presence of pain, and determine whether a capsular or noncapsular pattern of movement is present (see Fig. 1-23). After this assessment of the PROM, the therapist repeats the PROM to measure and record the PROM using a goniometer (Fig. 1-24).

The following concepts and terms are important to understanding joint motion restriction when assessing PROM.

Normal Limiting Factors and End Feels

The unique anatomical structure of a joint determines the direction and magnitude of its PROM. The factors that normally limit movement and determine the range of the PROM at a joint include:

The stretching of soft tissues (i.e., muscles, fascia, and skin).

The stretching of ligaments or the joint capsule.

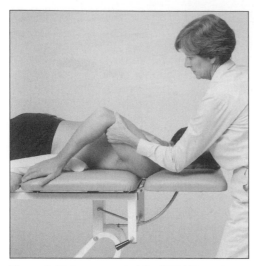

Figure 1-23 Assessment of the PROM to estimate the joint ROM, determine the end feels, establish the presence or absence of pain, and determine the presence of a capsular or noncapsular pattern of movement.

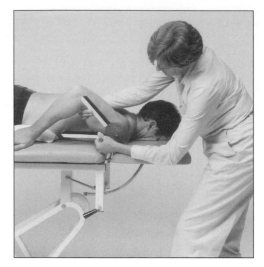

Figure 1-24 Using an instrument (e.g., universal goniometer) to measure the PROM.

The apposition of soft tissues.

Bone contacting bone.

When assessing the PROM of a joint, observe whether the range is full, restricted, or excessive, and by feel determine which structure(s) limits the movement. The end feel is the sensation transmitted to the therapist's hands at the extreme end of the PROM and indicates the structures that limit the joint movement (18). The end feel may be normal (physiological) or abnormal (pathological) (19).

A normal end feel exists when there is full PROM at the joint and the normal anatomy of the joint stops movement. An abnormal end feel exists when there is either a decreased or an increased passive joint ROM or when there is a normal PROM but structures other than the

normal anatomy stop joint movement. Normal and abnormal end feels are presented in Tables 1-3 and 1-4. The end feel(s) for joint movements are documented in subsequent chapters based on a knowledge of the anatomy of the region, clinical experience, and available references. Although several different end feels may be possible for a particular joint motion, only one end feel will be present. When several different end feels are possible at a joint, this will be indicated using a "/" between each possible end feel. For example, the end feel for elbow flexion may be soft/firm/hard (i.e., soft, firm, or hard).

Method to Assess End Feel

Movement is isolated to the joint being assessed (see Fig. 1-23). With the patient relaxed, stabilize the proximal joint segment and apply slight traction to and move the

TABLE 1-3   Normal (Physiological) End Feels[18-20]

End Feel General Terminology (Specific Terminology)	Description
Hard (Bony)	An abrupt, hard stop to movement when bone contacts bone; for example, passive elbow extension, the olecranon process contacts the olecranon fossa.
Soft (Soft tissue apposition)	When two body surfaces come together a soft compression of tissue is felt; for example, in passive knee flexion, the posterior aspects of the calf and thigh come together.
Firm (Soft tissue stretch)	A firm or springy sensation that has some give when muscle is stretched; for example, passive ankle dorsiflexion performed with the knee in extension is stopped due to tension in the gastrocnemius muscle.
(Capsular stretch)	A hard arrest to movement with some give when the joint capsule or ligaments are stretched. The feel is similar to stretching a piece of leather; for example, passive shoulder external rotation.

TABLE 1-4 Abnormal (Pathological) End Feels[18-20]

End Feel	Description
Hard	An abrupt hard stop to movement, when bone contacts bone, or a bony grating sensation, when rough articular surfaces move past one another, for example, in a joint that contains loose bodies, degenerative joint disease, dislocation, or a fracture.
Soft	A boggy sensation that indicates the presence of synovitis or soft tissue edema.
Firm	A springy sensation or a hard arrest to movement with some give, indicating muscular, capsular, or ligamentous shortening.
Springy block	A rebound is seen or felt and indicates the presence of an internal derangement; for example, the knee with a torn meniscus.
Empty	If considerable pain is present, there is no sensation felt before the extreme of passive ROM as the patient requests the movement be stopped, this indicates pathology such as an extra-articular abscess, a neoplasm, acute bursitis, joint inflammation, or a fracture.
Spasm	A hard sudden stop to passive movement that is often accompanied by pain, is indicative of an acute or subacute arthritis, the presence of a severe active lesion, or fracture. If pain is absent a spasm end feel may indicate a lesion of the central nervous system with resultant increased muscular tonus.

distal joint segment to the end of its ROM for the test movement. Traction consists of a very gentle pull applied along the longitudinal axis of the bone of the moving joint segment (13). The pull is so small that only the compression effect of the joint is released to neutralize the joint pressure (13). Apply gentle overpressure at the end of the ROM and note the end feel.

Capsular and Noncapsular Patterns

When assessing the PROM at a joint, visually estimate the available PROM for each movement at the joint, determine the end feels, and establish the presence or absence of pain (Fig. 1-23). If there is a decreased PROM, assess the *pattern of joint movement restriction*. The description of capsular and noncapsular patterns is derived from the work of Cyriax (18).

Capsular Pattern. If a lesion of the joint capsule or a total joint reaction is present, a characteristic pattern of restriction in the PROM will occur: the capsular pattern. Only joints that are controlled by muscles exhibit capsular patterns. When painful stimuli from the region of the joint provoke involuntary muscle spasm, a restriction in motion at the joint in the capsular proportions results. Each joint capsule resists stretching in selective ways; therefore, in time, certain aspects of the capsule become more contracted than others do. The capsular pattern manifests as a proportional limitation of joint motions that are characteristic to each joint; for example, the capsular pattern of the shoulder joint differs from the pattern of restriction at the hip joint. The capsular pattern at each joint is similar between individuals. Joints that rely primarily on ligaments for their stability do not exhibit capsular patterns, and the degree of pain elicited when the joint is strained at the extreme of movement indicates the severity of the total joint reaction or arthritis. The capsular pattern for each joint is provided in each chapter, with movements listed in order of restriction (most restricted to least restricted).

Noncapsular Pattern. A noncapsular pattern exists when there is limitation of movement at a joint but not in the capsular pattern of restriction. A noncapsular pattern indicates the absence of a total joint reaction. Ligamentous adhesions, internal derangement, or extra-articular lesions may result in a noncapsular pattern at the joint.

Ligamentous adhesions affect specific regions of the joint or capsule. Motion is restricted and there is pain when the joint is moved in a direction that stretches the affected ligament. Other movements at the joint are usually full and pain-free.

Internal derangement occurs when loose fragments of cartilage or bone are present within a joint. When the loose fragment impinges between the joint surfaces, the movement is suddenly blocked and there may be localized pain. All other joint movements are full and pain-free. Internal derangements occur in joints such as the knee, jaw, and elbow.

Extra-articular lesions that affect nonarticular structures, such as muscle adhesions, muscle spasm, muscle strains, hematomas, and cysts, may limit joint ROM in one direction while a full and painless PROM is present in all other directions.

Measurement of ROM

Instrumentation

A *goniometer* is an apparatus used to measure joint angles or movements (7). The goniometer chosen to assess joint ROM depends on the degree of accuracy required in the measurement, the time and resources available to the clinician, and the patient's comfort and well-being.

Radiographs, photographs, photocopies, and the use of the electrogoniometer, flexometer, or plumb line may give objective, valid, and reliable measures of ROM but are not always practical or available in the clinical setting. When doing clinical research, the therapist should investigate alternative instruments that will offer a more stringent assessment of joint ROM.

In the clinical setting, the universal goniometer (Figs. 1-25 and 1-26) is the goniometer most frequently used to measure ROM for the extremity joints. In this text, the universal goniometer is described and illustrated for the measurement of the ROM for the joints of the extremities. The OB "Myrin" goniometer (21) (OB Rehab, Solna, Sweden) (Fig. 1-27), although less commonly used in the clinic, is a useful tool and is described and illustrated for the measurement of selected ROM at the forearm, hip, knee, and ankle.

The universal goniometer, tape measure (Fig. 1-28), standard inclinometer (Fig. 1-29), and the Cervical Range-of-Motion Instrument (CROM) (22) (Performance Attainment Associates, Roseville, MN) (Fig. 1-30), are the tools used to measure spinal AROM as presented in this text. AROM measurements of the temporomandibular joints (TMJs) are performed using a ruler or calipers. These instruments and the measurement procedures employed when using these instruments to measure spinal and TMJ AROM are described and illustrated in Chapter 9.

Validity and Reliability

Validity

Validity is "the degree to which an instrument measures what it is supposed to measure" (23, p. 171). Validity indicates the accuracy of a measurement. The therapist uses a goniometer, inclinometer, or tape measure to provide measurements of the number of degrees or distance in centimeters of movement or the position of a joint. Measurements must be accurate because the results, taken to be valid representations of actual joint angles, are used to plan treatment and to determine treatment effectiveness, patient progress, and degree of disability.

Criterion-related validity is one means of assessing the accuracy of the instruments for assessing joint angles or positions. To establish this validity, the measures of the instrument being assessed are compared to the measures obtained with an instrument that is an accepted standard (criterion) for the measurement of joint angles; for example, a radiograph. When the supporting evidence from the accepted standard is collected at the same time as the measurement from the test instrument, concurrent validity can be assessed. If a close relationship is found between the measures obtained with the instrument and the accepted standard, the instrument measures are valid.

Reliability

Reliability is "the extent to which the instrument yields the same measurement on repeated uses either by the same operator (intraobserver reliability) or by different operators (interobserver reliability)" (24, p. 49). Reliability indicates the consistency of a measurement.

The therapist measures ROM and compares measurements taken over time to evaluate treatment effectiveness and patient progress. It is important for the therapist to know that joint position and ROM can be measured consistently (i.e., with minimal deviation due to measurement error). If this is possible, then in comparing ROM measurements the similarity or divergence between the measures can be relied on to indicate when a true change has occurred that is not due to measurement error or lack of measurement consistency.

The universal goniometer and OB "Myrin" goniometer are described here, along with the validity and reliability of the universal goniometer. The validity and reliability research pertaining to the tape measure/ruler, inclinometry, and the CROM is presented in Chapter 9, along with the description and application of these instruments.

Universal Goniometer

The *universal goniometer* (see Figs. 1-25 and 1-26) is a 180° or 360° protractor with one axis that joins two arms. One arm is stationary and the other arm is movable around the axis or fulcrum of the protractor. The size of universal goniometer used is determined by the size of the joint being assessed. Larger goniometers are usually used for measurement of joint range at large joints.

Validity and Reliability—Universal Goniometer. Radiographs, "the most accurate means of assessing joint motion," (25, p. 116) and photographs are accepted standards used for comparison to determine the accuracy of the universal goniometer. When the supporting evidence from the radiographs or photographs is collected at the same time as the measurement from the universal goniometer, concurrent validity can be assessed.

There has been little study of the criterion-related validity of the universal goniometer. Using x-ray bone angle measurements compared to goniometric measurements of knee joint position (26), high criterion-related validity has been found, along with disparate findings of goniometric accuracy in only a small part of the range, thought to be due to the increased complexity of movement in approaching terminal extension. Using a photographic reference standard to assess elbow joint positions, the "results indicate that relatively inexperienced raters should be able to use goniometers accurately to measure elbow position when given standardized methods to follow" (28, p. 1666).

Reliability of joint position and ROM using the universal goniometer depends on the joint being assessed but has generally been found to be good to excellent. Reliability study results indicate that:

1. The universal goniometer is more reliable than visual estimation of joint ROM (29–32).

2. The reliability of goniometric measurement varies depending on the joint and motion assessed (31,34–37).

3. Intratester reliability is better than intertester reliability; therefore, the same therapist should perform all measures when possible (29,30,33,34,37–39). Different therapists should not be used interchangeably to obtain ROM measurements on the same patient unless the intertester reliability is known (40).

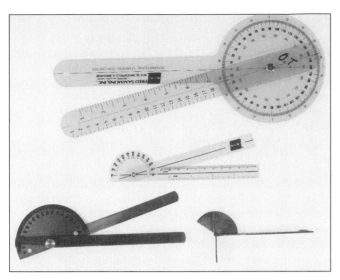

Figure 1-25 Various sizes of 180° and 360° universal goniometers.

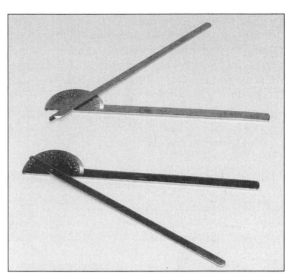

Figure 1-26 Universal goniometer with a 180° protractor. *(top)* ROM cannot be read as the cutaway portion of the movable arm is off the scale. *(bottom)* With the cutaway portion of the movable arm on the scale, the ROM can be read.

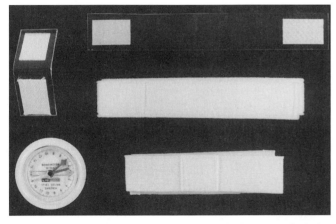

Figure 1-27 The OB goniometer, a compass/inclinometer, includes Velcro straps and plastic extension plates used to attach the goniometer to the body part being measured.

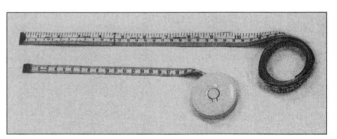

Figure 1-28 Tape measures used to measure joint ROM.

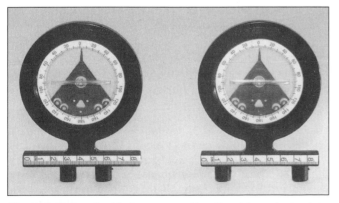

Figure 1-29 Standard inclinometers with adjustable contact points to facilitate placement on the surface of the body.

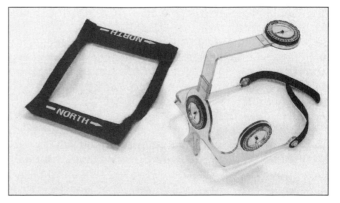

Figure 1-30 The Cervical-Range-of-Motion Instrument (CROM) consists of two gravity inclinometers, a magnetic compass inclinometer, and a magnetic yoke.

4. The size of the goniometer selected to assess ROM at a joint does not affect measurement reliability (41,42).

5. The findings are mixed on whether taking the average of repeated measures improves (30,38,43) or makes no difference to (35,36,41,44) the reliability of goniometric measures.

6. In the case of mild spastic diplegia in children, spasticity was found not to influence the intratester reliability of goniometric measurements (44); however, most researchers (45–47) conclude that reliability is low for ROM measurements in the presence of spasticity.

Joint ROM can be measured reliably using a universal goniometer when preferably the same therapist performs the repeated measures using a "rigid standardized measurement protocol" (37, p. 57) in the absence of spasticity. Miller (25) provides a method for clinicians to determine the intratester and intertester reliability within their clinical facility. Knowing the measurement error factor allows therapists to better determine patient progress.

Joint ROM Assessment and Measurement Procedure

Expose the Area

Explain to the patient the need to expose the area to be assessed. Adequately expose the area and drape the patient as required.

Explanation and Instruction

Briefly explain the ROM assessment and measurement procedure to the patient. Explain and demonstrate the movement to be performed and/or passively move the patient's uninvolved limb through the ROM.

Assessment of the Normal ROM

Initially assess and record the ROM of the uninvolved limb to determine the patient's normal ROM and normal end feels, and to demonstrate the movement to the patient before performing the movement on the involved side. If there is bilateral limb involvement, use your clinical knowledge and experience to judge the patient's normal PROM, keeping in mind that the PROM is usually slightly greater than the AROM. The therapist can use the tables of normal AROM values provided by the American Academy of Orthopaedic Surgeons (48) and the suggested normal AROM values derived from an evaluation of the research literature by Berryman Reese and Bandy (49) as a guide to normal AROM. These "normal" AROMs are presented in table form at the beginning of each chapter. "Normal" ranges can be misleading because joint ROM can vary between individuals depending on gender, age, occupation, and health status (50). Therefore, "normal" ranges should be used only as a guide when assessing and treating patients. More importantly, determine the essential functional ROM required by the patient to perform activities of daily living (ADL) and the patient's ability to meet these requirements.

Assessment and Measurement Procedure

Patient Position. Ensure that the patient is comfortable and well supported, with the joint to be assessed in the anatomical position. Position the patient so the proximal joint segment can be stabilized to allow only the desired motion, movement can occur through the full ROM unrestricted, and the goniometer can be properly placed to measure the ROM. If the patient's position varies from the standard assessment position outlined in this text, make a special note on the ROM assessment form.

Substitute Movements. When assessing and measuring AROM and PROM, ensure that only the desired movement occurs at the joint being assessed. Substitute movements may take the form of additional movements at the joint being assessed or at other joints, thus giving the appearance of having a greater joint ROM than is actually present.

When assessing and measuring AROM and PROM, try to eliminate substitute movements. For AROM this may be accomplished through adequate explanation and instruction to the patient regarding the movement to be performed and the substitute movement(s) to be avoided. Additionally, substitute motion(s) may be avoided for AROM and PROM by using proper patient positioning, adequately stabilizing the proximal joint segment as required, and acquiring substantial practice in assessing AROM and PROM. To assess joint ROM accurately the therapist must know and recognize the possible substitute movements. If the presence of substitute movements results in inaccurate AROM or PROM assessment and measurement, the treatment plan may be inappropriate.

Stabilization. Stabilize the proximal joint segment to limit movement to the joint being assessed or measured and prevent substitute movement for lack of joint range by making use of:

1. The patient's body weight (used to help stabilize the shoulder or pelvic girdles).

2. The patient's position. For instance, when assessing hip abduction ROM with the patient supine, at the end of the hip abduction ROM the pelvis may move toward the side being assessed and give the appearance of a greater range of hip abduction than actually exists. If the contralateral leg is positioned over the opposite side of the plinth with the foot resting on a stool, this leg will act to prevent the unwanted shift of the pelvis.

3. External forces (external pressure applied directly by the therapist and devices such as belts or sandbags). In stabilizing, ensure that manual contacts or devices avoid tender or painful areas; for example, in some viral diseases (i.e., poliomyelitis) muscle bellies may be tender.

Assessment of Passive Range and End Feel. Movement is isolated to the joint being assessed. With the patient relaxed, stabilize the proximal joint segment and apply slight (i.e., gentle) traction to and move the distal joint segment to the end of the PROM for the test movement (see Fig. 1-23). Apply slight (i.e., gentle) overpressure at the end of the PROM and note the magnitude of the ROM and end feel. Then return the limb to the start position.

Following the assessment of the PROM for all movements at a joint, determine the presence of a capsular or noncapsular pattern of movement.

Measurement. The method used to assess joint ROM is called the *neutral zero method* (48). All joint motions are measured from a defined zero position, either the anatomical position or a position specified as zero. Any movement on either side of zero is positive and moves toward 180°.

If the involved joint has a full AROM and PROM, the joint ROM does not have to be measured. The full ROM is recorded as full, N (normal), or WNL (within normal limits).

Measurement Procedure—Universal Goniometer

* *Goniometer placement:* The preferred placement of the goniometer is lateral to the joint, just off the surface of the limb (see Figs. 1-22 and 1-24), but it may also be placed over the joint (see Figs. 5-29 and 5-32) using only light contact between the goniometer and the skin. If joint swelling is present, placing the goniometer over the joint may give erroneous results when assessing joint ROM.
* *Axis:* The axis of the goniometer is placed over the axis of movement of the joint. A specific bony prominence or anatomical landmark can be used to represent the axis of motion, even though this may not represent the exact location of the axis of movement throughout the entire ROM.
* *Stationary arm:* The stationary arm of the goniometer usually lies parallel to the longitudinal axis of the fixed proximal joint segment and/or points toward a distant bony prominence on the proximal segment.
* *Movable arm:* The movable arm of the goniometer usually lies parallel to the longitudinal axis of the moving distal joint segment and/or points toward a distant bony prominence on the distal segment. If careful attention is paid to the correct positioning of the two goniometer arms and the positions are maintained as the joint moves through the ROM, the goniometer axis will be aligned approximately with the axis of motion (50).

The goniometer is first aligned to measure the defined zero position for the ROM at a joint. If it is not possible to attain the defined zero position, the joint is positioned as close as possible to the zero position, and the distance the movable arm is positioned away from the 0° start position on the protractor is recorded as the start position. To measure the AROM, have the patient move actively through the full AROM and either move the moveable arm at the goniometer along with the limb through the entire range of movement to the end of the AROM, or realign the goniometer at the end of the AROM. One of the following two techniques is then used to measure the PROM at a joint:

i. Have the patient actively move through the joint ROM and relax at the end of the ROM. Realign the goniometer at the end of the AROM and passively move the goniometer and the body part through the final few degrees of the PROM.

ii. Move the movable arm of the goniometer and the limb segment through the entire range of movement to the end of the PROM.

Using either technique, the distance the movable arm moves away from the 0° start position on the protractor is recorded as the joint ROM. When using a goniometer with a 180° protractor (see Fig. 1-26), ensure the goniometer is positioned such that the cutaway portion of the moving arm remains on the protractor so that the ROM can be read at the end of the assessed joint ROM.

To avoid parallax when reading a goniometer, look directly onto the scale and view the scale with both eyes open or by closing one eye. The methodology should be consistent on subsequent readings.

Proficiency in assessing and measuring joint ROM is gained through practice. It is also important to practice the techniques on as many persons as possible to become familiar with the variation between individuals.

OB "Myrin" Goniometer

The OB "Myrin" goniometer (see Fig. 1-27), a compass inclinometer, consists of a fluid-filled rotatable container mounted on a plate (21). The container has:

* A compass needle that reacts to Earth's magnetic field and measures movements in the horizontal plane.
* An inclination needle that is influenced by the force of gravity and measures movements in the frontal and sagittal planes.
* A scale on the container floor marked in 2° increments.

Two straps with Velcro fastenings are supplied to attach the goniometer to the body segment, and two plastic extension plates are also supplied to position the goniometer for certain joint measurements (21). When using the OB goniometer, magnetic fields other than those of the earth will cause the OB goniometer compass needle to deviate and therefore must be avoided.

The advantages of using the OB goniometer for measuring joint ROM are:

* It is not necessary to align the inclinometer with the joint axis.
* Rotational movements using a compass inclinometer are measured with ease.
* Assessment of trunk and neck ROM is measured with ease.
* There is little change in the alignment of the goniometer throughout the ROM.
* PROM is more easily assessed using the OB goniometer, as the therapist does not have to hold the goniometer and can stabilize the proximal joint segment with one hand and passively move the distal segment with the other.

The disadvantages of the OB goniometer are that it is expensive and bulky compared to the universal goniometer and it cannot be used to measure the small joints of the hand and foot. As noted above, magnetic fields other than those of the earth will cause the compass needle to deviate and must be avoided.

Measurement Procedure—OB "Myrin" Goniometer

- *Velcro strap and/or plastic extension plate:* Apply the Velcro strap to the limb segment proximal or distal to the joint being assessed. Attach the appropriate plastic extension plate to the Velcro strap for some ROM measurements.

- *OB Goniometer:* Attach the goniometer container to the Velcro strap or the plastic extension plate. The goniometer is positioned in relation to bony landmarks and placed in the same location on successive measurements (52). With the patient in the start position, rotate the fluid-filled container until the 0° arrow lines up directly underneath either the inclination needle, if the movement occurs in a vertical plane (i.e., the frontal or sagittal planes) (see Figs. 4-26, 4-27, 8–21, and 8-22), or the compass needle, if the movement occurs in the horizontal plane (21) (see Figs. 7-16 and 7–17).

- Ensure the needle is free to swing during the measurement (21). Do not deviate the goniometer during the measurement by touching the strap or goniometer dial or by applying hand pressure to change the contour of the soft tissue mass near the OB goniometer.

- At the end of the AROM or PROM, the number of degrees the inclination needle (see Figs. 4-28, 4-29, and 8-20) or the compass needle (see Fig. 7-17) moves away from the 0° arrow on the compass dial is recorded as the joint ROM.

- Forearm supination and pronation, tibial rotation, and hamstring and gastrocnemius muscle length are described and illusrated in this text as examples of how to apply the OB goniometer.

Sources of Error in Measuring Joint ROM.

The goniometer scale must be read carefully to avoid erroneous ROM measurements. Sources of error to avoid when measuring joint ROM are (52):

- Reading the wrong side of the scale on the goniometer (e.g., when the goniometer pointer is positioned midway between 40° and 50°, reading the value of 55° rather than 45°).

- A tendency to read values that end in a particular digit, such as zero (i.e., "_0°").

- Having expectations of what the reading "should be" and allowing this to influence the recorded result. For example, the patient has been attending treatment for 2 weeks and the therapist expects and sees an improvement in the ROM that is not actually present.

- A change in the patient's motivation to perform.

- Taking successive ROM measurements at different times of the day.

- Measurement procedure error: Make sure that sources of error do not occur or are minimized, so that ROM measurements are reliable and the patient's progress will be

accurately monitored. For reliable measurements, ROM should be assessed at the same time each day, by the same therapist, using the same measuring tool, using the same patient position, and following a standard measurement protocol (50). Treatment may affect ROM; therefore, ROM should be assessed in a consistent manner relative to the application of treatment techniques.

If upper or lower extremity ROM is measured by the same therapist, a 3° or 4° increase in the ROM indicates improvement (36). If different therapists measure the ROM, an increase of more than 5° for the upper extremity and 6° for the lower extremity would be needed to indicate progress (36).

Recording of Measurement

Standard information to be included on a ROM recording form includes patient name, date of birth or age, diagnosis, date of examination, assessing therapist, and whether the AROM or PROM is recorded. Different conventions are used internationally when listing the date numerically (either day/month/year or month/day/year); to ensure clear communication when recording dates, the month is written in full or abbreviated form, as shown in Figures 1-31 and 1-32.

Pictorial or numerical charts are used to record ROM. Figure 1-31 gives samples of selected joint motion recordings from a pictorial recording form; see Appendix A for a sample of a numerical recording form. If the AROM and PROM are full, the joint ROM does not have to be measured with a goniometer or tape measure and the ROM may be recorded as full, N (normal), WNL (within normal limits), or numerically.

If the PROM is either decreased or increased from the normal ROM, the existing ROM is indicated on a pictorial chart, or the number of degrees of motion is recorded on a numerical chart.

Every space on the ROM recording form should include an entry (8). If the measurement was not performed, NT (not tested) should be entered and a line may be drawn from the first such entry to the end of several adjacent entries so that NT does not have to be recorded in every space (8).

Any changes from the standard method of assessing joint ROM as presented in this text should be noted on the assessment form.

The ranges of motion are recorded on the numerical chart as follows (Fig. 1-32).

- When it is possible to begin the movement at the 0° start position, the ROM is recorded by writing the number of degrees the joint has moved away from 0°—for example, right shoulder elevation through flexion 160° or 0°–160°, right knee flexion 75° or 0°–75°, right knee extension 0°.

- When it is not possible to begin the movement from the 0° start position, the ROM is recorded by writing the number of degrees the joint is away from the 0° at the beginning of the ROM followed by the number of degrees the joint is away from 0° at the end of the ROM—for example, the patient cannot achieve 0° right elbow extension due to a contracture (abnormal short-

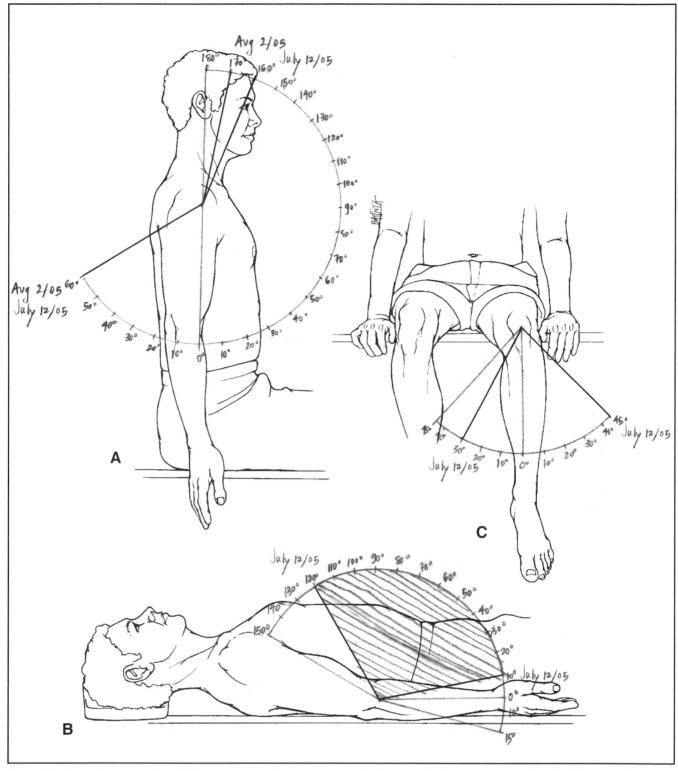

Figure 1-31 Examples of recording ROM using a pictorial recording form: **(A)** right shoulder flexion and extension, **(B)** right elbow flexion and extension/hyperextension, and **(C)** left hip internal and external rotation. The use of shading to show the available elbow flexion ROM is illustrated in **B**.

ening) of the elbow flexor muscles; the end feel is firm. More specifically, the right elbow cannot be extended beyond 10° of elbow flexion and can be flexed to 120°. The ROM would be recorded as right elbow flexion 10°–120°.

• For a joint that is in a fixed position or ankylosed, this is recorded on the chart along with the position of the joint.

On pictorial charts, the therapist extends lines from the joint axis on the diagram to the appropriate number

RANGE OF MOTION MEASUREMENT

Patient's Name	Jane Donner	Age	31
Diagnosis	#Ⓡ distal humerus shaft, depressed, #Ⓛ tibial plateau	Date of Onset	July 10/05
Therapist	Tom Becker	AROM or PROM	PROM

Recording:

1. The Neutral Zero Method defined by the American Academy of Orthopaedic Surgeons[1] is used for measurement and recording.

2. Average ranges defined by the American Academy of Orthopaedic Surgeons[1] are provided in parentheses.

3. The columns designated with asterisks are used for indicating limitation of range of motion and referencing for summarization.

4. Space is left at the end of each section to record hypermobile ranges and comments regarding positioning of the patient or body part, edema, pain, and/or end feel.

	Left Side				Right Side		
*	Oct 8/05	*	**Date of Measurement**	*	Oct 8/05	*	
			Shoulder Complex				
	0–180°		Elevation through flexion (0–180°)	*	0–160°		
	N		Elevation through abduction (0–180°)		N		
			Shoulder Glenhumeral Joint				
			Extension (0–60°)				
			Horizontal abduction (0–45°)				
			Horizontal adduction (0–135°)				
			Internal rotation (0–70°)				
	↓		External rotation (0–90°)		↓		
			Hypermobility:				
			Comments: end feel: Ⓡ shoulder flexion firm				
			Elbow and Forearm				
	0–150°		Flexion (0–150°)	*	10–120°		
	N		Supination (0–80°)		N		
	↓		Pronation (0–80°)		↓		
			Hypermobility: Ⓛ elbow hyperextension 5°				
			Comments: end feels: Ⓡ elbow extension firm; flexion firm				
			Knee				
	0–135°		Flexion (0–135°)	*	0–75°		
	NT		Tibial rotation		NT		
			Hypermobility:				
			Comments: end feel: Ⓛ knee flexion firm				

Figure 1-32 Example of recording ROM using a numeric recording form.

of degrees marked on the arc of movement at the start and end positions for the movement. The area between the two lines may be shaded in to provide a visual image of the ROM (see Fig. 1-31B). The date is recorded at the end of each line drawn to a degree marking on the arc of movement.

Figure 1-31 provides examples of ranges of motion recorded using a pictorial chart for the following:

- Right shoulder elevation through flexion 160° or 0°–160° and right shoulder extension 60° or 0°–60° as assessed on July 12, 2005. The patient was reassessed on August 2, 2005, and the ROM for right shoulder elevation through flexion increased to 170° or 0°–170°, and there was no change in the ROM for right shoulder extension.
- Right elbow flexion 10°–120° assessed on July 12, 2005.
- The July 12, 2005, assessment of left hip external rotation of 30° or 0°–30° and left hip internal rotation of 45° or 0°–45°.

The SFTR method (53) is a less commonly used method of recording joint ROM. The letters S, F, and T represent the plane of motion (sagittal, frontal, and transverse, respectively); (see Fig. 1-16) of the joint ROM assessed the R represents rotational motions. To record ROM, the letter identifying the plane of motion or rotational motion is noted. The letter is followed by three numbers that represent the start position, 0° with normal movement, and the ROM present on either side of the start position. The start position is recorded as the middle number. The ROM present on either side of the start position is recorded before and after the start position using the conventions indicated below (53). If a joint is ankylosed, only two numbers are recorded, 0° and the joint position to either the right or left of 0° using the conventions.

Conventions and examples of recording ROM using the SFTR Method are as follows:

- Motion occurring in the S (i.e., sagittal plane) is extension and flexion. The number to the left of the start position represents extension ROM, and the number to the right represents flexion ROM.

Example: Shoulder left S:60-0-180° right S:60-0-80°.

Interpretation: Left shoulder ROM is WNL, with 60° extension and 180° shoulder elevation through flexion. Right shoulder extension is 60° and shoulder elevation through flexion 80°.

- Motion occurring in the F (i.e., frontal plane) is abduction and adduction. The number to the left of the start position represents abduction, eversion, or left spinal lateral flexion ROM and the number to the right of the start position represents adduction, inversion, or right spinal lateral flexion ROM.

Example: Hip right F:45-0-30°.

Interpretation: Right hip abduction is 45° and adduction is 30°.

- Motion occurring in the T (i.e., transverse plane) is horizontal abduction and horizontal adduction, and retraction and protraction. The number to the left of the start position represents horizontal abduction or retraction ROM and the number to the right of the start position represents horizontal adduction or protraction ROM.

Example: Shoulder left T(F90):35-0-90°.

Interpretation: (F90) following the T indicates frontal plane 90°, meaning the motions of horizontal abduction and adduction were performed with the left shoulder in a start position of 90° abduction. Left shoulder horizontal abduction is 35° and horizontal adduction is 90°.

- An R indicates rotational motion. The number left of the start position represents external rotation, forearm supination, or spinal rotation to the left. The number right of the start position represents internal rotation, forearm pronation, or spinal rotation to the right.

Example: Hip right R(S90):45-0-30°.

Interpretation: The (S90) after the R indicates hip rotation was measured with the hip in the sagittal plane 90° (i.e., with the hip flexed 90°). Right hip external rotation ROM is 45° and internal rotation is 30°.

Example: Elbow left S:0-0-150° right S: 0-10-120°.

Interpretation: The ROM recorded indicates motion in the sagittal plane. Left elbow ROM is WNL with a start position of 0°, 0° extension, and 150° flexion. Right elbow extension and flexion has a start position of 10°, elbow flexion is 10° to 120°, or right elbow flexion is 120°.

Example: Knee right S: 0-15°.

Interpretation: The use of only two numbers indicates the knee joint is ankylosed. The S indicates the ankylosed position is in the sagittal plane; therefore, the joint is in either an extended or flexed position. The number is to the right of the 0 and by convention represents flexion. Thus, the knee is ankylosed in 15° flexion.

Assessing Joint ROM with a Two- or Multijoint Muscle in the Region

If during the assessment of joint ROM the movement will lengthen or stretch a two- or multijoint muscle, move the nontest joint crossed by the muscle into position so that the two-joint or multijoint muscle is placed on slack. This prevents the muscle from becoming passively insufficient and restricting the assessed joint ROM. For example, when the hip is flexed to assess hip flexion ROM with the knee in extension (see Fig. 1-18), the two-joint hamstring muscles will be stretched and the passive insufficiency of the hamstrings may limit the hip flexion ROM. Therefore, the knee is positioned in flexion to place the hamstrings on slack and prevent restriction of the hip flexion ROM due to passive insufficiency of the hamstrings.

ASSESSMENT AND MEASUREMENT OF MUSCLE LENGTH

To assess and measure the length of a muscle, the muscle is passively stretched (i.e., lengthened) across the joints crossed by the muscle. When the muscle is on full stretch, the patient will report a pulling sensation or pain in the region of the muscle and the therapist will assess a firm end feel. A universal goniometer, inclinometer (e.g., OB goniometer), or tape measure is used to measure the PROM possible at the last joint moved to place the muscle on full stretch, or the therapist observes and notes a limitation in joint PROM due to muscle tightness. The PROM measurement indirectly represents the length of the shortened muscle. Placing the muscle on slack and retesting the joint PROM will normally result in an increased PROM. The procedure of assessing or measuring muscle length is described and illustrated for each joint complex at the end of the joint ROM section of Chapters 3 through 9.

One-Joint Muscle. To assess and measure the length of a muscle that crosses one joint, the joint crossed by the muscle is positioned so that the muscle is lengthened across the joint. The final position of the joint is assessed and measured; this represents an indirect measure of the muscle length. An example of assessing and measuring the length of a one-joint muscle is described for the hip adductors on page 160.

Two-Joint Muscle. To assess and measure the length of a two-joint muscle, one of the joints crossed by the muscle is positioned so that the muscle is lengthened across the joint. The therapist then moves the second joint through a PROM until the muscle is on full stretch and prevents further motion at the joint. The final position of the second joint is assessed and measured; this represents an indirect measure of the muscle length. An example of assessing and measuring the length of a two-joint muscle is described for the gastrocnemius on page 214.

Multijoint-Muscle. To assess and measure the length of a multijoint muscle, all but one of the joints crossed by the muscle are positioned so that the muscle is lengthened across the joints. The therapist then moves the one remaining joint crossed by the muscle through a PROM until the muscle is on full stretch and prevents further motion at the joint. The final position of the joint is assessed and measured; this represents an indirect measure of the muscle length. An example of assessing and measuring the length of a multijoint muscle is described for the long finger extensors on page 127.

Summary—Joint ROM Assessment and Measurement

The main steps in the assessment and measurement of joint ROM are outlined in Figures 1-21 through 1-24, using shoulder extension as an example.

Passive joint ROM must be assessed before assessing muscle strength. The full available PROM at the joint then becomes the range the muscle(s) can be expected to move the limb through and is therefore defined as the full available ROM for the purpose of grading muscle strength.

FUNCTIONAL APPLICATION OF ASSESSMENT OF JOINT ROM

Evaluation of functional activities, through task analysis and observation of the patient's performance in activities, can guide the therapist in proceeding with a detailed assessment and provide objective and meaningful treatment goals. Ask the patient about his or her ability to perform activities. It is essential to observe the patient performing functional activities (54) such as dressing, sitting, and walking during the initial assessment.

After completing the ROM evaluation, consider the impact of deficit on the patient's daily life. Knowledge of functional anatomy of the musculoskeletal system is required to integrate the assessment findings into meaningful and practical information. The knowledge of functional anatomy assists the therapist in gaining insight into the effect of joint ROM limitations in the patient's daily life.

Outline of the Assessment Process

"An Outline of the Assessment Process," located on the inside front cover of this text, serves as an overview of the assessment process and a review of some of the main points presented in this chapter.

References

1. Basmajian JV. *Surface Anatomy: An Instructional Manual.* Baltimore: Williams & Wilkins; 1983.
2. Neumann DA. *Kinesiology of the Musculoskeletal System: Foundations for Physical Rehabilitation.* Philadelphia: Mosby; 2002.
3. Hollis M. *Safer Lifting for Patient Care.* 2nd ed. Oxford, England: Blackwell Scientific Publications; 1985.
4. MacConaill MA, Basmajian JV. *Muscles and Movements: A Basis for Human Kinesiology.* 2nd ed. New York: Robert E. Krieger; 1977.
5. Kapandji IA. *The Physiology of the Joints.* Vol 1. 5th ed. New York: Churchill Livingstone; 1982.
6. Standing S, ed. Gray's Anatomy: The Anatomical Basis of Clinical Practice. 39th ed. London: Elsevier Churchill Livingstone; 2005.
7. Venes D (ed). *Taber's Cyclopedic Medical Dictionary.* 19th ed. Philadelphia: FA Davis; 2001.
8. Duesterhaus Minor MA, Duesterhaus Minor S. *Patient Evaluation Methods for the Health Professional.* Reston, VA: Reston Publishing; 1985.
9. Soderberg GL. *Kinesiology: Application to Pathological Motion.* 2nd ed. Baltimore: Williams & Wilkins; 1997.
10. Perry J. Shoulder function for the activities of daily living. In: Matsen FA, Fu FH, Hawkins RJ. *The Shoulder: A Balance of Mobility and Stability.* Rosemont, IL: American Academy of Orthopaedic Surgeons; 1993.
11. Kendall FP, McCreary EK, Provance PG, et al. *Muscles Testing and Function with Posture and Pain.* 5th ed. Baltimore: Lippincott Williams & Wilkins; 2005.
12. Gowitzke BA, Milner M. *Understanding the Scientific Bases of Human Movement.* 2nd ed. Baltimore: Williams & Wilkins; 1980.

13. Kaltenborn FM. *Mobilization of the Extremity Joints. Examination and Basic Treatment Techniques.* 3rd ed. Oslo: Olaf Norlis Bokhandel; 1985.
14. Lundon K, Hampson D. Acquired ectopic ossification of soft tissues: implications for physical therapy. *Can J Rehabil.* 1997;10:231–246.
15. Hall CM, Brody LT. *Therapeutic Exercise: Moving Toward Function.* Philadelphia: Lippincott Williams & Wilkins; 1999.
16. Kisner C, Colby LA. *Therapeutic Exercise: Foundations and Techniques.* 4th ed. Philadelphia: FA Davis; 2002.
17. O' Connor P, Sforzo GA, Frye P. Effect of breathing instruction on blood pressure responses during isometric exercise. *Phys Ther.* 1989;69: 55–59.
18. Cyriax J. *Textbook of Orthopaedic Medicine: vol 1. Diagnosis of Soft Tissue Lesions.* 8th ed. London: Bailliere Tindall; 1982.
19. Norkin CC, White DJ. *Measurement of Joint Motion: A Guide to Goniometry.* 3rd ed. Philadelphia: FA Davis; 2003.
20. Magee DJ. *Orthopaedic Physical Assessment.* 4th ed. Philadelphia: WB Saunders; 2002.
21. Instruction Manual: OB Goniometer "Myrin." Available from OB Rehab, Solna, Sweden.
22. Performance Attainment Associates. *CROM Procedure Manual: Procedure for Measuring Neck Motion with the CROM.* St. Paul, MN: Univ. of Minn.; 1988.
23. Currier DP. *Elements of Research in Physical Therapy.* 3rd ed. Baltimore: Williams & Wilkins; 1990.
24. Sim J, Arnell P. Measurement validity in physical therapy research. *Phys Ther.* 1993;73:48–56.
25. Miller PJ. Assessment of joint motion. In: Rothstein JM, ed. *Measurement in Physical Therapy.* New York: Churchill Livingstone;1985.
26. Gogia PP, Braatz JH, Rose SJ, Norton BJ. Reliability and validity of goniometric measurements at the knee. *Phys Ther.* 1987;67:192–195.
27. Enwemeka CS. Radiographic verification of knee goniometry. *Scand J Rehabil Med.* 1986;18:47–49.
28. Fish DR, Wingate L. Sources of goniometric error at the elbow. *Phys Ther.* 1985;65:1666–1670.
29. Youdas JW, Carey JR, Garrett TR. Reliability of measurements of cervical spine range of motion—comparison of three methods. *Phys Ther.* 1991;71:23–29.
30. Low J. The reliability of joint measurement. *Physiotherapy.* 1976;62:227–229.
31. Baldwin J, Cunningham K. Goniometry under attack: a clinical study involving physiotherapists. *Physiother Can.* 1974;26:74–76.
32. Watkins MA, Riddle DL, Lamb RL, Personius WJ. Reliability of goniometric measurements and visual estimates of knee range of motion obtained in a clinical setting. *Phys Ther.* 1991;71:15–22.
33. Bovens AMPM, van Baak MA, Vrencken JGPM, et al. Variability and reliability of joint measurements. *Am J Sports Med.* 1990;18:58–63.
34. Pandya S, Florence JM, King WM, et al. Reliability of goniometric measurements in patients with Duchenne muscular dystrophy. *Phys Ther.* 1985;65:1339–1342.
35. Elveru RA, Rothstein JM, Lamb RL. Goniometric reliability in a clinical setting: subtalar and ankle joint measurements. *Phys Ther.* 1988;68:672–677.
36. Boone DC, Azen SP, Lin C-M, et al. Reliability of goniometric measurements. *Phys Ther.* 1978;58:1355–1360.
37. Dijkstra PU, deBont LGM, van der Weele LTh, Boering G. Joint mobility measurements: reliability of a standardized method. *J Craniomandibular Practice.* 1994;12:52–57.
38. Youdas JW, Bogard CL, Suman VJ. Reliability of goniometric measurements and visual estimates of ankle joint active range of motion obtained in a clinical setting. *Arch Phys Med Rehabil.* 1993;74:1113–1118.
39. Horger MM. The reliability of goniometric measurements of active and passive wrist motions. *Am J Occup Ther.* 1990;44:342–348.
40. Hellebrant FA, Duvall EN, Moore ML. The measurement of joint motion: Part III, reliability of goniometry. *Phys Ther Rev.* 1949;29:302–307.
41. Rothstein JM, Miller PJ, Roettger RF. Goniometric reliability in a clinical setting: elbow and knee measurements. *Phys Ther.* 1983;63:1611–1615.
42. Riddle DL, Rothstein JM, Lamb RL. Goniometric reliability in a clinical setting: shoulder measurements. *Phys Ther.* 1987;67:668–673.
43. Watkins B, Darrah J, Pain K. Reliability of passive ankle dorsiflexion measurements in children: comparison of universal and biplane goniometers. *Pediatr Phys Ther.* 1995;7:3–8.
44. Kilgour G, McNair P, Stott NS. Intrarater reliability of lower limb sagittal range-of-motion measures in children with spastic diplegia. *Develop Med Child Neurol.* 2003;45: 385–390.
45. Stuberg WA, Fuchs RH, Miedaner JA. Reliability of goniometric measurements of children with cerebral palsy. *Develop Med Child Neurol.* 1988;30:657–666.
46. Ashton B, Pickles B, Roll JW. Reliability of goniometric measurements of hip motion in spastic cerebral palsy. *Develop Med Child Neurol.* 1978;20:87–94.
47. Harris SR, Smith LH, Krukowski L. Goniometric reliability for a child with spastic quadriplegia. *J Pediatr Orthop.* 1985;5:348–351.
48. American Academy of Orthopaedic Surgeons. *Joint Motion: Method of Measuring and Recording.* Chicago: AAOS; 1965.
49. Berryman Reese N, Bandy WD. *Joint Range of Motion and Muscle Length Testing.* Philadelphia: WB Saunders; 2002.
50. Moore ML. Clinical assessment of joint motion. In: Basmajian JV, ed. *Therapeutic Exercise.* 4th ed. Baltimore: Williams & Wilkins; 1984.
51. Ekstrand J, Wiktorsson M, Oberg B, Gillquist J. Lower extremity goniometric measurements: a study to determine their reliability. *Arch Phys Med Rehabil.* 1982;63:171–175.
52. Stratford P, Agostino V, Brazeau C, Gowitzke BA. Reliability of joint angle measurement: a discussion of methodology issues. *Physiother Can.* 1984;36:5–9.
53. Gerhardt JJ, Cocchiarella L, Randall LD. *The Practical Guide to Range of Motion Assessment.* American Medical Association; 2002.
54. Smith LK. Functional tests. *Phys Ther Rev.* 1954;34:19–21.

EXERCISES AND QUESTIONS

See the Answer Guide in Appendix F for suggested answers to the following exercises and questions.

1. JOINT MOVEMENTS

Define the following movements and identify the opposite movement. Starting from anatomical position, demonstrate each movement and the opposite movement at one joint. Identify the plane and axis of each movement.

i.   Flexion
ii. Abduction
iii. Internal rotation
iv. Lateral flexion
v.   Horizontal adduction

2. OSTEOKINEMATICS AND ARTHROKINEMATICS

A. Define the terms *osteokinematics* and *arthrokinematics*.
B. Explain how a therapist applies osteokinematics and arthrokinematics when assessing restricted knee flexion PROM.

3. CONTRAINDICATIONS AND PRECAUTIONS FOR ROM ASSESSMENT

A. When are AROM and PROM assessment techniques contraindicated?
B. Case: Mrs. Smith, a frail 76-year-old, was involved in a car accident and suffered a fracture of the midshaft of her left humerus. She is just out of cast and is referred for physical therapy. On her initial visit, Mrs. Smith appears to be slightly intoxicated and protects her left upper extremity. Would the therapist assess Mrs. Smith's ROM? Explain.

4. THE RATIONALE FOR THE ASSESSMENT OF AROM AND PROM

A. Case: Mr. Fitzgerald, a 30-year-old teacher, suffered a fracture of his right distal femur. The femoral fracture is now well united. The therapist assesses the AROM of Mr. Fitzgerald's lower extremities with the patient high sitting (i.e., sitting on a plinth with his feet off the ground). The therapist assesses and measures all AROM of the lower extremities and finds all AROM to be normal bilaterally except for the following right knee and ankle AROM:

AROM	Left	Right
Knee flexion	135°	20–60° (R knee pain)
Knee extension	0°	20° flexion
Ankle dorsiflexion	20°	0°

i.   When measuring joint ROM using the neutral zero method, identify the defined zero position for measuring knee and ankle ROM.

ii. Assume the high sitting position and demonstrate the following:

a) Mr. Fitzgerald's left knee AROM

Identify any two- or multijoint muscle(s) in the region that could restrict knee ROM with Mr. Fitzgerald in the high sitting position. Explain why the muscle(s) would restrict the ROM. Identify an alternate start position that could be used for the assessment of Mr. Fitzgerald's left knee AROM that would eliminate any two- or multijoint muscle(s) identified above from restricting knee ROM.

b) Mr. Fitzgerald's right knee AROM

iii. What information can the therapist gather from the assessment of Mr. Fitzgerald's AROM?

iv. From the AROM assessment, can the therapist determine the reason for Mr. Fitzgerald's decreased right knee and ankle ROM? Explain.

v. Explain why the therapist would go on to assess Mr. Fitzgerald's PROM.

B. The therapist assesses Mr. Fitzgerald's PROM and finds all PROM of the lower extremities to be normal bilaterally except for the following right knee and ankle PROM:

PROM	Left	Right
Knee flexion	135° soft end feel	60° empty end feel (pain R knee)
Knee extension	0° firm end feel	0° firm end feel
Ankle dorsiflexion	20° firm end feel	5° firm end feel (pulling sensation over calf muscles)

Comparing only the AROM and PROM findings, what could the therapist conclude regarding Mr. Fitzgerald's right knee and ankle?

5. ASSESSMENT AND MEASUREMENT OF AROM AND PROM USING THE UNIVERSAL GONIOMETER

The following exercises are designed to facilitate learning of the AROM and PROM assessment and measurement process. The assessment and measurement of elbow flexion and extension/hyperextension serve as an example of the process as described and illustrated on pages 85 and 86.

Working in a group of three persons:

- One person, having normal elbow joints (i.e., no history of pathology/injury), serves as the patient.
- The second person is the therapist, who carries out the assessment and measurement of AROM and PROM.
- The third person assists the therapist by reading the instructions below and the description of the assessment and measurement of elbow flexion-extension/hyperextension on pages 85 and 86 to guide the therapist through the assessment and measurement process.

Before beginning the assessment and measurement of AROM and/or PROM, the therapist:

- Tells the patient about the assessment and measurement process and may demonstrate the movement(s) to be performed to the patient.
- Explains the need to expose the area to be assessed and drapes the patient as required.

A. Demonstrate assessment of AROM for elbow flexion and extension/hyperextension.

i. Whenever possible, observe the AROM by having the patient perform the movements bilaterally and symmetrically. Ask the patient to communicate any pain or other symptoms during the performance of the test movements.

Start Position. The patient is sitting on a chair or stool with the arms hanging by the side with the shoulder, elbow, and forearm in anatomical position.

Stabilization. The patient is instructed to sit up straight, keep the upper arms in at his or her sides, and move only the forearms and hands.

End Positions. Flexion—The patient is instructed, "Bend your elbows to bring the palms of your hands towards your shoulders as far as you can." Extension/Hyperextension—The patient is instructed, "Straighten your elbows as far as you can." The therapist may also demonstrate these movements to the patient.

The therapist observes the AROM to determine:

- The patient's willingness to move and ability to follow directions, perform well-coordinated movement, and move the part through the full AROM.
- Movement(s) that cause or increase pain.

ii. All three persons in the group can perform the following exercise.

- Assume the start position for the assessment of elbow flexion AROM as described above.
- Next, position your elbow in 90° flexion and assume this is as far as you can actively flex your elbow.

- Without allowing further elbow flexion, try to give the appearance that your elbow flexion is greater than 90° ROM.
    a) What substitute movement(s) did you use to give the appearance of a greater AROM than was actually possible?
    b) Substitute movement(s) should be avoided when performing the assessment and measurement of AROM. How can this be accomplished?
    c) Assume the supine position and repeat the above exercise. Did the change in position affect the substitute movement(s) possible when performing elbow flexion AROM? Explain.

B. <u>Demonstrate measurement of AROM</u> for elbow flexion and extension/hyperextension using the universal goniometer.

Start Position. The patient is sitting on a chair or stool with the arms hanging by the side in anatomical position. The goniometer is aligned at the start position of 0°.

Goniometer Alignment. The goniometer alignment for AROM is the same as that for the measurement of PROM as described and illustrated on pages 85 and 86. The surface anatomy required for the alignment of the goniometer is described and illustrated on page 84.

Stabilization. The patient is instructed to sit up straight, keep the upper arms in at his or her sides, and move only the forearms and hands.

End Positions. Flexion—The patient is instructed, "Bend your elbows to bring the palms of your hands towards your shoulders as far as you can." Extension/Hyperextension—The patient is instructed, "Straighten your elbows as far as you can." The therapist may also demonstrate the above movements to the patient.

As the patient moves through the AROM, the goniometer is either moved through the range along with the limb to the end of the AROM, or realigned at the end of the movement. The ROM, in degrees, is read from the goniometer at the end of the AROM and recorded.

C. <u>Demonstrate assessment of PROM</u> for elbow flexion and extension/hyperextension.
- Assess the PROM carefully and slowly.
- Ask the patient to communicate any pain or other symptoms during the test movements.
- Reassure the patient that you will stop the movement at any time if there is pain.

The patient must be relaxed during the assessment of PROM, but it is often difficult for the patient to relax. Tell the patient, "Relax, and let me do all the work to move your arm." If the patient continues to have difficulty relaxing, support the forearm and hand and instruct the patient, "Let your arm drop into my hand so that I can feel the whole weight of your arm." When performing passive elbow flexion, instruct the patient, "Relax while I bring your hand toward your shoulder." When performing passive elbow extension/hyperextension, instruct the patient, "Relax while I straighten your elbow."
Refer to pages 85 and 86 and follow the description and illustrations to demonstrate the assessment of PROM. The therapist:
- Observes the amount of movement possible at the joint.
- Determines the quality of movement throughout the PROM.
- Notes the presence or absence of pain.
- Assesses and records the end feels.

D. <u>Demonstrate measurement of PROM</u> for elbow flexion and extension/hyperextension using the universal goniometer. Refer to pages 85 and 86 and follow the description and illustrations to demonstrate and record the measurement of PROM.

E. When carrying out the assessment/measurement procedures, did the therapist:
- Ensure the patient was comfortable and well supported?
- Communicate well with the patient?
- Assume an appropriate position and stance, and appear comfortable (see Fig. 1-1)?
- Adequately stabilize the humerus (i.e., proximal joint segment)?
After completion of the above exercises, change roles and repeat the exercises.

6. VALIDITY AND RELIABILITY—UNIVERSAL GONIOMETER

A. Define the terms *validity* and *reliability*.
B. Explain how the therapist would obtain reliable joint ROM measurements using the universal goniometer.

7. ASSESSMENT AND MEASUREMENT OF MUSCLE LENGTH

Work in a group of three as described in Exercise 5 above. Before beginning an assessment and measurement of muscle length, the therapist:

- Tells the patient about the assessment and measurement process and demonstrates the movement(s) to be performed.
- Explains the need to expose the area to be assessed and drapes the patient as required.

Refer to pages 156 and 157 and follow the description and illustrations to demonstrate the assessment and measurement of muscle length using the hamstrings as an example. The person serving as the patient should have normal back and hip joints (i.e., no history of pathology or injury in these regions).

8. USING THE OB "MYRIN" GONIOMETER TO MEASURE JOINT ROM

A. Briefly describe the OB "Myrin" goniometer, a compass/inclinometer, and explain how it is applied to measure joint ROM.
B. Identify the advantages and disadvantages of using the OB "Myrin" goniometer compared to the universal goniometer to measure joint ROM.

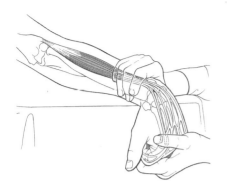

Relating Treatment to Assessment

Chapter Rationale

Although the guidelines for diagnosis and treatment protocols are beyond the scope of this text, this chapter links the general procedure used to assess deficiencies in active range of motion (AROM), passive range of motion (PROM), and muscle length with the general procedure, used when appropriate, to treat these deficiencies. Through illustrations and descriptions, the reader is provided with an overview of the similarities and differences between clinical assessments presented in this textbook and similar treatments. Understanding the similarities between assessment and treatment, and using the knowledge and skills for assessing active and passive ROM and muscle length, the reader will be able to demonstrate similar treatments using active and passive movement. Understanding the link between assessment and treatment is essential for the reader to be able to integrate patient assessment and treatment in the clinical setting.

Chapter Objectives

Upon completion of Chapter 2: Relating Treatment to Assessment, for treatment and assessment using active and passive movement, the reader should be able to:

- List the key steps for applying the assessment and treatment.
- Describe the fundamental difference between similar assessments and treatments.

- Identify the key steps that are the same and the key steps that are different when comparing similar assessments and treatments.
- Identify the treatments that are similar to the assessments of AROM, PROM, and muscle length.
- Identify and demonstrate the treatment a therapist would use when presented with assessment findings of deficiencies in AROM, PROM, or muscle length.

SIMILAR ASSESSMENT AND TREATMENT METHODS

Similar assessments and treatments are categorized according to the type of movement used (i.e., active and passive movement) as set out in Table 2-1.

When used for assessment, active movement is called active range of motion (AROM). When AROM is used specifically to assess muscle strength, it is called manual muscle testing (MMT). Active movement used for treatment is called active exercise and may be used to maintain or increase joint ROM and/or muscle strength.

When used for assessment, passive movement is called passive range of motion (PROM) or muscle length assessment. The therapist uses PROM to determine the ROM at a joint, end feel, and the length of muscles. When used for treatment to maintain or increase joint ROM and muscle length, this movement is called relaxed passive movement and prolonged passive stretch.

KEY STEPS WHEN APPLYING ASSESSMENTS AND TREATMENTS

The key steps used when applying assessments and treatments are listed in order in the first column of Table 2-1. These steps are set out in detail for assessment in Chapter 1 and are summarized here and in Table 2-1 to compare with those for treatment.

Purpose

The therapist performs an assessment to evaluate how an injury or disease affects the patient's status. Treatment, if appropriate, is then used to eliminate or lessen the effects of an injury or disease. Assessment is repeated as required to evaluate the outcome of treatment.

General Procedure

The general procedure is the same when using active or passive movement for similar assessment and treatment.

Explanation and Instruction

Before carrying out an assessment or treatment, explain to the patient the assessment or treatment and obtain the patient's consent. When applying a specific assessment or treatment for the first time, explain and/or demonstrate the movement to be performed and/or ask the patient to relax and passively move the patient's limb through the movement.

Expose Region. For assessment and treatment, expose the area to be assessed or treated and drape the patient as required.

Start Position. For assessment and treatment, ensure the patient is in a safe, comfortable position and is adequately supported. When positioning the patient, the effect of gravity on the movement or position held may be relevant.

Stabilization. For assessment and treatment, provide adequate stabilization to ensure that only the required movement occurs. For assessment and treatment, either (a) the proximal joint segment or site of attachment of the origin of the muscle(s) is stabilized or (b) the distal joint segment or site of insertion of the muscle(s) is stabilized.

Movement. For assessment and treatment, either (a) the distal joint segment or site of attachment of the insertion of the muscle(s) is moved or (b) the proximal joint segment or site of origin of the muscle(s) is moved.

Assistance. For passive movements used in assessment and treatment, the therapist usually applies assistance at the distal end of either the distal joint segment or the segment into which the muscle(s) is/are inserted.

End Position. For assessment and treatment, either passively move or instruct the patient to move the body segment(s) through either a selected part of or the full ROM possible. For prolonged passive stretch, the therapist passively moves the body segment(s) to the point in the ROM that provides maximal stretch of the muscle(s).

Substitute Movement. For assessment and treatment, ensure there are no substitute movements that may exaggerate the actual joint ROM and/or muscle length and the patient's capacity to perform an exercise. To avoid unwanted movements, explain/demonstrate to the patient how the movement is to be performed and the substitute movements to be avoided. Pay attention to positioning and stabilizing the patient. Experience and careful observation enables the therapist to prevent substitute movements and detect any that may occur.

Purpose-Specific Procedure

After applying the general procedure, specific procedure is used to provide outcomes that meet the specific purpose of the assessment or treatment. Purpose-specific procedures include measuring active or passive ROM, noting the end feel, grading muscle strength, changing the number of times a movement is performed, changing the length of time a position is held, and/or changing the magnitude of the resistance used.

Charting

For assessment, deviations from standardized testing procedure and the findings are noted in the chart. For treatment, details of the procedures used and any change in the patient's condition are noted in the chart.

TABLE 2-1 **Comparing Assessment and Treatment**

Key Steps	Active Movement		Passive Movement			
	Assessment	Treatment	Assessment	Treatment	Assessment	Treatment
	Active ROM (AROM)	*Active Exercise*	*Passive ROM (PROM)*	*Relaxed Passive Movement*	*Muscle Length*	*Prolonged Passive Stretch*
PURPOSE	Assessment of:	Treatment to maintain/ increase:	Assessment of:	Treatment of maintain/ increase:	Assessment of:	Treatment to maintain/ increase:
	• AROM • muscle strength • ability to perform ADL	• joint ROM • muscle strength • ability to perform ADL	• joint ROM • end feel	• joint ROM	• muscle length	• muscle length
GENERAL PROCEDURE Explanation/ Instruction	← Verbal (clear, concise), demonstration and/or passive movement →					
Expose Area	← Expose area and drape as required →					
Start Position	• safe, comfortable, adequate support • consider effect of gravity		← • safe, comfortable, adequate support, relaxed →			
Stabilization*	• proximal joint segment(s) • muscle origin(s)		• proximal joint segment(s)		• muscle origin(s)	
Movement*	• distal joint segment(s)		• distal joint segment(s)		• other joints crossed by muscle(s)	
Assistance	n/a		• applied at distal end of distal joint segment(s)		• applied at distal end of segment(s) muscle(s) inserted on	
End Position	• end of selected portion of full AROM		• end of selected portion of full AROM		• muscle(s) on full stretch	
Substitute Movement	← Ensure no substitute movement →					
PURPOSE-SPECIFIC PROCEDURE	• usually estimate and/or measure AROM	• active movement performed according to exercise prescription	• observe and/or measure joint PROM • note end feel	• passive movement performed according to treatment prescription	• visually observe and/or measure joint position at maximum stretch of muscle	• joint held at position of maximal muscle stretch for prescribed length of time

(continues)

TABLE 2-1 *Continued*

| Key Steps | Active Movement | | | Passive Movement | | | |
	Assessment	Treatment	Assessment	Treatment	Assessment	Treatment
CHARTING	• joint AROM • MMT grade	• describe exercise prescribed • note any change in patient's condition	• joint PROM • end feel	• describe treatment prescribed • note any change in patient's condition	• joint position • end feel	• descri position of stretch and length of time stretch applied • note any change in patient's condition

*For ease of explanation and understanding, the proximal joint segment or site of attachment of the origin of the muscle is stabilized and the distal joint segment or site of attachment of the insertion of the muscle described as the moving segment.

ADL, activities of daily living; MMT, manual muscle testing

Note: The shaded area highlights "General Procedure" that is the same for similar assessment and treatment.

EXAMPLES OF SIMILAR ASSESSMENT AND TREATMENT METHODS

Examples of similar assessments and treatments using active and passive movement are described and illustrated. These examples apply to other joints and muscles in the body.

Note that for similar assessments and treatments, the "General Procedure" is the same, but the "Purpose," "Purpose-Specific Procedure," and "Charting" are different.

In Table 2-1 and in these examples, for ease of explanation and understanding, the proximal joint segment or site of attachment of the origin of the muscle is stabilized and the distal joint segment or site of attachment of the insertion of the muscle is described as the moving segment.

Knee Extension:* AROM Assessment and Treatment Using Active Exercise

Assessment	**Treatment**
AROM	**Active Exercise**

PURPOSE
To assess AROM, quadriceps muscle strength and determine the ability to perform ADL.

PURPOSE
To maintain or increase AROM, quadriceps muscle strength, and the ability to perform ADL.

GENERAL PROCEDURE

Explanation/Instruction. The therapist explains, demonstrates, and/or passively moves the limb through knee extension. The therapist instructs the patient to straighten the knee as far as possible.

Expose Region. The patient wears shorts.

Start Position. The patient is sitting, grasps the edge of the plinth, and has the nontest foot supported on a stool (Fig. 2-1).

Stabilization. The patient is instructed to maintain the thigh in the start position or the therapist may stabilize the thigh.

Movement. The patient performs knee extension.

End Position. The knee is extended as far as possible through the ROM (Fig. 2-2). The hamstrings may restrict knee extension in this position.

Substitute Movement. The patient leans back to posteriorly tilt the pelvis and extend the hip joint.

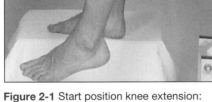

Figure 2-1 Start position knee extension: AROM assessment and active exercise.

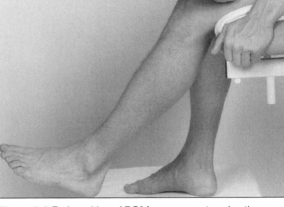

Figure 2-2 End position: AROM assessment and active exercise. The therapist may stabilize the femur and/or palpate for contraction of the knee extensors.

PURPOSE-SPECIFIC PROCEDURE
AROM is visually assessed or measured using the universal goniometer. Following the assessment of PROM, the therapist grades the strength of the knee extensors using AROM.

PURPOSE-SPECIFIC PROCEDURE
Knee extension is performed actively by the patient a predetermined number of times according to the exercise prescription.

CHARTING
Knee extension AROM is recorded in degrees and/or the knee extensors are assigned a grade for strength.

CHARTING
The prescribed exercise is described, and any change in the patient's condition is noted.

*To show an example of movement performed against gravity.

Note: Movement performed with gravity eliminated could also be used to illustrate the similarity between AROM assessment and active exercise.

Hip Flexion: PROM Assessment and Treatment Using Relaxed Passive Movement

Assessment
PROM

Treatment
Relaxed Passive Movement

PURPOSE
To assess hip flexion PROM and determine an end feel.

PURPOSE
To maintain or increase hip flexion ROM.

GENERAL PROCEDURE

Explanation/Instruction. The therapist explains, demonstrates, and/or passively moves the limb through hip flexion. The therapist instructs the patient to relax as the movement is performed.

Expose Region. The patient wears shorts and is draped as required.

Start Position. The patient is supine. The hip and knee on the test side are in the neutral position. The other hip is extended on the plinth (Fig. 2-3).

Stabilization. The therapist stabilizes the pelvis. The trunk is stabilized through body positioning.

Movement. The therapist raises the lower extremity off the plinth and applies slight traction to and moves the femur anteriorly to flex the hip.

End Position. The femur is moved to the limit of hip flexion (Fig. 2–4).

Substitute Movement. Posterior pelvic tilt and flexion of the lumbar spine.

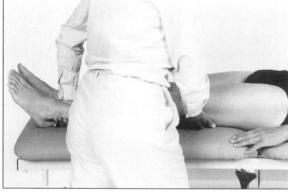

Figure 2-3 Start position hip flexion: PROM assessment and relaxed passive movement.

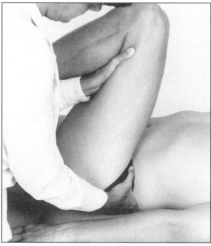

Figure 2-4 End position hip flexion: PROM assessment and relaxed passive movement.

PURPOSE-SPECIFIC PROCEDURE
The therapist applies slight overpressure at the end of the PROM to identify the end feel. The therapist observes and measures the joint PROM.

CHARTING
The end feel and number of degrees of hip flexion PROM are recorded.

PURPOSE-SPECIFIC PROCEDURE
The hip is passively moved into flexion a predetermined number of times according to the treatment prescription.

CHARTING
The prescribed treatment is described, and any change in the patient's condition is noted.

Long Finger Extensors: Muscle Length Assessment and Treatment Using Prolonged Passive Stretch

Assessment **Muscle Length**	**Treatment** **Prolonged Passive Stretch**
PURPOSE To assess the length of the long finger extensor muscles.	**PURPOSE** To maintain or increase the length of the long finger extensor muscles.

GENERAL PROCEDURE

Explanation/Instruction. The therapist explains, demonstrates, and/or passively positions the patient in the stretch position. The therapist instructs the patient to relax as the movement is performed and held.

Expose Region. The patient wears short-sleeved shirt.

Start Position. The patient is sitting. The elbow is extended, the forearm is pronated, and the fingers are flexed (Fig. 2-5).

Stabilization. The therapist stabilizes the radius and ulna.

Movement. The therapist applies slight traction to and flexes the wrist.

End Position. The wrist is flexed to the limit of motion so that the long finger extensors are fully stretched (Figs. 2-6 and 2-7).

Substitute Movement. Finger extension.

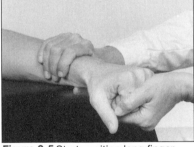

Figure 2-5 Start position long finger extensors: muscle length assessment and prolonged passive stretch.

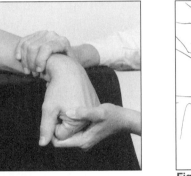

Figure 2-6 End position long finger extensors on stretch: muscle length assessment and prolonged passive stretch.

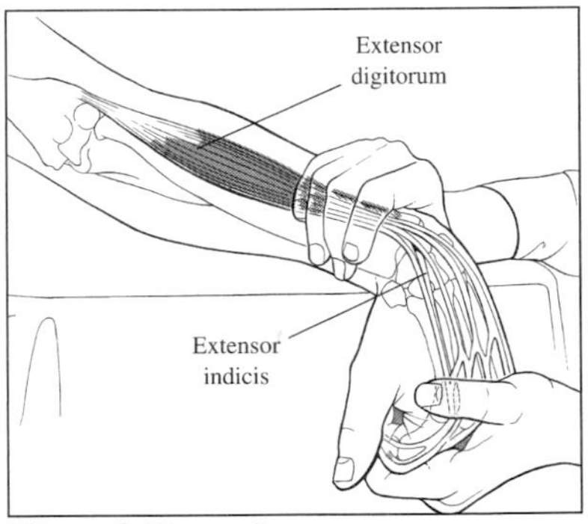

Figure 2-7 Long finger extensors on stretch.

PURPOSE-SPECIFIC PROCEDURE

With the long finger extensors on full stretch, the angle of wrist flexion is observed and/or measured, and the therapist identifies the end feel.

CHARTING

The long finger extensors may be described as being shortened, and the angle of wrist flexion may be recorded. The end feel is noted.

PURPOSE-SPECIFIC PROCEDURE

The position of maximum wrist flexion is maintained so that the long finger flexors are placed on full stretch for a prescribed length of time, and the therapist identifies the end feel.

CHARTING

The stretch position and the length of time the stretch is applied to the long finger extensors are recorded. Any change in the patient's condition is noted.

EXERCISES AND QUESTIONS

See the Answer Guide in Appendix F for suggested answers to the following exercise and questions.

1. **LIST THE KEY STEPS USED TO APPLY THE SIMILAR ASSESSMENTS AND TREATMENTS THAT USE ACTIVE AND PASSIVE MOVEMENTS.**

2. **DESCRIBE THE FUNDAMENTAL DIFFERENCE BETWEEN ASSESSMENT AND TREATMENT.**

3. **IDENTIFY THE KEY STEPS THAT ARE THE SAME AND THE KEY STEPS THAT ARE DIFFERENT WHEN APPLYING SIMILAR ASSESSMENTS AND TREATMENTS.**

4. **IDENTIFY THE TREATMENTS THAT ARE SIMILAR TO THE FOLLOWING ASSESSMENTS:**

A. Active ROM (AROM): _____

B. Passive ROM (PROM): _____

C. Muscle length: _____

5. **ASSESSMENT FINDING: SHORTENED TENSOR FASCIA LATAE**

A. Identify the assessment a therapist uses to assess this muscle length deficiency.

B. Identify the treatment that is similar to the assessment identified in 5.A. and would be used to treat the shortened muscle.

C. Demonstrate the general procedure for the treatment identified in 5.B. that would be used to lengthen the tensor fascia latae.

6. **ASSESSMENT FINDING: HIP MUSCLE PARALYSIS, DECREASED HIP FLEXION PROM WITH SOFT END FEEL**

A. Identify the assessment the therapist used to assess this PROM deficiency.

B. Identify the treatment that is similar to the assessment identified in 6.A. and would be used to maintain hip flexion ROM.

C. Demonstrate the general procedure for the treatment identified in 6.B. that would be used to maintain the hip flexion PROM.

7. **ASSESSMENT FINDING: DECREASED ELBOW FLEXION AROM**

A. Identify the assessment the therapist used to assess this AROM deficiency.

B. Identify the treatment that is similar to the assessment identified in 7.A. and would be used to maintain or increase elbow flexion AROM.

C. Demonstrate the general procedure for the treatment identified in 7.B. that would be used to maintain or increase the elbow flexion AROM.

SECTION II

Section Rationale

Through illustration and description, and the use of exercises and questions, the reader is provided with the knowledge and practical instruction required to gain proficiency in the clinical skills of assessment and measurement of active and passive range of motion (ROM) and muscle length at the extremity joints and the active ROM at the temporomandibular and spinal articulations. This knowledge and these skills are essential for the reader to accurately assess a patient's present status, plan treatment, and assess the patient's progress, effectiveness of the treatment program, and the patient's ability to perform activities of daily living (ADL).

Section Objectives

Upon completion of Chapters 3 through 9, for all articulations and movements, the reader should be able to:

- Identify and describe the
  a. shape of each articulation;
  b. components of each physiological or functional joint.
- Demonstrate, define, and describe* each joint movement.
- Demonstrate palpation of the anatomical structures used to assess and measure ROM and muscle length.
- Demonstrate the assessment and measurement of
  a. active ROM (AROM);
  b. passive ROM (PROM)**;
  c. muscle length.

- List the
  a. substitute movements to avoid when assessing AROM;
  b. normal limiting factor(s) and end feel(s);
  c. capsular pattern(s);
  d. function(s) of the joint complex in ADL.
- Identify and describe the rationale for the direction of glide of the articular surfaces.
- Identify
  a. the "normal" AROM;
  b. ADL that require specified joint movement(s);
  c. the ROM required for selected ADL.

*Identify the axis/plane of movement.
**Note: For Chapter 9, the assessment and measurement of the PROM of the temporomandibular joint (TMJ), cervical, thoracic, and lumbar spines, are beyond the scope of this text.

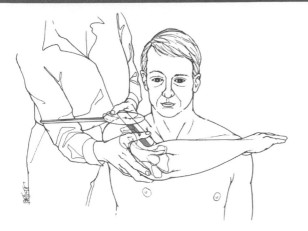

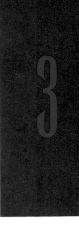

Shoulder Complex

ARTICULATIONS AND MOVEMENTS

The articulations of the shoulder complex and the joint axes of the scapula and glenohumeral joint are illustrated in Figures 3-1 through 3-4. The sternoclavicular, acromioclavicular, scapulothoracic, and glenohumeral joints make up the shoulder complex. The shoulder complex can be divided into two components: (a) the shoulder girdle, which includes the sternoclavicular, acromioclavicular, and scapulothoracic joints; and (b) the glenohumeral joint.

The joints and movements of the shoulder complex are described below and summarized in Tables 3-1, 3-2, and 3-3. The integrated movement patterns of these joints, associated with the normal function of the shoulder complex, are discussed at the end of this chapter in the "Functional Application" section.

The Joints of the Shoulder Girdle

The shoulder girdle is connected directly to the trunk via the sternoclavicular joint, a saddle joint. The articular surfaces of the joint are formed medially by the lateral aspect of the manubrium sternum and the adjacent superior surface of the first costal cartilage, and laterally by the medial end of the clavicle. An articular disc is located between the joint surfaces. The articulating surface of the clavicle is convex vertically and concave horizontally and articulates with the reciprocal surfaces on the medial aspect of the manubrium part of the sternum and first costal cartilage (2). The movements at the sternoclavicular joint include elevation, depression, protraction, retraction, and rotation of the clavicle. During elevation and depression, the lateral end of the clavicle moves superiorly and inferiorly, respectively, in the frontal plane around a sagittal axis. The lateral end of the clavicle moves in an anterior direction with protraction and in a posterior direction with retraction, and these movements take place in the horizontal plane about a vertical axis. Rotation of the clavicle occurs in the sagittal plane around a frontal axis (i.e., an axis that passes along the long axis of the clavicle). Clavicular elevation and rotation are essential components to the normal performance of shoulder elevation through flexion or abduction (5). Mobility at the sternoclavicular joint is essential to enable scapular motion.

The acromioclavicular joint, linking the clavicle and scapula, is classified as a plane joint formed by the relatively flat articular surfaces of the lateral end of the clavicle and the acromion process of the scapula. In some instances, the joint surfaces are partially separated by an articular disc (2). The acromioclavicular joint permits limited gliding motion between the clavicle and scapula during shoulder girdle movement.

A physiological or functional joint, the scapulothoracic joint consists of flexible soft tissues (i.e., subscapularis and serratus anterior) sandwiched between the scapula and the chest wall that allow the scapula to move over the thorax. Scapular motions are accompanied by movement of the clavicle via the acromioclavicular and sternoclavicular joints. Scapular motions include elevation, depression, retraction, protraction, lateral (upward) rotation, and medial (downward) rotation. Movement of the scapula in a cranial direction is called elevation and is accompanied by elevation of the clavicle. The scapula and clavicle move in a caudal direction with scapular depression. Scapular retraction and protraction occur in the horizontal plane around a vertical axis as the medial border of the scapula moves toward (retraction) or away from (protraction) the vertebral column. Scapular retraction and protraction are accompanied by retraction and protraction of the clavicle, respectively. The scapula rotates laterally and medially, with reference to the movement of the inferior angle, so that the glenoid cavity moves in either an upward (cranial) or a downward (caudal) direction, respectively (see Fig. 3-2).

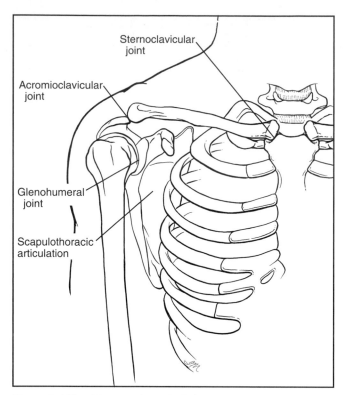

Figure 3-1 Shoulder complex articulations.

In the clinical setting, motion at the sternoclavicular joint and scapula is not easily measured, and it is not possible to measure motion at the acromioclavicular joint. Therefore, scapular and clavicular motions are normally assessed by visual observation of active movement and through passive movement.

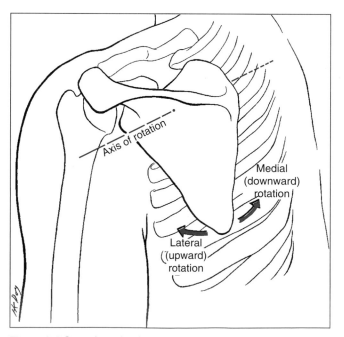

Figure 3-2 Scapular axis of rotation.

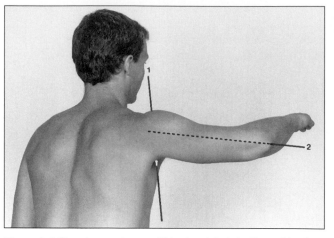

Figure 3-3 Glenohumeral axes: *(1)* horizontal abduction-adduction; *(2)* internal-external rotation.

The Glenohumeral Joint

The glenohumeral or shoulder joint is a ball-and-socket joint formed medially by the concave surface of the scapular glenoid cavity and laterally by the convex surface of the head of the humerus. From the anatomical position, the glenohumeral joint may be flexed and extended in the sagittal plane with movement occurring around a frontal axis (see Fig. 3-4). The movements of shoulder abduction and adduction occur in the frontal plane around a sagittal axis, and shoulder internal rotation and external rotation occur in a horizontal plane around a vertical axis (see Figs. 3-3 and 3-4). The glenohumeral movements are accompanied at varying points in the range of motion (ROM) by scapular, clavicular, and trunk motion. Thus, motion at the scapulothoracic, acromioclavicular, and sternoclavicular articulations extends the ROM capabilities of the glenohumeral joint.

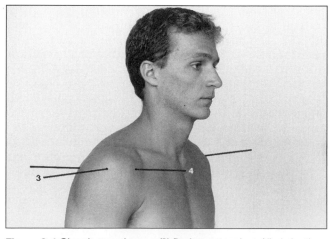

Figure 3-4 Glenohumeral axes: *(3)* flexion-extension; *(4)* abduction-adduction.

TABLE 3-1   Joint Structure: Scapular Movements

	Elevation	Depression	Abduction (Protraction)	Abduction (Retraction)
Articulation[1,2]	Scapulothoracic Acromioclavicular Sternoclavicular	Scapulothoracic Acromioclavicular Sternoclavicular	Scapulothoracic Acromioclavicular Sternoclavicular	Scapulothoracic Acromioclavicular Sternoclavicular
Plane	Frontal	Frontal	Horizontal	Horizontal
Axis	Sagittal	Sagittal	Vertical	Vertical
Normal limiting factors[1,3–6]* (See Figs. 3-5 and 3-6)	Tension in the costoclavicular ligament, inferior sternoclavicular joint capsule, lower fibers of trapezius, pectoralis minor, and subclavius	Tension in the interclavicular ligament, inferior sternoclavicular ligament, articular disk, upper fibers of trapezius, and levator scapulae; bony contact between the clavicle and the superior aspect of the first rib	Tension in the trapezoid ligament, posterior sternoclavicular ligament, posterior lamina of the costoclavicular ligament, trapezius, and rhomboids	Tension in the conoid ligament, anterior lamina of the costoclavicular ligament, anterior sternoclavicular ligament, pectoralis minor, and serratus anterior
Normal end feel[3,7]	Firm	Firm/hard	Firm	Firm
Normal AROM[1]†	10–12 cm (total range for elevation—depression)		15 cm (total range for abduction—adduction)	

	Medial Rotation (Downward Rotation)	Lateral Rotation (Upward Rotation)		
Articulation[1,2]	Scapulothoracic Acromioclavicular Sternoclavicular	Scapulothoracic Acromioclavicular Sternoclavicular		
Plane	Frontal	Frontal		
Axis	Sagittal	Sagittal		
Normal limiting factors[1,3-6]* (See Figs. 3-5 and 3-6)	Tension in the conoid ligament and serratus anterior	Tension in the trapezoid ligament, the rhomboid muscles and the levator scapulae		
Normal end feel[3,7]	Firm	Firm		
Normal AROM[1]	60° displacement of inferior angle is 10–12 cm (total range for medial-lateral rotation)			

Note: Medial and lateral rotations of the scapula are associated with extension and/or adduction and flexion and/or abduction of the shoulder, respectively.

*Note: There is a paucity of definitive research that identifies the normal limiting factors (NLF) of joint motion. The NLF and end feels listed here are based on knowledge of anatomy, clinical experience, and available references.
†AROM, active range of motion.

TABLE 3-2 Joint Structure: Glenohumeral Joint Movements

	Extension	Internal Rotation	External Rotation	Horizontal Abduction	Horizontal Adduction
Articulation[1,2]	Glenohumeral	Glenohumeral	Glenohumeral	Glenohumeral	Glenohumeral
Plane	Sagittal	Horizontal	Horizontal	Horizontal	Horizontal
Axis	Frontal	Longitudinal	Longitudinal	Vertical	Vertical
Normal limiting factors[1,3–6]* (See Fig. 3-6)	Tension in the anterior band of the coracohumeral ligament, the anterior joint capsule, and clavicular fibers of pectoralis major	Tension in the posterior joint capsule, infraspinatus, and teres minor	Tension in all bands of the glenohumeral ligament, coracohumeral ligament, the anterior joint capsule, subscapularis, pectoralis major, teres major, and latissimus dorsi	Tension in the anterior joint capsule, the glenohumeral ligament, and pectoralis major	Tension in the posterior joint capsule Soft tissue apposition
Normal end feel[3,7]	Firm	Firm	Firm	Firm	Firm/soft
Normal AROM[8] (AROM[9])	0–60° (0–60°)	0–70° (0–70°)	0–90° (0–90°)	0–45° (−)	0–135° (−)

*Note: There is a paucity of definitive research that identifies the normal limiting factors (NLF) of joint motion. The NLF and end feels listed here are based on knowledge of anatomy, clinical experience, and available references.

TABLE 3-3 Joint Structure: Shoulder Complex Movements

	Elevation Through Flexion	Elevation Through Abduction
Articulation[1,2]	Glenohumeral Acromioclavicular Sternoclavicular Scapulothoracic	Glenohumeral Acromioclavicular Sternoclavicular Scapulothoracic Subdeltoid[1]
Plane	Sagittal	Frontal
Axis	Frontal	Sagittal
Normal limiting factors[1,3–6]* (See Fig. 3-6)	Tension in the posterior band of the coracohumeral ligament, posterior joint capsule, shoulder extensors, and external rotators; scapular movement limited by tension in rhomboids, levator scapulae, and the trapezoid ligament	Tension in the middle and inferior bands of the glenohumeral ligament, inferior joint capsule, shoulder adductors; greater tuberosity of the humerus contacting the upper portion of the glenoid and glenoid labrum or the lateral surface of the acromion; scapular movement limited by tension in rhomboids, levator scapulae, and the trapezoid ligament
Normal end feel[3,7]	Firm	Firm/hard
Normal AROM[1,2,8] (AROM[9])	0–180° (0–165°) 0–60°, glenohumeral 60–180°, glenohumeral, scapular movement, and trunk movement	0–180° (0–165°) 0–30°, glenohumeral 30–180°, glenohumeral, scapular movement, and trunk movement
Capsular pattern[7,10]	Glenohumeral: external rotation, abduction (only through 90–120° range), internal rotation Sternoclavicular/acromioclavicular: pain at extreme range of motion notably horizontal adduction and full elevation	

*Note: There is a paucity of definitive research that identifies the normal limiting factors (NLF) of joint motion. The NLF and end feels listed here are based on knowledge of anatomy, clinical experience, and available references.

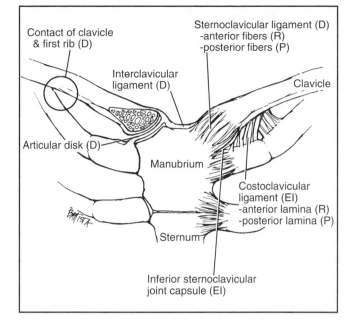

Figure 3-5 Anterior view of sternoclavicular joints showing noncontractile structures that normally limit motion.*

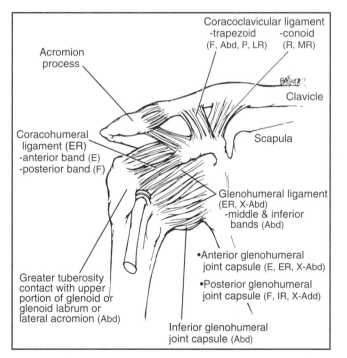

Figure 3-6 Anterior view of the shoulder showing noncontractile structures that normally limit motion.*

*Motion limited by structure is identified in brackets, using the following abbreviations for (1) Scapular movements, (2) Glenohumeral joint movements, and (3) shoulder complex movements:

(1) Scapular movements:
  El, elevation;   P, protraction;
  D, depression;   R, retraction;
  MR, medial (downward) rotation;   LR, lateral (upward) rotation.
(2) Glenohumeral joint movements:
  E, extension;   X-Add, horizontal adduction;
  IR, internal rotation;   X-Abd, horizontal abduction.
  ER, external rotation;
(3) Shoulder complex movements:
  F, elevation through flexion;   Abd, elevation through abduction.
Muscles normally limiting motion are not illustrated.

SURFACE ANATOMY

(Figs. 3-7 through 3-12)

Structure	Location
1. Inion	Dome-shaped process that marks the center of the superior nuchal line.
2. Vertebral border of the scapula	Approximately 5 to 6 cm lateral to the thoracic spinous processes covering ribs 2 to 7.
3. Inferior angle of the scapula	At the inferior aspect of the vertebral border of the scapula.
4. Spine of the scapula	The bony ridge running obliquely across the upper four fifths of the scapula.
5. Acromion process	Lateral aspect of the spine of the scapula at the tip of the shoulder.
6. Clavicle	Prominent S-shaped bone on the anterosuperior aspect of the thorax.
7. Coracoid process	Approximately 2 cm distal to the junction of the middle and lateral thirds of the clavicle in the deltopectoral triangle. Press firmly upward and laterally, deep to the anterior fibers of the deltoid.
8. Brachial pulse	Palpate pulse on the medial, proximal aspect of the upper arm posterior to the coracobrachialis.
9. Lateral epicondyle of the humerus	Lateral projection at the distal end of the humerus.
10. Olecranon process of the ulna	Posterior aspect of the elbow at the proximal end of the shaft of the ulna.
11. T12 spinous process	The most distal thoracic spinous process slightly above the level of the olecranon process of the ulna when the body is in the anatomical position.
12. Sternum	Flat bone surface along the midline of the anterior aspect of the thorax.

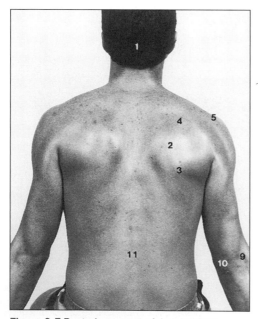

Figure 3-7 Posterior aspect of the shoulder complex.

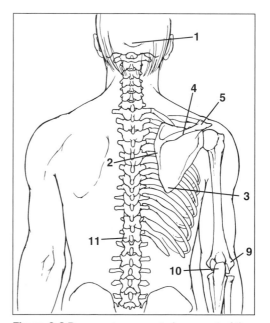

Figure 3-8 Bony anatomy, posterior aspect of the shoulder complex.

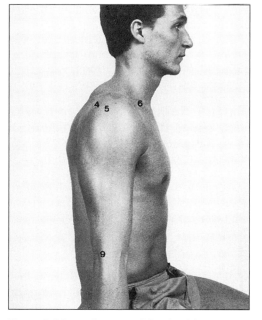

Figure 3-9 Lateral aspect of the shoulder complex.

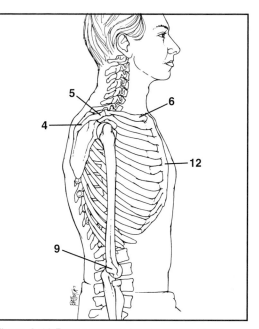

Figure 3-10 Bony anatomy, lateral aspect of the shoulder complex.

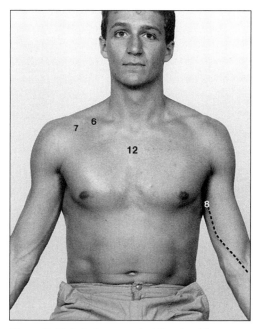

Figure 3-11 Anterior aspect of the shoulder complex.

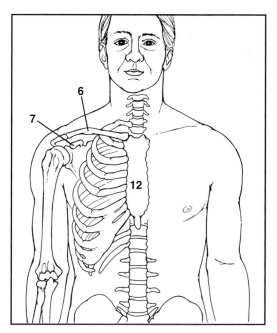

Figure 3-12 Bony anatomy, anterior aspect of the shoulder complex.

RANGE OF MOTION ASSESSMENT AND MEASUREMENT

General Scan: Upper Extremity Active Range of Motion

The AROM of the upper extremity joints is scanned, starting with the patient in the sitting or standing position with the arms at the sides (Fig. 3-13). The patient places the left hand behind the neck, then reaches down the spine to the limit of movement (Fig. 3-14A). Observe the ROM of scapular abduction and lateral (upward) rotation, shoulder elevation and external rotation, elbow flexion, forearm supination, wrist radial deviation, and finger extension. The patient places the right hand on the low back, and then reaches up the spine to the limit of movement. Observe the ROM of scapular adduction and medial (downward) rotation, shoulder extension and internal rotation, elbow flexion, forearm pronation, wrist radial deviation, and finger extension. The vertebral levels reached at the levels of the tips of the middle fingers as the patient reaches behind the neck or up the back may be used as a measure of AROM of the upper extremity joints.

The patient returns to the start position and the scan is carried out as the patient places the right hand behind the neck, then reaches down the spine to the limit of movement and places the left hand on the low back, then reaches up the spine to the limit of movement (see Fig. 3-14B). There is often an appreciable difference in the ROM between sides, as shown in Figure 3-14.

When performing the general scan of upper extremity AROM in the presence of restricted left glenohumeral joint mobility, observe the normal ROM on the right side and the restricted left shoulder joint ROM and substitute movements at the left shoulder girdle and other articulations (Fig. 3-15). In an attempt to reach behind the neck with the left hand (see Fig. 3-15A), the patient uses substitute movements to compensate for the decreased left glenohumeral joint abduction and external rotation ROM. The substitute movements include neck lateral flexion; wrist extension; increased scapular abduction, elevation, posterior tilt, and lateral (upward) rotation; and trunk lateral flexion. In an attempt to place the left hand on the low back (see Fig. 3-15B), the patient uses substitute movements to compensate for the lack of left glenohumeral joint extension and internal rotation ROM. The substitute movements include trunk flexion, excessive scapular adduction, depression, anterior tilt, and medial (downward) rotation.

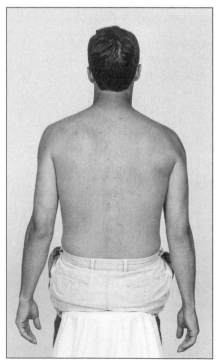

Figure 3-13 Start position: scan of AROM of the upper extremities.

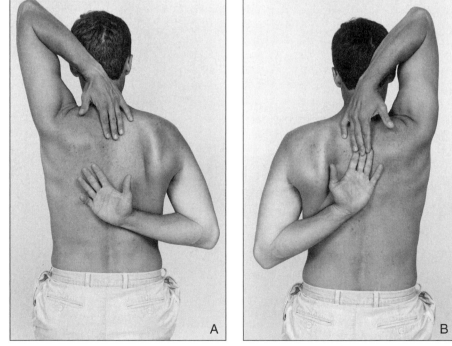

Figure 3-14 A and B. End positions: scan of AROM of the upper extremities.

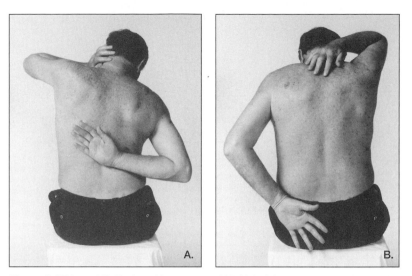

Figure 3-15 A and B. End positions: scan of AROM of the upper extremities with decreased left glenohumeral joint mobility. Substitute motions are observed at the left shoulder girdle and more distant joints.

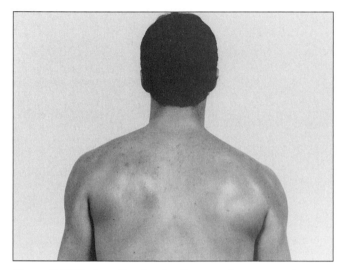

Figure 3-16 Start position for all active scapular movements.

Scapular Movements

Scapular movement (see Table 3-1) is assessed by visual observation of active movement and through passive movement. The ROM is estimated as either "full" or "restricted."

AROM Assessment

Start Position. The patient is sitting and assumes a relaxed, anatomical posture (Fig. 3-16). The therapist observes the motions from behind the patient.

Scapular Elevation

Movement. The patient moves the shoulders toward the ears in an upward or cranial direction (Fig. 3-17).

Scapular Depression

Movement. The patient moves the shoulders toward the waist in a downward or caudal direction (Fig. 3-18).

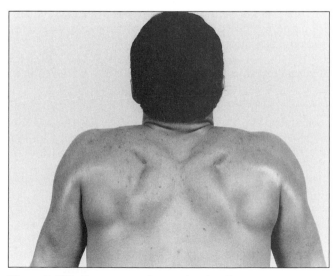

Figure 3-17 Active movement: scapular elevation.

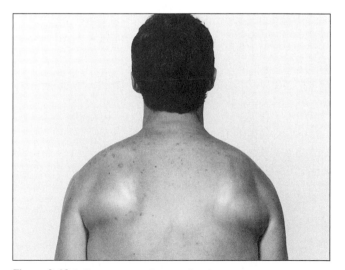

Figure 3-18 Active movement: scapular depression.

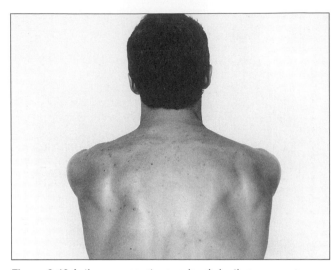

Figure 3-19 Active movement: scapular abduction.

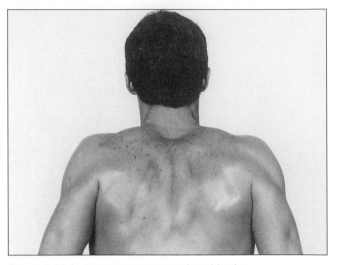

Figure 3-20 Active movement: scapular adduction.

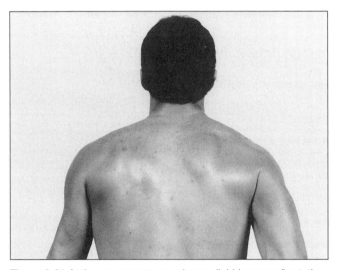

Figure 3-21 Active movement: scapular medial (downward) rotation.

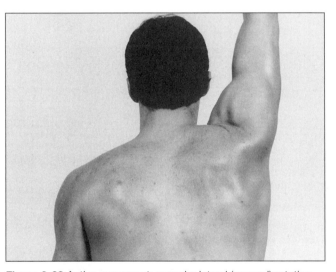

Figure 3-22 Active movement: scapular lateral (upward) rotation.

Scapular Abduction

Movement. From the start position, the patient flexes the arms to 90°, and scapular abduction is observed as the patient reaches forward (Fig. 3-19). The vertebral borders of the scapulae move away from the vertebral column.

Scapular Adduction

Movement. The patient moves the scapulae horizontally toward the vertebral column (Fig. 3-20).

Scapular Medial (Downward) Rotation

Movement. The patient extends and adducts the arm to place the hand across the small of the back and the inferior angle of the scapula moves in a medial direction (Fig. 3-21).

Scapular Lateral (Upward) Rotation

Movement. The patient elevates the arm through flexion or abduction (Fig. 3-22). During elevation, the inferior angle of the scapula moves in a lateral direction.

PROM Assessment

Start Position. The patient is in a side-lying position with the hips and knees flexed, with the head relaxed and supported on a pillow. This position remains unchanged for all scapular movements.

Stabilization. The weight of the trunk stabilizes the thorax.

Scapular Elevation

Procedure. The therapist's right hand cups the inferior angle of the scapula and elevates the scapula. The left hand assists in controlling the direction of movement (Fig. 3-23).

End Feel. Firm.

Joint Glides. *Scapular elevation*—the scapula glides in a cranial direction on the thorax. *Sternoclavicular joint:* elevation of the clavicle—the convex medial end of the clavicle glides inferiorly on the fixed concave surface of the manubrium. *Acromioclavicular joint*—gliding.

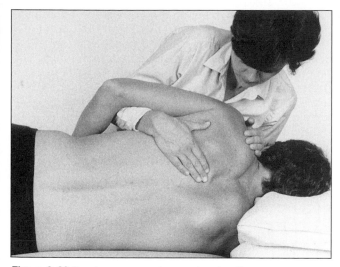

Figure 3-23 Passive movement: scapular elevation.

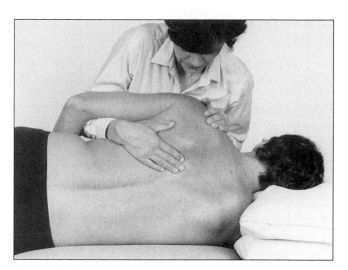

Figure 3-24 Passive movement: scapular depression.

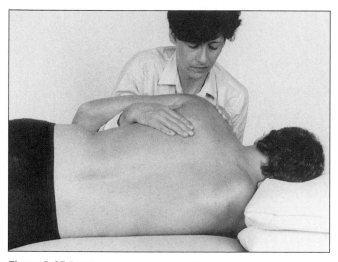

Figure 3-25 Passive movement: scapular abduction.

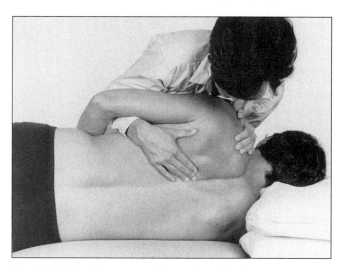

Figure 3-26 Passive movement: scapular adduction.

Scapular Depression

Procedure. The therapist's left hand is placed on the top of the shoulder girdle to depress the scapula. The right hand cups the inferior angle of the scapula to control the direction of movement (Fig. 3-24).

End Feel. Firm/hard.

Joint Glides. *Scapular depression*—the scapula glides in a caudal direction on the thorax. *Sternoclavicular joint:* depression of the clavicle—the convex medial end of the clavicle glides superiorly on the fixed concave surface of the manubrium. *Acromioclavicular joint*—gliding.

Scapular Abduction

Procedure. The therapist uses the thumb and index finger of the right hand to grasp the vertebral border and inferior angle of the scapula and abducts the scapula. The therapist's left hand is placed on top of the shoulder girdle to assist in abduction (Fig. 3-25).

End Feel. Firm.

Joint Glides. *Scapular abduction*—the scapula glides laterally on the thorax. *Sternoclavicular joint:* protraction of the clavicle—the concave medial end of the clavicle glides anteriorly on the fixed concave surface of the manubrium. *Acromioclavicular joint*—gliding.

Scapular Adduction

Procedure. The therapist uses the thumb and index finger of the right hand to grasp the axillary border and inferior angle of the scapula and adducts the scapula. The therapist's left hand is placed on top of the shoulder girdle to assist in adduction (Fig. 3-26).

End Feel. Firm.

Joint Glides. *Scapular adduction*—the scapula glides medially on the thorax. *Sternoclavicular joint:* retraction of the clavicle—the concave medial end of the clavicle glides posteriorly on the fixed concave surface of the manubrium. *Acromioclavicular joint*—gliding.

Shoulder Complex—Movements

The shoulder complex can be divided into two components: (a) the shoulder girdle, which includes the sternoclavicular, acromioclavicular, and scapulothoracic joints; and (b) the glenohumeral joint (see Tables 3-2 and 3-3). Restricted motion at the glenohumeral joint can be compensated for by movements at the shoulder girdle. Figures 3-27 and 3-28 illustrate the compensatory motions used, at the left shoulder girdle and more distant articulations, when left glenohumeral joint mobility is restricted.

In Figure 3-27A the patient combs his hair using the normal right upper extremity. In Figure 3-27B, the patient attempts to comb his hair using the left upper extremity with restricted glenohumeral joint mobility. The patient employs substitute motion at the left shoulder girdle (i.e., increased scapular abduction, depression, posterior tilt, and lateral [upward] rotation); trunk (i.e., extension and right lateral flexion); neck (i.e., flexion and right lateral flexion); and wrist (i.e., increased extension and radial deviation) to compensate for decreased glenohumeral joint abduction and external rotation ROM.

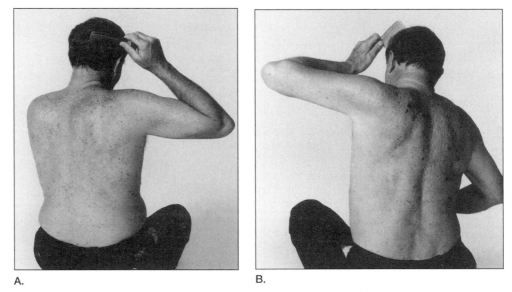

A.   B.

Figure 3-27 A. Patient combs hair using normal right upper extremity. **B.** Patient attempts to comb hair using left upper extremity with restricted glenohumeral joint movement. Substitute motions are observed at the left shoulder girdle and more distant joints.

The patient also has no difficulty reaching into his back pocket with his right hand with normal ROM at the joints of the right upper extremity (see Fig. 3-28A). However, when attempting to place his left hand in his back pocket (see Fig. 3-28B), the patient must use the substitute movements of increased scapular adduction, depression, posterior tilt, and medial (downward) rotation; trunk flexion and right lateral flexion; and wrist flexion and ulnar deviation to substitute for the decreased glenohumeral joint extension and internal rotation ROM.

When assessing and measuring PROM, it is important to differentiate between motion occurring at the shoulder girdle (scapular motion) and motion at the glenohumeral joint. To isolate the glenohumeral joint PROM, the therapist must stabilize the scapula and clavicle. To ensure adequate stabilization of the scapula and clavicle when performing PROM and measuring glenohumeral joint motion, a second therapist may assist to align the goniometer. To assess and measure movements that require motion at all articulations of the shoulder complex, the trunk is stabilized.

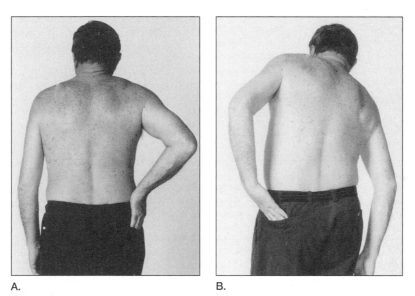

A.   B.

Figure 3-28 A. Patient reaches into back pocket using normal right upper extremity. **B.** Patient attempts to reach into back pocket using left upper extremity with restricted glenohumeral joint movement. Substitute motions are observed at the left shoulder girdle and more distant joints.

Shoulder Elevation Through Flexion (Glenohumeral Joint and Scapular Motion)

AROM Assessment

Substitute Movement. Trunk extension and shoulder abduction.

PROM Assessment

Start Position. The patient is in a crook-lying (Fig. 3-29) or a sitting position. The arm is at the side with the palm facing medially.

Stabilization. The weight of the trunk. The therapist stabilizes the thorax.

Therapist's Distal Hand Placement. The therapist grasps the distal humerus.

End Position. The therapist applies slight traction to and moves the humerus anteriorly and upward to the limit of motion for shoulder elevation through flexion (Fig. 3-30). The elbow is maintained in extension to prevent restriction of shoulder flexion ROM due to passive insufficiency of the two-joint triceps muscle (11).

End Feel. Firm.

Joint Glides/Spin. Shoulder elevation through flexion:

Scapular lateral (upward) rotation—the inferior angle of the scapula rotates in a lateral direction on the thorax.

Sternoclavicular joint: (a) elevation of the clavicle—the convex medial end of the clavicle glides inferiorly on the fixed concave surface of the manubrium, and (b) posterior rotation of the clavicle—the clavicle spins on the fixed surfaces of the manubrium.

Acromioclavicular joint—gliding.

Glenohumeral joint flexion—the convex humeral head spins (i.e., rotates around a fixed point) on the fixed concave glenoid cavity.

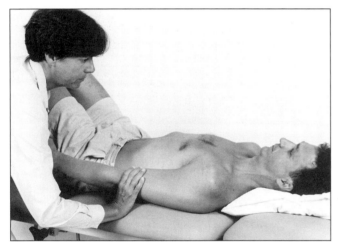

Figure 3-29 Start position for shoulder elevation through flexion.

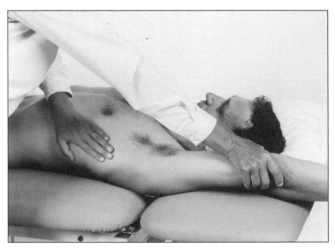

Figure 3-30 Firm end feel at limit of shoulder elevation through flexion.

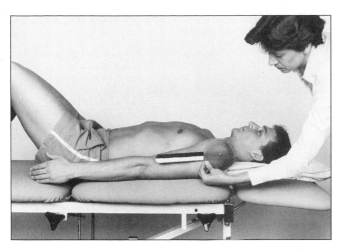

Figure 3-31 Start position for shoulder elevation through flexion: supine.

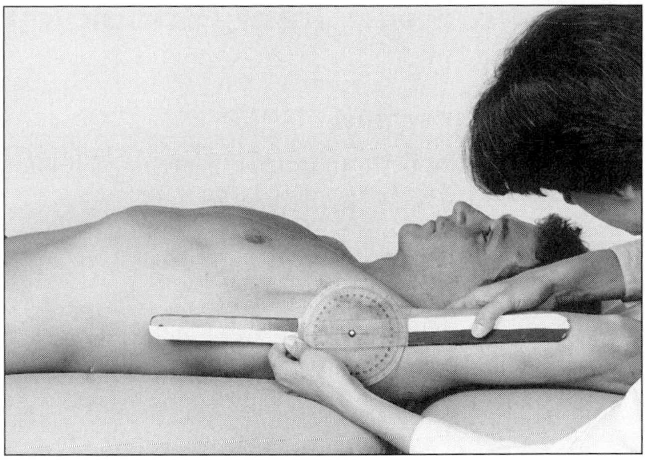

Figure 3-32 Shoulder elevation through flexion.

Measurement: Universal Goniometer

Start Position. The patient is in a crook-lying position (Fig. 3-31) or sitting (see Fig. 3-34). The arm is at the side, with the palm facing medially.

Stabilization. The weight of the trunk. The scapula is left free to move.

Goniometer Axis. The axis is placed at the lateral aspect of the center of the humeral head, about 2.5 cm inferior to the lateral aspect of the acromion process (see Fig. 3-36).

Stationary Arm. Parallel to the lateral midline of the trunk.

Movable Arm. Parallel to the longitudinal axis of the humerus.

End Position. The humerus is moved in an anterior and upward direction to the limit of motion in elevation (180°). This movement represents scapular and glenohumeral motion (Fig. 3-32).

Glenohumeral Joint (Shoulder) Flexion

AROM Assessment

The patient cannot perform isolated glenohumeral joint flexion ROM without the scapula being stabilized.

PROM Assessment

Start Position. The patient is in a crook-lying or a sitting position. The arm is at the side with the palm facing medially.

Stabilization. The therapist places one hand on the axillary border of the scapula to stabilize the scapula.

Therapist's Distal Hand Placement. The therapist grasps the distal humerus.

End Position. While stabilizing the scapula, the therapist applies slight traction to and moves the humerus anteri-

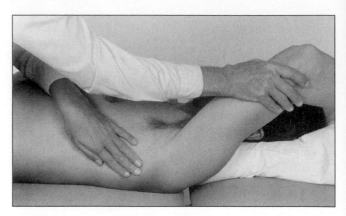

Figure 3-33 Firm end feel at limit of glenohumeral joint flexion.

orly and upward to the limit of motion to assess glenohumeral joint motion (Fig. 3-33).

End Feel. Firm.

Joint Spin. *Glenohumeral joint flexion*—the convex humeral head spins on the fixed concave glenoid cavity.

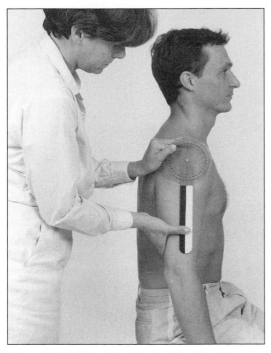

Figure 3-34 Start position for shoulder elevation through flexion: sitting.

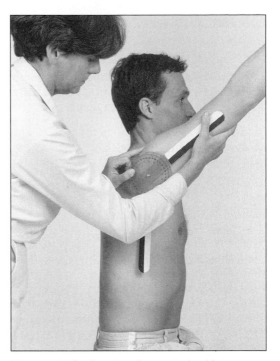

Figure 3-35 Goniometer alignment: shoulder elevation through flexion, glenohumeral joint flexion, and extension.

Measurement: Universal Goniometer

Start Position. The patient is in sitting (Fig. 3-34) or crook-lying position. The arm is at the side, with the palm facing medially.

Stabilization. The therapist stabilizes the scapula.

Goniometer Axis. The axis is placed at the lateral aspect of the center of the humeral head about 2.5 cm inferior to the lateral aspect of the acromion process (see Fig. 3-36).

Stationary Arm. Parallel to the lateral midline of the trunk.

Movable Arm. Parallel to the longitudinal axis of the humerus.

End Position. The humerus is moved in an anterior and upward direction to the limit of motion (120° [5]) to measure glenohumeral joint flexion (Figs. 3-35 and 3-36).

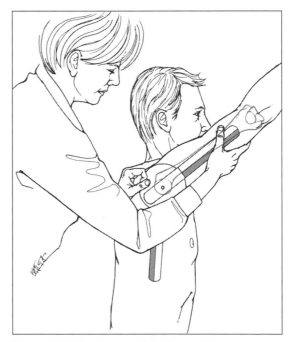

Figure 3-36 Glenohumeral joint flexion ROM.

Shoulder Extension

AROM Assessment

Substitute Movement. Scapular anterior tilting, scapular elevation, and shoulder abduction. In sitting, the patient may flex and ipsilaterally rotate the trunk.

PROM Assessment

Start Position. The patient is prone (Fig. 3-37) or sitting. The arm is at the side, with the palm facing medially.

Stabilization. The therapist stabilizes the scapula to isolate and assess glenohumeral joint motion.

Therapist's Distal Hand Placement. The therapist grasps the distal humerus.

End Position. The therapist applies slight traction to and moves the humerus posteriorly until the scapula begins to move (Fig. 3-38). The elbow is flexed to prevent restriction of shoulder extension ROM due to passive insufficiency of the two-joint biceps brachii muscle (11).

End Feel. Firm.

Joint Spin. *Glenohumeral joint extension*—the convex humeral head spins on the fixed concave glenoid cavity.

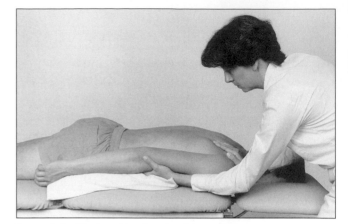

Figure 3-37 Start position for glenohumeral joint extension.

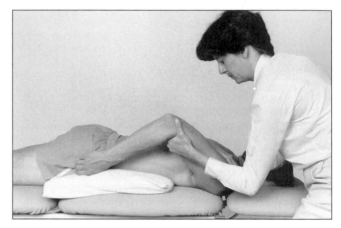

Figure 3-38 Firm end feel at limit of glenohumeral joint extension.

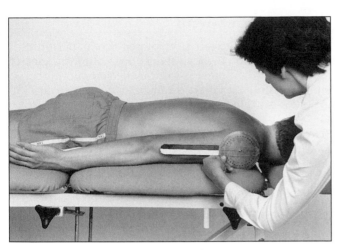

Figure 3-39 Start position for shoulder extension.

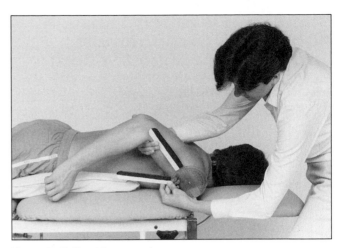

Figure 3-40 Shoulder extension: prone.

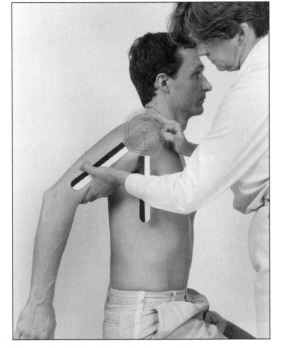

Figure 3-41 Shoulder extension: sitting.

Measurement: Universal Goniometer

Start Position. The patient is prone (Fig. 3-39) or sitting. The arm is at the side, with the palm facing medially.

Stabilization. The therapist's forearm may be used to stabilize the scapula.

Goniometer Axis. The axis is placed at the lateral aspect of the center of the humeral head about 2.5 cm inferior to the lateral aspect of the acromion process (see Fig. 3-36).

Stationary Arm. Parallel to the lateral midline of the trunk.

Movable Arm. Parallel to the longitudinal axis of the humerus, pointing toward the lateral epicondyle of the humerus.

End Position. The humerus is moved posteriorly to the limit of motion (60°) (Figs. 3-40 and 3-41).

Shoulder Elevation Through Abduction (Glenohumeral Joint and Scapular Motion)

AROM Assessment

Substitute Movement. Contralateral trunk lateral flexion, scapular elevation, and shoulder flexion.

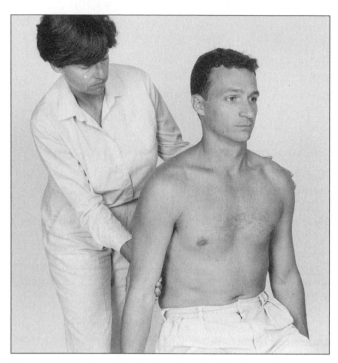

Figure 3-42 Start position for shoulder elevation through abduction.

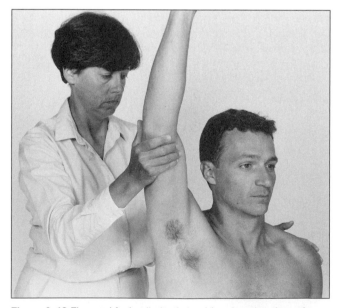

Figure 3-43 Firm end feel at limit of shoulder elevation through abduction.

PROM Assessment

The humerus is externally rotated when performing shoulder elevation through abduction to allow the greater tuberosity of the humerus to clear the acromion process. Prior to testing elevation through abduction, ensure the patient is capable of full shoulder external rotation.

Start Position. The patient is sitting (Fig. 3-42) or supine. The arm is at the side with the shoulder in external rotation. Ensure the patient sits in an upright posture, as the slouched sitting posture has been shown (12) to result in decreased shoulder abduction ROM.

Stabilization. The therapist stabilizes the trunk.

Therapist's Distal Hand Placement. The therapist grasps the distal humerus.

End Position. The therapist applies slight traction to and moves the humerus laterally and upward to the limit of motion for elevation through abduction (Fig. 3-43).

End Feel. Firm.

Joint Glides. Shoulder elevation through abduction:

Scapular lateral (upward) rotation—the inferior angle of the scapula rotates in a lateral direction on the thorax.

Sternoclavicular joint: (a) elevation of the clavicle—the convex medial end of the clavicle glides inferiorly on the fixed concave surface of the manubrium, and (b) posterior rotation of the clavicle—the clavicle spins on the fixed surface of the manubrium.

Acromioclavicular joint—gliding.

Glenohumeral joint abduction—the convex humeral head glides inferiorly on the fixed concave glenoid cavity.

Measurement: Universal Goniometer

Start Position. The patient is supine (Fig. 3-44) or sitting. The arm is at the side in adduction and external rotation.

Stabilization. The weight of the trunk.

Goniometer Axis. The axis is placed at the midpoint of the anterior or posterior aspect of the glenohumeral joint, about 1.3 cm inferior and lateral to the coracoid process (Figs. 3-45 and 3-46).

Stationary Arm. Parallel to the sternum.

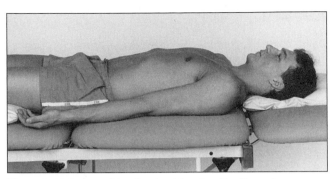

Figure 3-44 Start position for shoulder elevation through abduction.

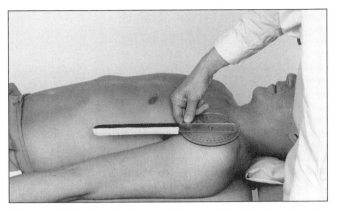

Figure 3-45 Goniometer placement for shoulder elevation through abduction.

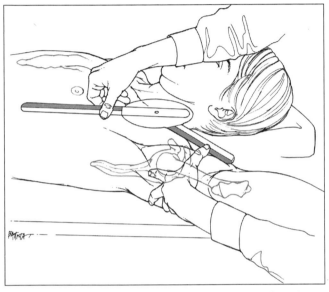

Figure 3-46 Goniometer alignment: shoulder elevation through abduction and glenohumeral joint abduction.

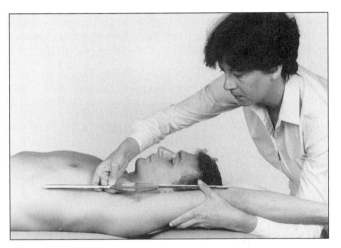

Figure 3-47 Shoulder elevation through abduction.

Movable Arm. Parallel to the longitudinal axis of the humerus.

End Position. The humerus is moved laterally and upward to the limit of motion in elevation (180°) (Fig. 3-47). This movement represents scapular and glenohumeral movement. The posterior aspect may be preferred for measurement of shoulder elevation through abduction range in women because the breast may interfere with the goniometer placement anteriorly (Fig. 3-48).

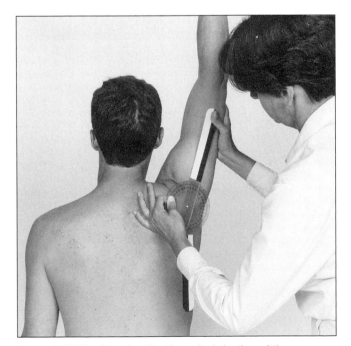

Figure 3-48 Shoulder elevation through abduction: sitting.

Glenohumeral Joint (Shoulder) Abduction

AROM Assessment

The patient cannot perform isolated glenohumeral joint abduction ROM without the scapula being stabilized.

PROM Assessment

Start Position. The patient is supine (Fig. 3-49) or sitting. The arm is at the side with the elbow flexed to 90°.

Stabilization. The therapist stabilizes the scapula.

Therapist's Distal Hand Placement. The therapist grasps the distal humerus.

End Position. The therapist applies slight traction to and moves the humerus laterally and upward to the limit of motion of glenohumeral joint abduction (Fig. 3-50).

End Feel. Firm or hard.

Joint Glide. *Glenohumeral joint abduction*—the convex humeral head glides inferiorly on the fixed concave glenoid cavity.

Measurement: Universal Goniometer (not shown)

Start Position. The patient is supine or sitting. The arm is at the side with the elbow flexed to 90° (see Fig. 3-49).

Goniometer Placement. The goniometer is placed the same as for shoulder elevation through abduction (see Figs. 3-45 and 3-46).

Stabilization. The therapist stabilizes the scapula and clavicle to isolate and measure glenohumeral joint abduction.

End Position. The humerus is moved laterally and upward to the limit of motion (90–120° [5]) to measure glenohumeral joint abduction.

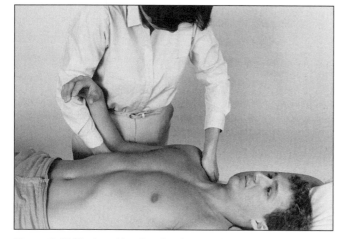

Figure 3-49 Start position for glenohumeral joint abduction.

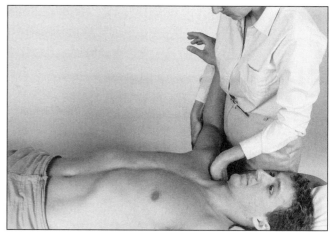

Figure 3-50 Firm or hard end feel at limit of glenohumeral joint abduction.

Shoulder Horizontal Abduction and Adduction

AROM Assessment

Substitute Movement. Scapular retraction (horizontal abduction), scapular protraction (horizontal adduction), and trunk rotation.

PROM Assessment

Start Position. The patient is sitting. The shoulder is in 90° of abduction and neutral rotation. The elbow is flexed and the forearm is in midposition (Fig. 3-51).

Stabilization. The therapist stabilizes the trunk and scapula to isolate and assess glenohumeral joint motion.

Therapist's Distal Hand Placement. The therapist supports the arm in abduction and grasps the distal humerus.

End Position. The therapist applies slight traction to and moves the humerus posteriorly to the limit of motion for horizontal abduction (Fig. 3-52) and anteriorly to the limit of motion for horizontal adduction (Fig. 3-53).

End Feels. Horizontal abduction—firm; horizontal adduction—firm/soft.

Joint Glides. *Glenohumeral joint horizontal abduction*—the convex humeral head glides anteriorly on the fixed concave glenoid cavity. *Glenohumeral joint horizontal adduction*—the convex humeral head glides posteriorly on the fixed concave glenoid cavity.

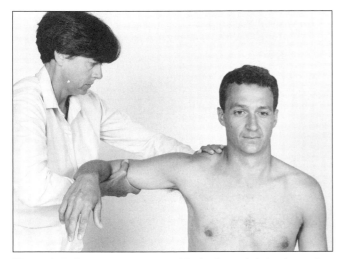

Figure 3-51 Start position for shoulder horizontal abduction and horizontal adduction.

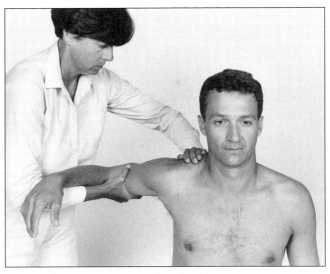

Figure 3-52 Firm end feel at limit of shoulder horizontal abduction.

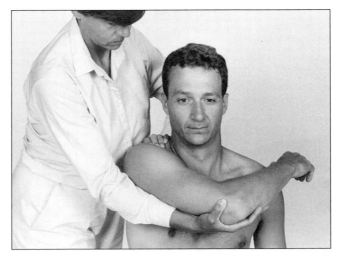

Figure 3-53 Firm or soft end feel at limit of shoulder horizontal adduction.

Measurement: Universal Goniometer

Start Position. The patient is sitting. The shoulder is in 90° of abduction and neutral rotation. The elbow is flexed and the forearm is in midposition (Fig. 3-54). An

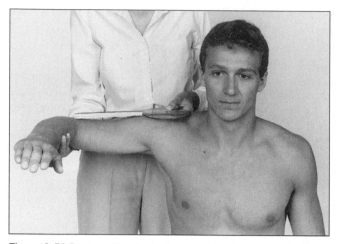

Figure 3-54 Start position for horizontal abduction and adduction.

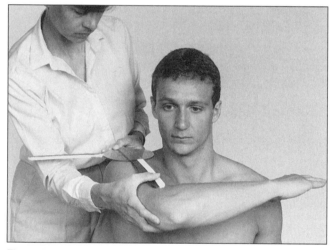

Figure 3-55 Shoulder horizontal adduction.

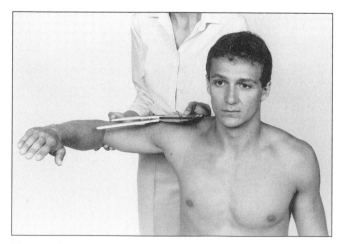

Figure 3-57 Shoulder horizontal abduction.

alternate start position has the shoulder in 90° of flexion, the elbow is flexed, and the forearm is in midposition (Fig. 3-58). The start position of the shoulder should be recorded.

Stabilization. The therapist stabilizes the trunk and scapula.

Goniometer Axis. The axis is placed on top of the acromion process (Figs. 3-55 and 3-56).

Stationary Arm. Perpendicular to the trunk.

Movable Arm. Parallel to the longitudinal axis of the humerus.

End Position. The therapist supports the arm in abduction. The therapist applies slight traction to and moves the humerus anteriorly across the chest to the limit of motion in horizontal adduction (135°) (Figs. 3-55 and 3-56) and posteriorly to the limit of motion in horizontal abduction (45°) (Fig. 3-57).

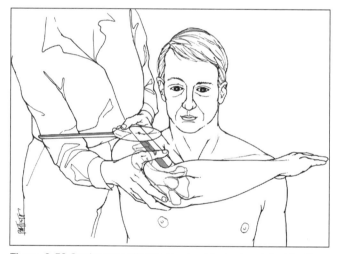

Figure 3-56 Goniometer alignment: shoulder horizontal adduction.

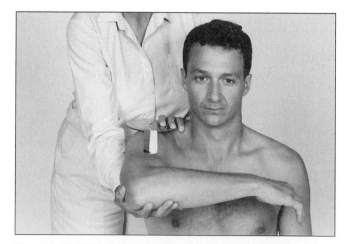

Figure 3-58 Alternate start position for horizontal abduction and adduction.

Shoulder Internal Rotation

AROM Assessment

Substitute Movement. In prone with the shoulder in 90° abduction: scapular elevation, shoulder abduction, and elbow extension. In supine with the shoulder in 90° abduction: scapular elevation, protraction and anterior tilt, shoulder abduction, and elbow extension. In sitting with the arm at the side: scapular elevation, shoulder abduction, and trunk rotation.

PROM Assessment

Start Position. The patient is prone or supine. In prone, the shoulder is in 90° of abduction, the elbow is flexed to 90°, and the forearm is in midposition (Fig. 3-59). A towel is placed under the humerus to achieve the abducted position. This start position is contraindicated if the patient has a history of posterior dislocation of the glenohumeral joint.

Stabilization. The therapist stabilizes the scapula and maintains the position of the humerus, without restricting movement. In prone, the plinth limits scapular protraction and anterior tilt. When assessing internal rotation ROM in supine with the shoulder in 90° of abduction, Boon and Smith (13) recommend the therapist place one hand over the clavicle and coracoid process to stabilize the scapula for more reliable and reproducible results.

Therapist's Distal Hand Placement. The therapist grasps the distal radius and ulna.

End Position. The therapist moves the palm of the hand toward the ceiling to the limit of internal rotation (Fig. 3-60);—that is, when scapular movement first occurs.

End Feel. Firm.

Joint Glide. *Glenohumeral joint internal rotation*—with the shoulder in the anatomical position, the convex humeral head glides posteriorly on the fixed concave glenoid cavity.

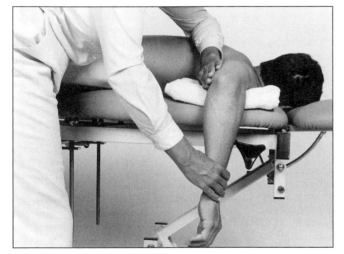

Figure 3-59 Start position for shoulder internal rotation.

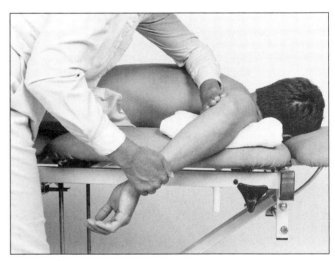

Figure 3-60 Firm end feel at limit of shoulder internal rotation.

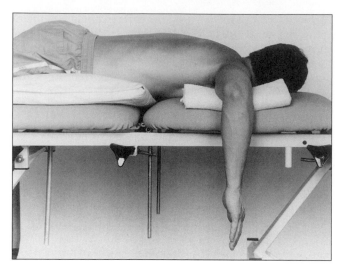

Figure 3-61 Start position for shoulder internal rotation.

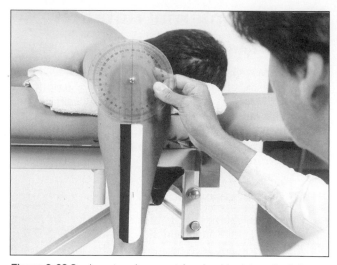

Figure 3-62 Goniometer placement for shoulder internal rotation.

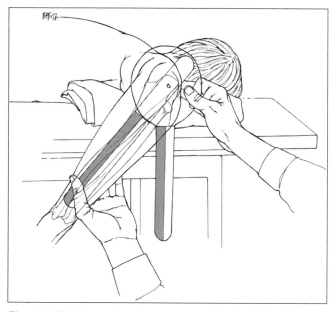

Figure 3-63 Shoulder internal rotation.

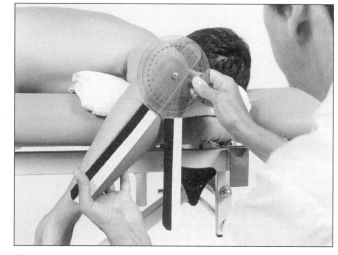

Figure 3-64 Goniometer alignment: shoulder internal and external rotation.

Measurement: Universal Goniometer

Start Position. The patient is prone or supine. The shoulder is in 90° of abduction, the elbow is flexed to 90°, and the forearm is in midposition (Fig. 3-61). A towel is placed under the humerus to achieve the abducted position. This start position is contraindicated if the patient has a history of posterior dislocation of the glenohumeral joint.

Goniometer Axis. The axis is placed on the olecranon process of the ulna (Figs. 3-62 and 3-63).

Stationary Arm. Perpendicular to the floor.

Movable Arm. Parallel to the longitudinal axis of the ulna, pointing toward the ulnar styloid process.

End Position. The palm of the hand is moved toward the ceiling to the limit of internal rotation (70°) (Figs. 3-63 and 3-64).

Shoulder External Rotation

AROM Assessment

Substitute Movement. In supine with the shoulder in 90° abduction: elbow extension, scapular depression, and shoulder adduction. In sitting with the arm at the side: scapular depression, shoulder adduction, and trunk rotation.

PROM Assessment

Start Position. The patient is supine. The shoulder is in 90° of abduction, the elbow is flexed to 90°, and the forearm is in midposition (Fig. 3-65). A towel is placed under the humerus to achieve the abducted position. This start position is contraindicated if the patient has a history of anterior dislocation of the glenohumeral joint.

Stabilization. The weight of the trunk. The therapist stabilizes the scapula.

Therapist's Distal Hand Placement. The therapist grasps the distal radius and ulna.

End Position. The therapist moves the dorsum of the hand toward the floor to the limit of external rotation (Fig. 3-66); —that is, when scapular movement first occurs.

End Feel. Firm.

Joint Glide. *Glenohumeral joint external rotation*—with the shoulder in the anatomical position, the convex humeral head glides anteriorly on the fixed concave glenoid cavity.

Measurement: Universal Goniometer

The measurement process is similar to that for internal rotation with the following exceptions.

Start Position. The patient is supine (Fig. 3-67). This start position is contraindicated if the patient has a history of anterior dislocation of the glenohumeral joint.

End Position. The dorsum of the hand moves toward the floor to the limit of motion in external rotation (90°) (Fig. 3-68).

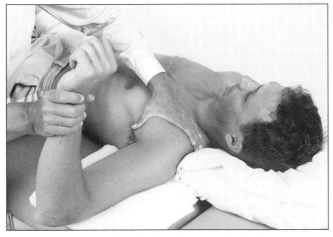

Figure 3-65 Start position for shoulder external rotation.

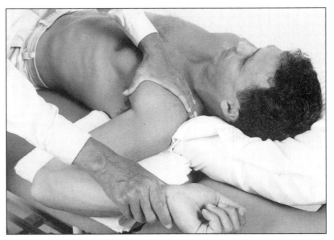

Figure 3-66 Firm end feel at limit of shoulder external rotation.

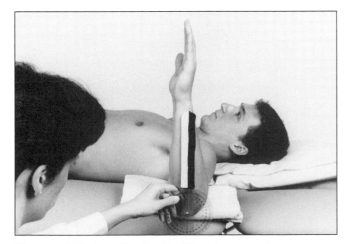

Figure 3-67 Start position for shoulder external rotation.

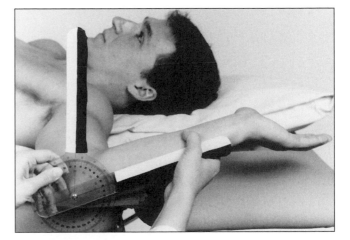

Figure 3-68 Shoulder external rotation.

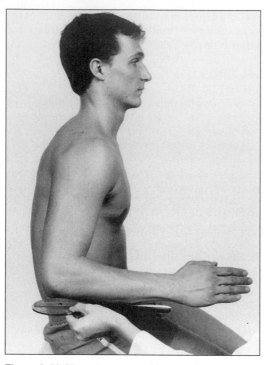

Figure 3-69 Alternate start position for shoulder internal rotation.

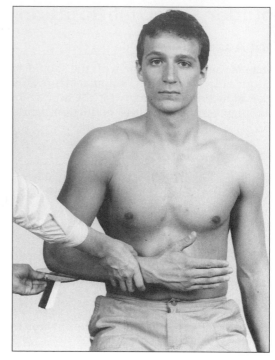

Figure 3-70 Shoulder internal rotation.

Alternate Assessment and Measurement: Internal/External Rotation

If the patient cannot achieve 90° of shoulder abduction, the end feel can be assessed (not shown) and the measurement can be taken while the patient is sitting. The starting position should be documented.

Start Position. The patient is sitting. To measure shoulder internal rotation, the shoulder is abducted to about 15°, the elbow is flexed to 90°, and the forearm is in midposition (Fig. 3-69). To measure external rotation (not

shown), the arm is at the side in adduction, the elbow is flexed to 90°, and the forearm is in midposition.

Goniometer Axis. The axis is placed under the olecranon process.

Stationary Arm. Perpendicular to the trunk.

Movable Arm. Parallel to the longitudinal axis of the ulna.

End Positions. The palm of the hand is moved toward the abdomen to the limit of shoulder internal rotation (Fig. 3-70). The therapist moves the hand away from the abdomen to the limit of external rotation.

MUSCLE LENGTH ASSESSMENT AND MEASUREMENT

Pectoralis Major

Origin (2)	Insertion (2)
Pectoralis Major	
a. Clavicular head: anterior border of the sternal half of the clavicle.	Lateral lip of the intertubercular groove of the humerus.
b. Sternal head: ipsilateral half of the anterior surface of the sternum; cartilage of the first 6 or 7 ribs; sternal end of the 6th rib; aponeurosis of the external abdominal oblique.	

This muscle length assessment technique is contraindicated if the patient has a history of anterior dislocation of the glenohumeral joint.

Start Position. The patient is supine with the shoulder in external rotation and 90° elevation through a plane midway between forward flexion and abduction. The elbow is in 90° flexion (Fig. 3-71).

Stabilization. The therapist stabilizes the trunk.

End Position. The shoulder is moved into horizontal abduction to the limit of motion, to put the pectoralis major on full stretch (Figs. 3-72 and 3-73).

Assessment. With shortness of the pectoralis major muscle, shoulder horizontal abduction will be restricted. The therapist either observes the available PROM or uses a goniometer to measure and record the available shoulder horizontal abduction PROM.

End Feel. Pectoralis major on stretch—firm.

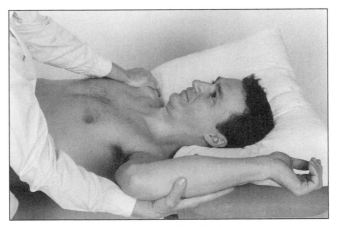

Figure 3-71 Start position: length of pectoralis major.

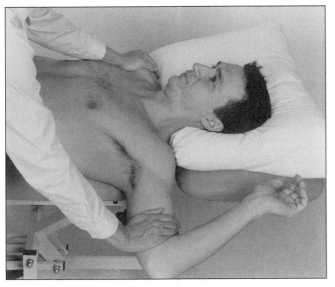

Figure 3-72 Pectoralis major on stretch.

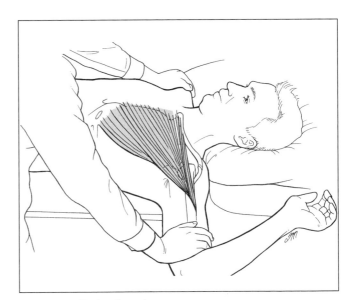

Figure 3-73 Pectoralis major.

Pectoralis Minor (14)

Origin (2)	Origin (2)
Pectoralis Minor	
Outer surfaces of ribs 2 to 4 or 3 to 5 near the costal cartilages; fascia over corresponding external intercostals.	Medial border and upper surface of the coracoid process of the scapula.

This muscle length assessment technique is contraindicated if the patient has a history of posterior dislocation of the glenohumeral joint.

Start Position. The patient is supine with the scapula over the side of the plinth, with the shoulder in external rotation and about 80° flexion. The elbow is flexed (Fig. 3-74).

Stabilization. The weight of the trunk.

End Position. The therapist applies force through the long axis of the shaft of the humerus to move the shoulder girdle in a cranial and dorsal direction to put the pectoralis minor on full stretch (Figs. 3-75 and 3-76).

Assessment. The therapist observes decreased scapular retraction ROM in the presence of a shortened length of pectoralis minor.

End Feel. Pectoralis minor on stretch—firm.

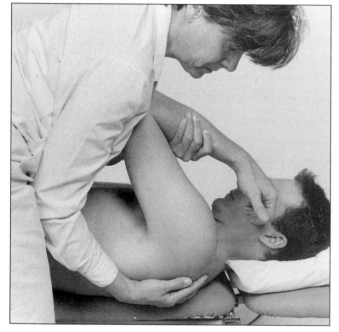

Figure 3-74 Start position: length of pectoralis minor.

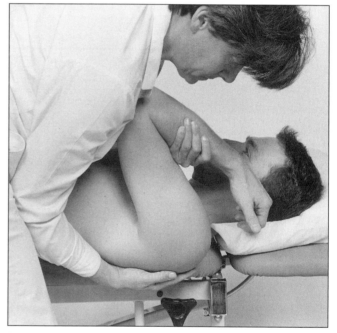

Figure 3-75 Pectoralis minor on stretch.

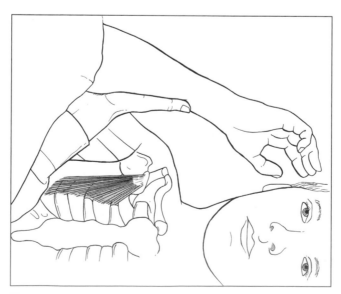

Figure 3-76 Pectoralis minor.

FUNCTIONAL APPLICATION

Joint Function

The function of the shoulder complex is to position or move the arm in space for the purpose of hand function. The shoulder complex is the most mobile joint complex in the body, providing a ROM that exceeds that of any other joint. Because of this mobility, stability is sacrificed (5,15–19).

Functional Range of Motion

The glenohumeral joint may be abducted and adducted, flexed and extended, and internally and externally rotated. In the performance of functional activities, the glenohumeral movements are accompanied at varying points in the ROM by scapular, clavicular, and trunk motion. These motions extend the functional range capabilities of the shoulder joint, and without their contribution, movement of the upper limbs would be severely restricted (16,18,19). The functional movements of the shoulder complex are described to emphasize the interdependence of the components of the shoulder complex and trunk throughout movement.

Elevation of the Arm Over the Head

This functional motion of elevation to 170° to 180° may be achieved through forward flexion in the sagittal plane or abduction in the frontal plane. Owing to the position of the scapula, which lies 30° to 45° anterior to the frontal plane (20), many daily functional activities are performed in the plane of the scapula. The plane of the scapula is the

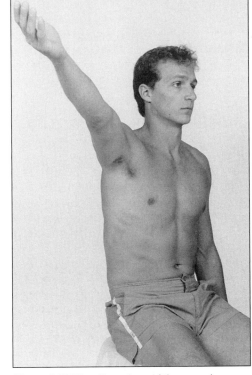

Figure 3-77 Elevation: plane of the scapula.

plane of reference for diagonal movements of shoulder elevation (Fig. 3-77). *Scaption* (21) is the term given to this midplane elevation. The plane used by an individual depends on the motion requirements of the activity and the position of the hand required for the task (Table 3-4).

To attain the full 180° of elevation through flexion or abduction, movement of the glenohumeral joint is accompanied by movement at the sternoclavicular,

TABLE 3-4	Shoulder Horizontal Adduction/Abduction and Other Shoulder ROM* Required for Selected Functional Activities†		
Activity	**Horizontal Adduction ROM (degrees)‡**	**Other Shoulder ROM (degrees)**	
Washing axilla	104 ± 12	flexion	52 ± 14
Eating	87 ± 29	flexion	52 ± 8
Combing hair	54 ± 27	abduction	112 ± 10
	Horizontal Abduction ROM (degrees)‡		
Reaching maximally up back	69 ± 11	extension	56 ± 13
Reaching perineum	86 ± 13	extension	38 ± 10

*Values are mean ± SD for eight normal subjects.

†This table was adapted from Master FA, Lippitt SB, Sidles JA, Harryman DT. *Practical Evaluation and Management of the Shoulder.* Philadelphia: WB Saunders; 1994:22, 23.[22]

‡The 0° start position for establishing the degrees of horizontal adduction and horizontal abduction is 90° shoulder abduction (see Fig. 3-41).

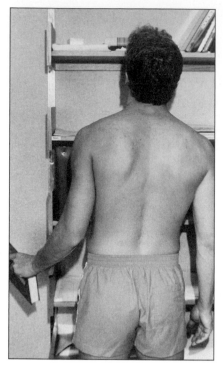

Figure 3-78 Setting phase of the scapula during elevation of the arm through abduction. The scapula remains stationary.

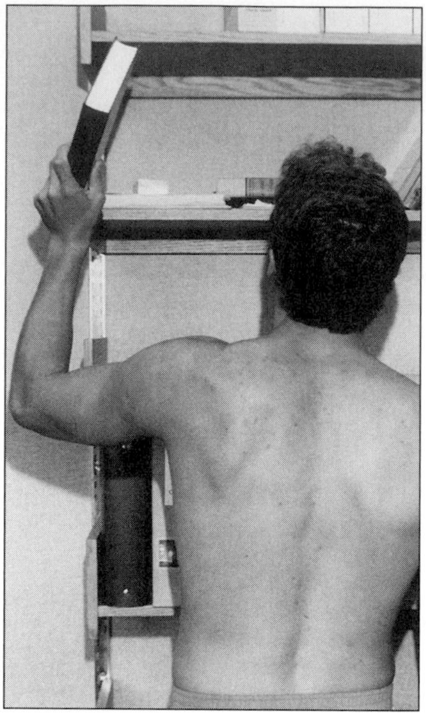

Figure 3-79 Scapulohumeral rhythm: during elevation beyond 60° of flexion or 30° of abduction, the scapula abducts and laterally (upward) rotates.

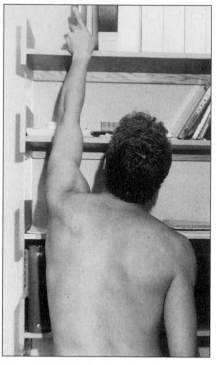

Figure 3-80 Full elevation through abduction: full range is achieved through contralateral trunk lateral flexion.

acromioclavicular, and scapulothoracic joints. The final degrees of motion can be achieved only through contribution of the spinal movement of trunk extension and/or contralateral lateral flexion (1,15,20). The total shoulder complex functions in a coordinated way to provide smooth movement and to gain a large excursion of movement for the upper extremity. The coordinated movement pattern achieved through scapulothoracic and glenohumeral movement is described as a "scapulohumeral rhythm" (5,15,17,20).

There are individual variations as to the contribution of all joints to the movement. Variation depends on the plane of elevation, the arc of elevation, the amount of load on the arm, and individual anatomical differences (19). Recognizing these variations, it is generally noted that the range of glenohumeral to scapular motion throughout elevation is in the ratio of 2:1; that is, 2° of glenohumeral motion to every degree of scapular motion (5,17,18,23). The scapulohumeral rhythm is described for elevation through flexion and for elevation through abduction. An understanding of the rhythm is essential in understanding the significance of limitations in joint range of motion at the shoulder complex.

Scapulohumeral Rhythm

During the initial 60° of shoulder flexion in the sagittal plane or the initial 30° of abduction in the frontal plane, there is an inconsistent scapulohumeral rhythm. It is during this phase that the scapula is seeking stability in relationship to the humerus (5,23–25). The scapula is in a setting phase where it may remain stationary, or it may slightly medially (downward) or laterally (upward) rotate

(23) (Fig. 3-78). The glenohumeral joint is the main contributor to movement in this phase. Feeding activities that are performed within this phase of shoulder elevation include using a spoon or a fork and drinking from a cup. These activities are carried out within the ranges of 5° to 45° shoulder flexion and 5° to 30° shoulder abduction (26).

Following the setting phase, there is a predictable scapulohumeral rhythm throughout the remaining arc of movement to 170° (Fig. 3-79). For every 15° of movement between 30° abduction or 60° flexion and 170° of abduction/flexion, 10° occurs at the glenohumeral joint and 5° occurs at the scapulothoracic joint. Movement of the scapula following the setting phase consists of the primary scapular movement of lateral (upward) rotation, accompanied by secondary rotations of posterior tilting (sagittal plane) and posterior rotation (transverse plane) as the humeral angle is increased with elevation of the arm in the scapular plane (27).

Range to 170° through abduction depends on a normal scapulohumeral rhythm and the ability to externally rotate the humerus fully through elevation. When the abducted arm reaches a position of 90°, movement through full range of elevation cannot continue because the greater tuberosity of the humerus contacts the superior margin of the glenoid fossa and the coracoacromial arch (1,25,28). External rotation of the humerus places the greater tuberosity posteriorly, allowing the humerus to move freely under the coracoacromial arch. Full shoulder elevation through flexion depends on scapulohumeral rhythm and the ability to rotate the humerus internally through range (29).

The final degrees of elevation are achieved through contralateral trunk lateral flexion (Fig. 3-80) and/or trunk extension. From the discussion of scapulohumeral rhythm, it becomes apparent that restriction in movement at any of the joints of the shoulder complex will limit the ability to position the hand for function.

Shoulder Extension

The range of 60° of shoulder extension is primarily obtained through the glenohumeral joint (28). A consistent scapulohumeral rhythm is not present in this movement. In the performance of functional activities, extension is often accompanied by adduction and medial (downward) rotation of the scapula (Fig. 3-81).

Forty-three degrees to 69° of shoulder extension is required to reach maximally up the back (22) (e.g., when hooking a bra; see Fig. 3-82), and 28° to 48° shoulder extension is necessary to reach the perineum (22) when performing toilet hygiene.

Horizontal Adduction and Abduction

The movements of horizontal adduction and abduction allow the arm to be moved around the body at shoulder level for such activities as washing the axilla or the back (Fig. 3-83), writing on a blackboard (Fig. 3-84), and sliding a window open or closed. Although by definition horizontal

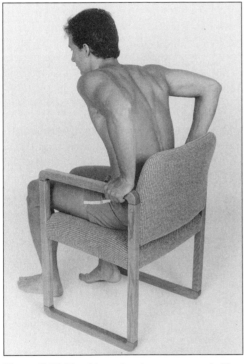

Figure 3-81 Shoulder extension accompanied by scapular adduction and medial (downward) rotation.

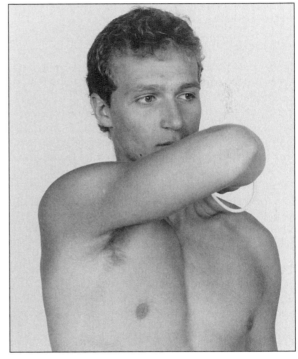

Figure 3-83 Horizontal adduction.

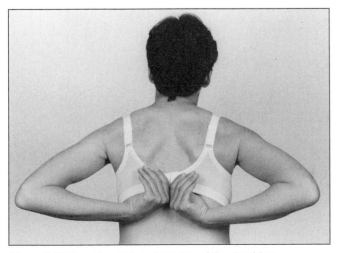

Figure 3-82 Functional internal rotation of the shoulders.

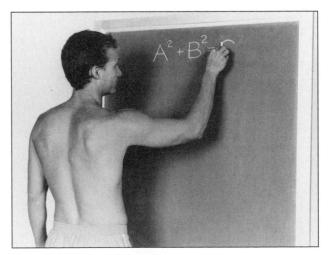

Figure 3-84 Horizontal abduction.

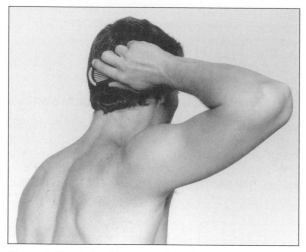

Figure 3-85 Full shoulder external rotation.

adduction and abduction movements take place in the transverse plane, many activities of daily living (ADL) require similar motions in planes located above or below shoulder level. These movements may also be referred to as horizontal adduction and abduction until the frontal plane is approached; the movements are then referred to as either adduction or abduction. Table 3-4 provides examples of the ROM required for selected ADL, to bring the arm in front of the body (horizontal adduction) or behind the body (horizontal abduction) and position the arm for other shoulder movements needed to perform these activities.

Internal and External Rotation

The range of movement varies with the position of the arm. Both ranges average 68° when the arm is at the side, whereas when the arm is abducted to 90°, 70° of internal rotation and 90° of external rotation can be achieved (8).

Full external rotation is required to place the hand behind the neck when performing self-care activities such as combing the hair (Fig. 3-85) and manipulating the clasp of a necklace.

Internal shoulder rotation is needed to do up the buttons on a shirt. Five degrees to 25° of shoulder internal rotation is required to use a spoon or fork and to drink from a cup (26). Full glenohumeral joint internal rotation, augmented by scapulothoracic and elbow joint motion, positions the hand behind the back to reach into a back pocket, perform toilet hygiene, and hook a bra (see Fig. 3-82). Mallon and colleagues (30) analyzed joint motions that occurred at the shoulder complex and elbow in placing the arm behind the back. The analysis revealed the presence of a coordinated pattern of motion occurring between scapular and glenohumeral joint motion. At the beginning of the ROM, internal rotation occurs almost exclusively at the glenohumeral joint as the hand is brought across in front of the body and to a position alongside the ipsilateral hip. As the movement continues and the hand is brought behind the low back, motion at the scapulothoracic joint augments glenohumeral joint internal rotation. The elbow is then flexed to reach up the spine to the level of the thorax.

Shoulder rotations have a functional link with forearm rotation (15). When the arm is away from the side, rotation at both joints is concerned with turning the palm·to

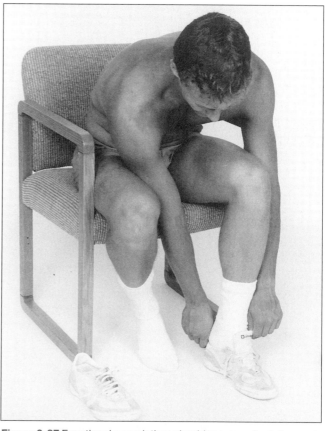

Figure 3-87 Functional association: shoulder external rotation and forearm supination.

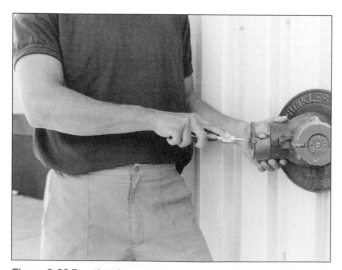

Figure 3-86 Functional association: shoulder internal rotation and forearm pronation.

face either the floor or the ceiling. Shoulder internal rotation is linked with pronation of the forearm, as both actions occur simultaneously with performance of many activities and pronation can be amplified by internal rotation of the shoulder (Fig. 3-86). Shoulder external rotation has a functional link with supination of the forearm when the elbow is extended. Examples of activities that illustrate this combined action are inserting a light bulb into a ceiling socket, releasing a bowling ball from the extended arm, and manipulating the foot into a shoe (Fig. 3-87).

References

1. Kapandji IA. *The Physiology of the Joints.* Vol 1. 5th ed. New York: Churchill Livingstone; 1982.
2. Standing S, ed. *Gray's Anatomy: The Anatomical Basis of Clinical Practice.* 39th ed. London: Elsevier Churchill Livingstone; 2005.
3. Norkin CC, White DJ. *Measurement of Joint Motion: A Guide to Goniometry.* 3rd ed. Philadelphia: FA Davis; 2003.
4. Daniels L, Worthingham C. *Muscle Testing: Techniques of Manual Examination.* 5th ed. Philadelphia: WB Saunders; 1986.
5. Levangie PK, Norkin CC. *Joint Structure & Function: A Comprehensive Analysis.* 3rd ed. Philadelphia: FA Davis; 2001.
6. Woodburne RT. *Essentials of Human Anatomy.* 5th ed. London: Oxford University Press; 1973.
7. Magee DJ. *Orthopaedic Physical Assessment.* 4th ed. Philadelphia: WB Saunders; 2002.
8. American Academy of Orthopaedic Surgeons. *Joint Motion: Method of Measuring and Recording.* Chicago: AAOS; 1965.
9. Berryman Reese N, Bandy WD. *Joint Range of Motion and Muscle Length Testing.* Philadelphia: WB Saunders; 2002.
10. Cyriax J. *Textbook of Orthopaedic Medicine,* vol. 1. *Diagnosis of Soft Tissue Lesions.* 8th ed. London: Bailliere Tindall; 1982.
11. Gajdosik RL, Hallett JP, Slaughter LL. Passive insufficiency of two-joint shoulder muscles. *Clin Biomech.* 1994;9:377–378.
12. Kebaetse M, McClure P, Pratt NA. Thoracic position effect on shoulder range of motion, strength, and three-dimensional scapular kinematics. *Arch Phys Med Rehabil.* 1999;80:945–950.
13. Boon AJ, Smith J. Manual scapular stabilization: its effect on shoulder rotational range of motion. *Arch Phys Med Rehabil.* 2000;81:978–983.
14. Evjenth O, Hamberg J. *Muscle Stretching in Manual Therapy A Clinical Manual: The Extremities.* Vol. 1. Alfta, Sweden: Alfta Rehab Forlag; 1984.
15. Smith LK, Lawrence Weiss E, Lehmkuhl LD. *Brunnstrom's Clinical Kinesiology.* 5th ed. Philadelphia: FA Davis; 1996.
16. MacConaill MA, Basmajian JV. *Muscles and Movements.* 2nd ed. New York: RE Kreiger; 1977.
17. Cailliet R: *Shoulder Pain.* 3rd ed. Philadelphia: FA Davis; 1991.
18. Rosse C. The shoulder region and the brachial plexus. In: Rosse C, Clawson DK, eds. *The Musculoskeletal System in Health and Disease.* New York: Harper & Row; 1980.
19. Zuckerman JD, Matsen FA. Biomechanics of the shoulder. In: Nordin M, Frankel VM. *Basic Biomechanics of the Musculoskeletal System.* 2nd ed. Philadelphia: Lea & Febiger; 1989.
20. Soderberg GL. *Kinesiology: Application to Pathological Motion.* 2nd ed. Baltimore: Williams & Wilkins; 1997.
21. Perry J. Shoulder function for the activities of daily living. In: Matsen FA, Fu FH, Hawkins RJ. *The Shoulder: A Balance of Mobility and Stability.* Rosemont, IL: American Academy of Orthopaedic Surgeons; 1993.
22. Matsen FA, Lippitt SB, Sidles JA, Harryman DT. *Practical Evaluation and Management of the Shoulder.* Philadelphia: WB Saunders; 1994.
23. Inman VT, Saunders M, Abbot LC. Observations on the function of the shoulder joint. *J Bone Joint Surg.* 1944;26:1–30.
24. Dvir Z, Berme N. The shoulder complex in elevation of the arm: a mechanism approach. *J Biomech.* 1978;11:219–225.
25. Kent BE. Functional anatomy of the shoulder complex: a review. *Phys Ther.* 1971;51:867–888.
26. Safaee-Rad R, Shwedyk E, Quanbury AO, Cooper JE. Normal functional range of motion of upper limb joints during performance of three feeding activities. *Arch Phys Med Rehabil.* 1990;71:505–509.
27. Ludewig PM, Cook TM, Nawoczenski DA. Three-dimensional scapular orientation and muscle activity at selected positions of humeral elevation. *J Orthop Sports Phys Ther.* 1996;24:57–65.
28. Peat M. The shoulder complex: a review of some aspects of functional anatomy. *Physiother Can.* 1977;29:241–246.
29. Blakey RL, Palmer ML. Analysis of rotation accompanying shoulder flexion. *Phys Ther* 1984;64:1214–1216.
30. Mallon WJ, Herring CL, Sallay PI, et al. Use of vertebral levels to measure presumed internal rotation at the shoulder: a radiologic analysis. *J Shoulder Elbow Surg.* 1996;5:299–306.

EXERCISES AND QUESTIONS

See the Answer Guide in Appendix F for suggested answers to the following exercises and questions.

1. PALPATION

A. For each anatomical structure or reference listed below, identify the shoulder complex ROM that would be measured using the structure or reference to align the universal goniometer. Also identify the part of the goniometer (i.e., axis, stationary arm, or moveable arm) that would be aligned with the anatomical structure or reference for the purpose of the measurement.

   i. Acromion process. _____

   ii. Lateral midline of the trunk. _____

   iii. Olecranon process. _____

   iv. Longitudinal axis of the humerus. _____

B. Palpate the following anatomical structures on a skeleton and on a partner.

Spine of the scapula	Coracoid process
Inferior angle of the scapula	Lateral epicondyle of the humerus
Vertebral border of the scapula	Clavicle
Acromion process	Sternum

2. ASSESSMENT OF AROM AT THE SHOULDER COMPLEX

A. List the articulations that make up the:
   i. Shoulder complex
   ii. Shoulder girdle
   iii. Shoulder joint.

B. Mobility at the sternoclavicular joint is essential to enable scapular motion. True or false?

C. With a partner, demonstrate how a therapist would perform a general scan of the AROM of the upper extremity joints.

D. i. List, define, and demonstrate the motions the therapist would observe when assessing scapular AROM.

   ii. What actions would a therapist instruct the patient to perform to observe scapular medial (downward) rotation and scapular lateral (upward) rotation?

- Instruct a partner to assume the anatomical position and use a grease pencil to mark the inferior angle of the scapula on the skin.
- Instruct the partner to perform the actions to observe scapular rotations.
- At the end of the full AROM of scapular medial [downward] rotation and lateral [upward] rotation, again mark the position of the inferior angle of the scapula on the skin. It may be necessary to support your partner's arm at the end of each action, and ask your partner to relax. This will enable you to more easily palpate and mark the inferior angle of the scapula.
- Observe the range of scapular motion.

   iii. Instruct a partner to perform the scapular AROM, and observe the movements.

E. For each of the shoulder movements listed below,
- Assume the start position for the assessment and measurement of the ROM
- Move your arm through half of the full AROM and hold the joint in this position to mimic a decreased AROM
- Without allowing further movement of the upper extremity, try to give the appearance of further movement or a greater than available AROM

- Identify the substitute movements used to give the appearance of a greater than available AROM for the movement being assessed. These should be the same substitute movement(s) a patient may use to augment a restricted AROM for each shoulder movement.

Shoulder AROM	Substitute Movement(s)
i. Extension	_____
ii. Abduction	_____
iii. External rotation	_____
iv. Horizontal abduction	_____

3. ASSESSMENT AND MEASUREMENT OF PROM AT THE SHOULDER COMPLEX

For each of the movements listed below, demonstrate the assessment and measurement of PROM on a partner and answer the questions that follow. Have a third partner evaluate your performance using the appropriate practical test form in Appendix E. Record your findings on the PROM recording form on page 78.

Scapular Elevation

i. Assume your partner presented with decreased AROM and PROM for scapular elevation. Identify the articulation(s) where motion could be decreased.

ii. What movement of the clavicle is associated with scapular elevation?

iii. If the movement of the clavicle identified in ii above is decreased, _____ glide of the medial end of the clavicle at the sternoclavicular joint would be restricted. Explain why the glide would be decreased in the direction indicated?

Shoulder Elevation Through Flexion and Through Abduction

i. What articulations of the shoulder complex participate in the movements of shoulder elevation through either flexion or abduction?

ii. Identify and describe the shape of the articular components that make up the glenohumeral joint and the sternoclavicular joint.

Glenohumeral (GH) Joint Abduction

i. When assessing GH joint abduction PROM, identify the stabilization procedure used by the therapist to isolate motion at the GH joint.

ii. Assume your partner has decreased GH joint abduction PROM and this was the result of decreased glide at the joint. What glide of the humeral head would be decreased? Explain the reason for the glide being decreased in the direction indicated.

Shoulder Extension

i. What position should the elbow be in when assessing shoulder extension ROM? Explain.

Shoulder Horizontal Adduction

i. Identify the two different start positions of the shoulder that a therapist may use when assessing horizontal adduction ROM. What other shoulder ROM would be assessed using these same start positions?

ii. Assume a patient presented with equally decreased shoulder horizontal adduction AROM and PROM. What restricted glide of the humeral head would result in decreased shoulder horizontal adduction ROM? Explain the reason for the glide being decreased in the direction(s) indicated.

Shoulder Internal Rotation

i. Assume a patient presented with decreased shoulder internal rotation PROM. Identify the joint(s) where motion would be decreased.

ii. Would the therapist assess AROM or PROM to determine end feel for shoulder internal rotation?

iii. When you assessed your partner's shoulder internal rotation PROM, was the PROM normal, hypomobile, or hypermobile? What end feel was present? Would this end feel be considered normal or abnormal? Explain.

iv. List the normal limiting factor(s) that would create a normal firm end feel for shoulder internal rotation.

Other Questions

A. If, when assessing and measuring ROM of the shoulder complex, the therapist stabilizes the scapula, what movements of the shoulder complex is the therapist able to assess?

B. Assume a patient's shoulder elevation through flexion is assessed in sitting position and the therapist finds:

   i.   an AROM of 80° and a PROM of 130°; why might the AROM be less than the PROM?

   ii. an AROM of 30° and the PROM of 30°, why might the patient present with these findings?

PROM RECORDING FORM

Patient's Name _____   Therapist _____

Left Side				Right Side			
*		*	**Date of Measurement**	*		*	
			Scapula				
			Elevation				
			Depression				
			Abduction				
			Adduction				
			Shoulder Complex				
			Elevation through Flexion (0–180°)				
			Elevation through Abduction (0–180°)				
			Shoulder (Glenohumeral) Joint				
			Flexion (0–120°)				
			Abduction (0–90° to 120°)				
			Extension (0–60°)				
			Horizontal abduction (0–45°)				
			Horizontal adduction (0–135°)				
			Internal rotation (0–70°)				
			External rotation (0–90°)				
			Hypermobility: Comments:				

4. MUSCLE LENGTH ASSESSMENT AND MEASUREMENT

For the pectoralis major and the pectoralis minor, demonstrate the assessment and measurement of muscle length on a partner and answer the questions below that pertain to the muscle assessed. Have a third partner evaluate your performance using the appropriate practical test form in Appendix E.

Pectoralis Major

i.   Identify the origin and insertion of the pectoralis major muscle.

ii. What movements of the upper extremity would position the origin and insertion of the pectoralis major muscle farther apart and thus place the muscle on stretch?

iii. If the pectoralis major is shortened, what end feel would the therapist note at the limit of the PROM when assessing pectoralis major muscle length?

iv. If the pectoralis major is shortened, what shoulder joint ROM would be restricted proportional to the decrease in muscle length? To assess this restriction using a universal goniometer, the goniometer axis is placed ____, the stationary arm is aligned _____, and the movable arm is aligned parallel to the _____.

Pectoralis Minor

i.   Identify the origin and insertion of the pectoralis minor muscle.

ii. What movement(s) of the scapula would move the origin and insertion of the pectoralis minor muscle farther apart and thus place the muscle on stretch?

iii. If the pectoralis minor is shortened and the patient is lying supine, what observation would indicate to the therapist that the pectoralis minor is shortened?

5. FUNCTIONAL ROM AT THE SHOULDER COMPLEX

A.   What is the function of the shoulder complex?

B.   i.   Hold your dominant arm at your side in anatomical position to simulate an immobile glenohumeral joint. With your dominant arm maintained in this position, attempt to carry out or simulate the following activities using your dominant upper extremity, using no compensatory movements of other body parts to assist. Identify those activities that are impossible to perform with an immobile glenohumeral joint fixed in anatomical position. (*Note:* You will not be able to perform shoulder internal or external rotation with the glenohumeral joint fixed in the anatomical position; therefore, while trying these activities, pay particular attention to restricting these motions.)

- Perform toilet hygiene activities.
- Reach to the midline of your chest to do up buttons.
- Comb your hair.
- Brush your teeth.
- Wash your axilla on the contralateral side.
- Drink a full cup of water.
- Eat cold soup with a spoon.

ii. Repeat the above activities and use compensatory movements of other body parts and shoulder internal and external rotation if necessary. Identify the tasks that could now be completed and identify the shoulder rotation and compensatory movement(s) used.

C.   For each of the following shoulder movements, identify two examples of ADL that require the movement:

i.   extension,

ii. elevation through flexion,

iii. flexion below shoulder level,

iv. external rotation, and

v.   horizontal adduction.

D. i. Explain the term "scapulohumeral rhythm."

   ii. What is the generally recognized ratio of glenohumeral motion to scapular motion through the complete range of shoulder elevation?

   iii. Identify the factors that effect variations as to the contribution of all joints to the scapulohumeral rhythm.

   iv. List the joints at which movement occurs to attain the full 180° elevation through flexion or abduction.

   v. Explain the main movement pattern(s) of the setting phase of shoulder elevation through flexion or abduction.

   vi. Explain the movement pattern through the ROM of shoulder elevation through flexion or abduction following the setting phase.

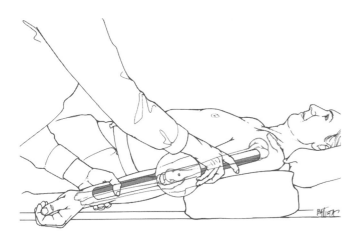

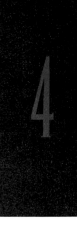

Elbow and Forearm

ARTICULATIONS AND MOVEMENTS

The elbow is made up of the humeroulnar and humeroradial joints, which are classified as hinge joints (Fig. 4-1). The humeroulnar joint is formed proximally by the trochlea of the humerus, which is convex anteroposteriorly (1), articulating with the concave surface of the trochlear notch of the ulna. The convex surface of the capitulum of the humerus articulates with the concave proximal aspect of the radial head to form the humeroradial joint.

From the anatomical position, the elbow may be flexed and extended in the sagittal plane with movement occur-

ring around a frontal axis (Fig. 4-2). The axis for elbow flexion and extension "passes through the center of the arcs formed by the trochlear sulcus and the capitellum (2, p.534)" of the humerus, except at the extremes of motion, when the axis is displaced anteriorly and posteriorly (2), respectively.

The forearm articulations (see Fig. 4-1) consist of the superior and inferior radioulnar joints and the syndesmosis formed by the interosseous membrane between the radius and ulna. The superior radioulnar joint is contained within the capsule of the elbow joint (1) and is a pivot joint formed between the convex surface of the radial head and the concave radial notch on the radial aspect of the proximal ulna. The annular ligament, lined with articular cartilage, encompasses the rim of the radial head (3). When motion occurs at the superior radioulnar joint, motion

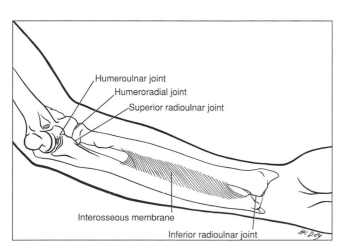

Figure 4-1 Elbow and forearm articulations.

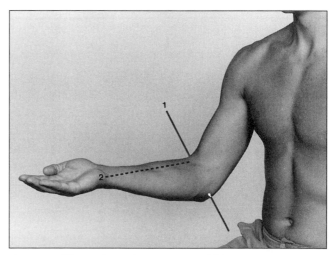

Figure 4-2 Elbow joint and forearm axes: (1) flexion-extension and (2) supination-pronation.

also occurs at the humeroradial joint as the head of radius spins on the capitulum. The inferior radioulnar joint is also a pivot joint. It is formed between the concave ulnar notch on the medial aspect of the distal radius and the convex ulnar head.

The forearm may be supinated and pronated. These movements occur around an oblique axis that passes through the head of the radius proximally and through the head of the ulna distally (4,5) (see Fig. 4-2). In supination, the radius lies alongside the ulna (Fig. 4-3). In pronation, the radius rotates around the relatively stationary ulna (Fig. 4-4). With the elbow in anatomical position, the movements of pronation and supination occur in the transverse plane around a longitudinal axis. The movements of the elbow and forearm joints are described in Table 4-1.

TABLE 4-1   Joint Structure: Elbow and Forearm Movements

	Flexion	Extension	Supination	Pronation
Articulation[1,6]	Humeroulnar, humeroradial	Humeroulnar, humeroradial	Humeroradial, superior radioulnar, inferior radioulnar, interosseous membrane	Humeroradial, superior radioulnar, inferior radioulnar, interosseous membrane
Plane	Sagittal	Sagittal	Transverse	Transverse
Axis	Frontal	Frontal	Longitudinal	Longitudinal
Normal limiting factors[3,6-8*]	Soft tissue apposition of the anterior forearm and upper arm; coronoid process contacting the coronoid fossa and the radial head contacting the radial fossa; tension in the posterior capsule and triceps	Olecranon process contacting the olecranon fossa; tension in the elbow flexors and anterior joint capsule and medial collateral ligament	Tension in the pronator muscles, quadrate ligament, palmar radioulnar ligament of the inferior radioulnar joint and oblique cord	Contact of the radius on the ulna; tension in the quadrate ligament, the dorsal radioulnar ligament, of the inferior radioulnar joint, the distal tract of the interosseous membrane[9], supinator, and biceps brachii muscles with elbow in extension
Normal end feel[7,10,11*]	Soft/hard/firm	Hard/firm	Firm	Hard/firm
Normal AROM[12†] (AROM[13])	0–150° (0–140°)	150–0° (140–0°)	0–80–90° (0–80°)	0–80–90° (0–80°)
Capsular pattern[10,11]	Elbow joint: flexion, extension, and rotation full and painless Superior radioulnar joint: equal limitation of supination and pronation Inferior radiolunar joint: full rotation with pain at extremes of rotation			

*Note: There is a paucity of definitive research that identifies the normal limiting factors (NLF) of joint motion. The NLF and end feels listed here are based on knowledge of anatomy, clinical experience, and available references. NLF are illustrated in Figures 4-3 and 4-4.
†AROM, active range of motion.

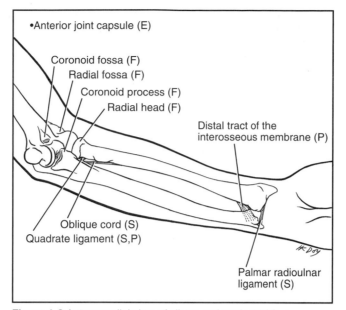

•Anterior joint capsule (E)

Coronoid fossa (F)
Radial fossa (F)
Coronoid process (F)
Radial head (F)

Distal tract of the
interosseous membrane (P)

Oblique cord (S)
Quadrate ligament (S,P)

Palmar radioulnar
ligament (S)

Figure 4-3 Anteromedial view of elbow and supinated forearm showing noncontractile structures that normally limit motion.*

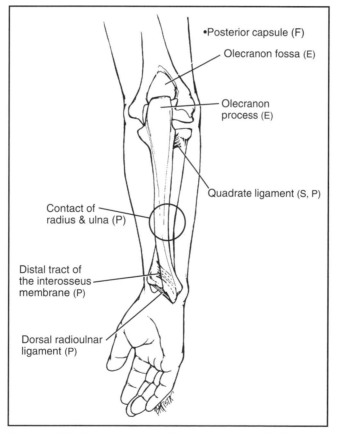

•Posterior capsule (F)
Olecranon fossa (E)

Olecranon
process (E)

Quadrate ligament (S, P)

Contact of
radius & ulna (P)

Distal tract of
the interosseus
membrane (P)

Dorsal radioulnar
ligament (P)

Figure 4-4 Posteromedial view of the elbow and pronated forearm showing noncontractile structures that normally limit motion.*

Motion limited by structure is identified in parentheses, using the following abbreviations: F, flexion; S, supination; E, extension; P, pronation. Muscles normally limiting motion are not illustrated.

SURFACE ANATOMY

(Figs. 4-5 through 4-7)

Structure	Location
1. Acromion process	Lateral aspect of the spine of the scapula at the tip of the shoulder.
2. Medial epicondyle of the humerus	Medial projection at the distal end of the humerus.
3. Lateral epicondyle of the humerus	Lateral projection at the distal end of the humerus.
4. Olecranon process	Posterior aspect of the elbow; proximal end of the shaft of the ulna.
5. Head of the radius	Distal to the lateral epicondyle of the humerus.
6. Styloid process of the radius	Bony prominence on the lateral aspect of the forearm at the distal end of the radius.
7. Head of the third metacarpal	Bony prominence at the base of the third digit.
8. Head of the ulna	Round bony prominence on the posteromedial aspect of the forearm at the distal end of the ulna.
9. Styloid process of ulna	Bony projection on the posteromedial aspect of the distal end of the ulna.

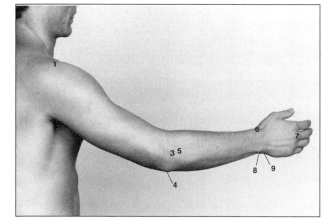

Figure 4-5 Posterolateral aspect of the arm.

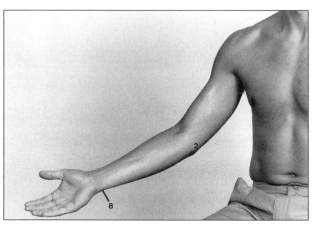

Figure 4-6 Anteromedial aspect of the arm.

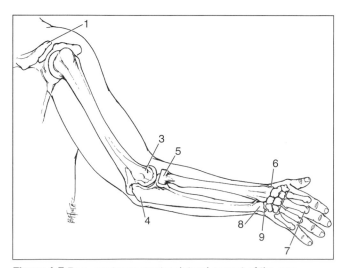

Figure 4-7 Bony anatomy, posterolateral aspect of the arm.

RANGE OF MOTION ASSESSMENT AND MEASUREMENT

Elbow Flexion-Extension/Hyperextension

AROM Assessment

Substitute Movement. *Flexion*—trunk extension, shoulder flexion, scapular depression, and wrist flexion. *Extension*—trunk flexion, shoulder extension, scapular elevation, and wrist extension.

PROM Assessment

Start Position. The patient is supine or sitting. The arm is in the anatomical position with the elbow in extension (Fig. 4-8). A towel is placed under the distal end of the humerus to accommodate the range of motion (ROM). Owing to biceps muscle tension, unusually muscular men may not be able to achieve 0°. Up to 15° of hyperextension is not uncommon in women (12,14,15) or children because the olecranon is smaller (15).

Stabilization. The therapist stabilizes the humerus.

Therapist's Distal Hand Placement. The therapist grasps the distal radius and ulna.

End Positions. The therapist applies slight traction to and moves the forearm in an anterior direction, applying slight overpressure at the limit of elbow flexion (Fig. 4-9). The therapist applies slight traction to and moves the forearm in a posterior direction, applying slight overpressure at the limit of elbow extension/hyperextension (Fig. 4-10).

End Feels. Flexion—soft/hard/firm; extension/hyperextension—hard/firm.

Joint Glides. *Flexion*—concave trochlear notch and concave radial head glide anteriorly on the fixed convexities of the trochlea and capitulum, respectively. *Extension*—concave trochlear notch and concave radial head glide posteriorly on the fixed trochlea and capitulum, respectively.

Measurement: Universal Goniometer

Start Position. The patient is supine or sitting. The arm is in the anatomical position with the elbow in extension (0°) (Fig. 4-11). A towel is placed under the distal end of the humerus to accommodate the ROM. Owing to biceps muscle tension, unusually muscular men may not be able to achieve 0°.

Stabilization. The therapist stabilizes the humerus.

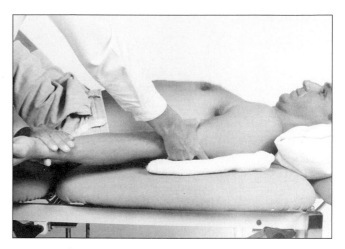

Figure 4-8 Start position for elbow flexion and extension/hyperextension PROM.

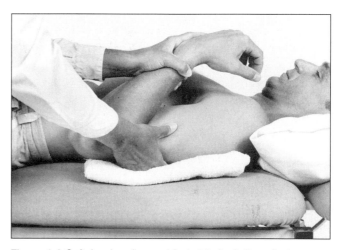

Figure 4-9 Soft, hard, or firm end feel at limit of elbow flexion.

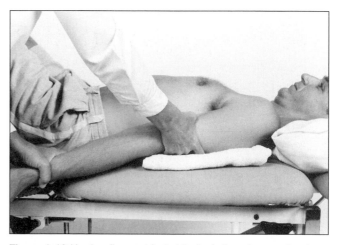

Figure 4-10 Hard or firm end feel at limit of elbow hyperextension.

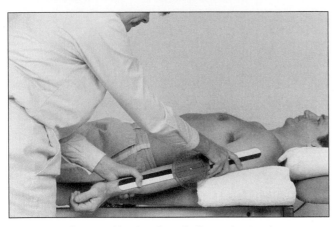

Figure 4-11 Start position for elbow flexion and extension.

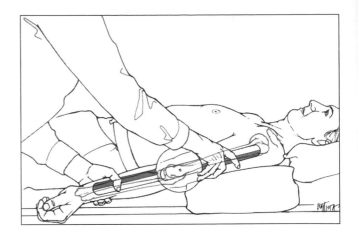

Figure 4-12 Goniometer alignment for elbow flexion and extension.

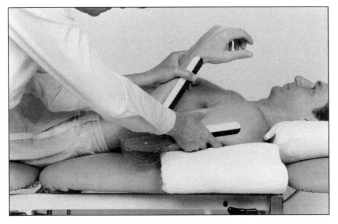

Figure 4-13 End position for elbow flexion.

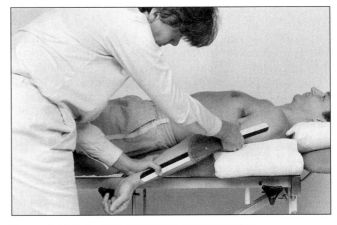

Figure 4-14 End position for elbow hyperextension.

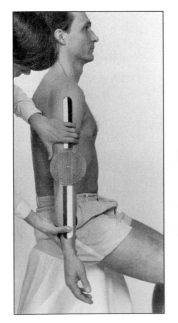

Figure 4-15 Elbow extension 0°.   Figure 4-16 Elbow flexion.

Goniometer Axis. The axis is placed over the lateral epicondyle of the humerus (Figs. 4-11 and 4-12).

Stationary Arm. Parallel to the longitudinal axis of the humerus, pointing toward the tip of the acromion process.

Movable Arm. Parallel to the longitudinal axis of the radius, pointing toward the styloid process of the radius.

End Position. From the start position of elbow extension, the forearm is moved in an anterior direction so that the hand approximates the shoulder to the limit of elbow flexion (150°) (Fig. 4-13).

Hyperextension. The forearm is moved in a posterior direction beyond 0° of extension (Fig. 4-14).

Alternate Measurement

The patient is sitting (Figs. 4-15 and 4-16).

Supination-Pronation

AROM Assessment

Substitute Movement. Supination—adduction and external rotation of the shoulder and ipsilateral trunk lateral flexion. Pronation—abduction and internal rotation of the shoulder and contralateral trunk lateral flexion.

PROM Assessment

Start Position. The patient is sitting. The arm is at the side, and the elbow is flexed to 90° with the forearm in midposition (Fig. 4-17A).

Stabilization. The therapist stabilizes the humerus.

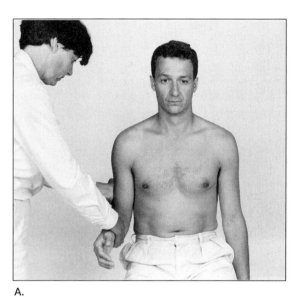

A.

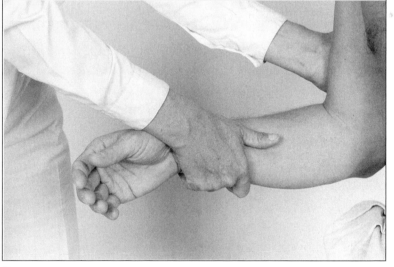

B.

Figure 4-17 A. Start position for supination and pronation. **B**. Therapist's hand position for PROM.

Therapist's Distal Hand Placement. The therapist grasps the distal radius and ulna (see Fig. 4-17).

End Positions. The forearm is rotated externally from midposition so that the palm faces upward and toward the ceiling to the limit of forearm supination (Fig. 4-18). The forearm is rotated internally so that the palm faces downward and toward the floor to the limit of forearm pronation (Fig. 4-19).

End Feels. Supination—firm; pronation—hard/firm.

Joint Glides. *Supination*—convex radial head spins (i.e., rotates around a fixed point) in the fixed concave radial notch, and the concave ulnar notch glides posteriorly on the fixed convex ulnar head (16). *Pronation*—convex radial head spins in the fixed concave radial notch, and the

concave ulnar notch glides anteriorly on the fixed convex ulnar head (16). *Humeroradial joint*—the head of the radius spins on the fixed capitulum during supination and pronation.

Four methods of measuring forearm supination and pronation are presented. Two methods use the universal goniometer and the other two methods use the OB "Myrin" goniometer to measure forearm ROM. Most activities of daily living (ADL) combine forearm rotation with hand use (e.g., gripping) (17). Two of the four methods (one using the universal goniometer and one the OB "Myrin" goniometer) measure forearm rotation with the hand in a gripping posture that simulates functional movements (see Figs. 4-20 and 4-26). The measurement performed using the OB "Myrin" goniometer attached proximal to the wrist (see Fig. 4-29) measures isolated forearm ROM.

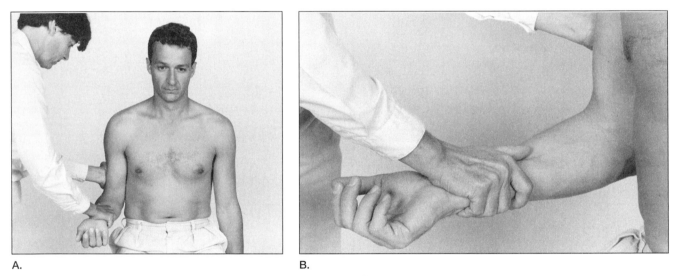

A.

B.

Figure 4-18 A. Firm end feel at limit of supination. **B**. Therapist's hand position.

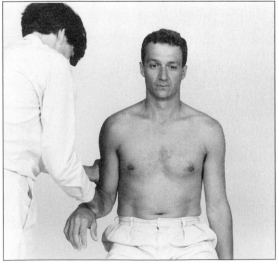
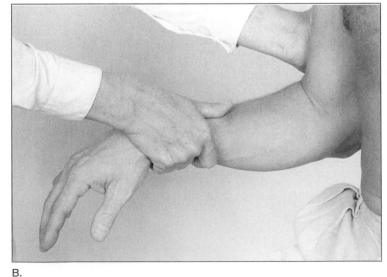

A.

B.

Figure 4-19 A. Hard or firm end feel at limit of pronation. **B**. Therapist's hand position.

Measurement: Universal Goniometer

Start Position. The patient is sitting. The arm is at the side, and the elbow is flexed to 90° with the forearm in midposition. A pencil is held in the tightly closed fist with the pencil protruding from the radial aspect of the hand (14), and the wrist in the neutral position (Fig. 4-20). The fist is tightly closed to stabilize the 4th and 5th metacarpals, thus avoiding unwanted movement of the pencil as the test movements are performed.

Stabilization. The patient stabilizes the humerus using the nontest hand.

Goniometer Axis. The axis is placed over the head of the third metacarpal.

Stationary Arm. Perpendicular to the floor.

Movable Arm. Parallel to the pencil.

End Position. The forearm is rotated externally from midposition so the palm faces upward and toward the ceiling (80° to 90° from midposition) (Fig. 4-21).

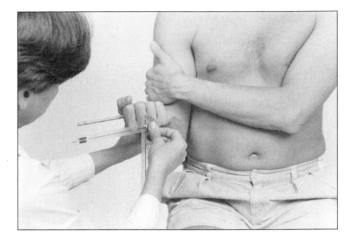

Figure 4-21 Supination.

Substitute Movement. Altered grasp of the pencil if the fist is not tightly closed during testing, thumb touching and moving the pencil, wrist extension and/or radial deviation.

End Position. The forearm is rotated internally so that the palm faces downward and toward the floor (80° to 90° from midposition) (Fig. 4-22).

Substitute Movement. Altered grasp of the pencil, wrist flexion and/or ulnar deviation.

High intratester (17,18) and intertester (17) reliability has been reported for the functional measurement method using the universal goniometer and the pencil held in the hand to measure active supination and pronation ROM.

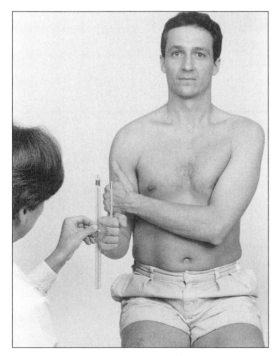

Figure 4-20 Functional measurement method: start position for supination and pronation.

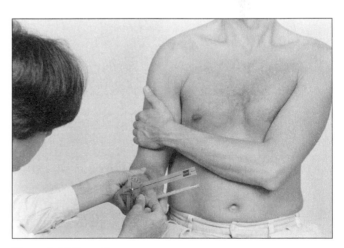

Figure 4-22 Pronation.

Alternate Measurement

This measurement is indicated if the patient cannot grasp a pencil.

Start Position. The arm is at the side, and the elbow is flexed to 90° with the forearm in midposition. The wrist is in neutral, and the fingers are extended (Fig. 4-23).

Stabilization. The patient stabilizes the humerus using the nontest hand.

Goniometer Axis. The axis is placed at the tip of the middle digit.

Stationary Arm. Perpendicular to the floor.

Movable Arm. Parallel to the tips of the four extended fingers.

End Position. The forearm is rotated externally so that the palm faces upward and toward the ceiling (80° to 90° from midposition) (Fig. 4-24).

Substitute Movement. Finger hyperextension, wrist extension, and wrist deviations.

End Position. The forearm is rotated internally so that the palm faces downward and toward the floor (80° to 90° from midposition) (Fig. 4-25).

Substitute Movement. Finger flexion, wrist flexion, and wrist deviations.

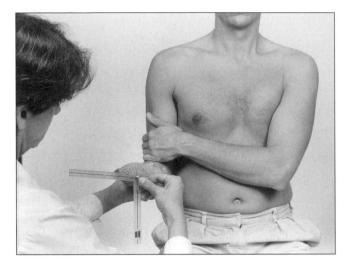

Figure 4-24 Supination.

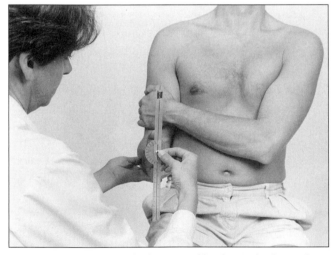

Figure 4-23 Alternate method: start position for supination and pronation.

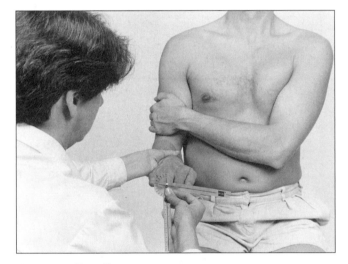

Figure 4-25 Pronation.

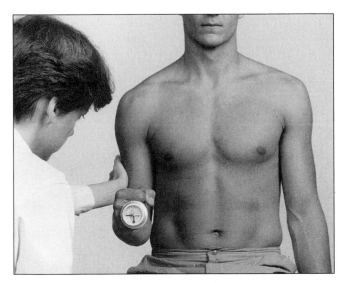

Figure 4-26 Start position for supination and pronation using the OB goniometer.

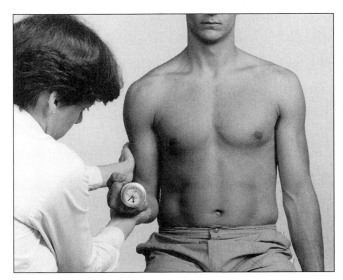

Figure 4-27 End position for supination.

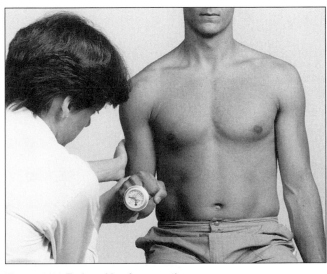

Figure 4-28 End position for pronation.

Measurement: OB Goniometer

Start Position. The patient is sitting. The shoulder is adducted, and the elbow is flexed to 90° with the forearm in midposition. The wrist is in neutral, and the fingers are flexed (Fig. 4-26).

Goniometer Placement. The dial is placed on the right-angled plate. The plate is held between the patient's index and middle fingers.

Stabilization. The therapist stabilizes the humerus.

End Position. The forearm is rotated externally from midposition to the limit of motion for supination (Fig. 4-27).

Substitute Movement. Wrist extension and deviations, shoulder adduction with external rotation, and ipsilateral trunk lateral flexion.

End Position. The forearm is rotated internally from midposition to the limit of motion for pronation (Fig. 4-28).

Substitute Movement. Wrist flexion and deviations, shoulder abduction with internal rotation, and contralateral trunk lateral flexion.

Alternate Placement

The strap is placed around the distal forearm. The dial is placed on the right-angled plate and attached on the radial side of the forearm (Fig. 4-29). This goniometer placement measures isolated forearm rotation ROM.

Substitute Movement. Using this alternate goniometer placement, substitute movements for supination are limited to shoulder adduction, shoulder external rotation, and ipsilateral trunk lateral flexion. Substitute movements for pronation are limited to shoulder abduction, shoulder internal rotation, and contralateral trunk lateral flexion.

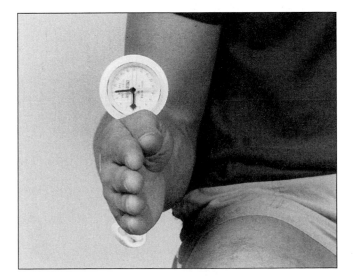

Figure 4-29 Alternate OB goniometer placement for supination and pronation.

MUSCLE LENGTH ASSESSMENT AND MEASUREMENT

Biceps Brachii

Origin (I)	Insertion (I)
Biceps Brachii	
a. Short head: apex of the coracoid process of the scapula.	Posterior aspect of the radial tuberosity and via the bicipital aponeurosis fuses with the deep fascia covering the origins of the flexor muscles of the forearm.
b. Long head: supraglenoid tubercle of the scapula.	

Start Position. The patient is supine with the shoulder in extension over the edge of the plinth, the elbow is flexed, and the forearm is pronated (Fig. 4-30).

Stabilization. The therapist stabilizes the humerus.

End Position. The elbow is extended to the limit of motion so that the biceps brachii is put on full stretch (Figs. 4-31 and 4-32).

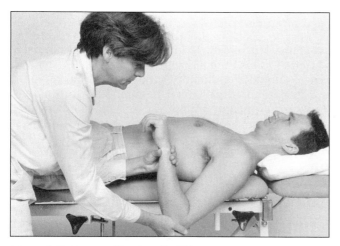

Figure 4-30 Start position: length of biceps brachii.

End Feel. Biceps brachii on stretch—firm.0

Measurement. The therapist uses a goniometer to measure and record the available elbow extension PROM. If the biceps is shortened, elbow extension PROM will be restricted proportional to the decrease in muscle length.

Universal Goniometer Placement. The goniometer is placed the same as for elbow flexion-extension.

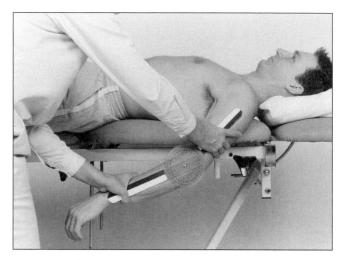

Figure 4-31 Goniometer measurement: length of biceps brachii.

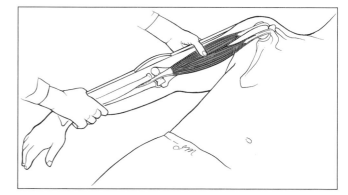

Figure 4-32 Biceps brachii on stretch.

Triceps

Start Position. The patient is sitting with the shoulder in full elevation through forward flexion and external rotation. The elbow is in extension and the forearm is in supination (Fig. 4-33).

Stabilization. The therapist stabilizes the humerus.

End Position. The elbow is flexed to the limit of motion so that the triceps is put on full stretch (Figs. 4-34 and 4-35).

End Feel. Triceps on stretch—firm.

Measurement. The therapist uses a goniometer to measure and record the available elbow flexion PROM. If the triceps is shortened, elbow flexion PROM will be restricted proportional to the decrease in muscle length.

Goniometer Placement. The goniometer is placed the same as for elbow flexion-extension.

Origin (1)	Insertion (1)
Triceps	
a. Long head: infraglenoid tubercle of the scapula.	Posteriorly, on the proximal surface of the olecranon; some fibers continue distally to blend with the antebrachial fascia.
b. Lateral head: posterolateral surface of the humerus between the radial groove and the insertion of teres minor; lateral intermuscular septum.	
c. Medial head: posterior surface of the humerus below the radial groove between the trochlea of the humerus and the insertion of teres major; medial and lateral intermuscular septum.	

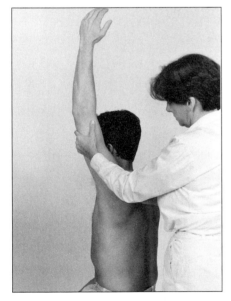

Figure 4-33 Start position: length of triceps.

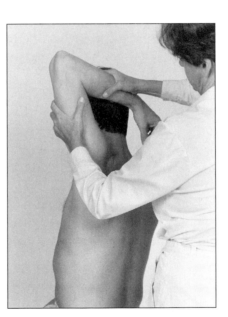

Figure 4-34 End position: triceps on stretch.

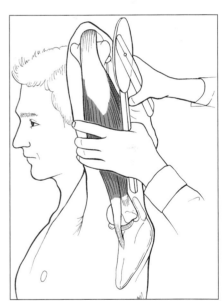

Figure 4-35 Goniometer measurement: length of triceps.

Alternate Measurement: Supine

This position is used if the patient has decreased shoulder flexion ROM.

Start Position. The patient is supine with the shoulder in 90° flexion and the elbow in extension (Fig. 4-36).

Stabilization. The therapist stabilizes the humerus.

End Position. The elbow is flexed to the limit of motion to put the triceps on stretch (Fig. 4-37).

Universal Goniometer Placement. The goniometer is placed the same as for elbow flexion-extension.

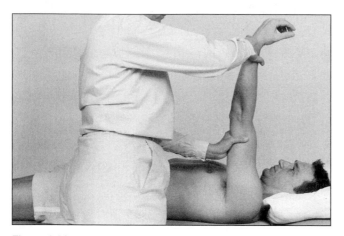

Figure 4-36 Alternate start position: triceps length.

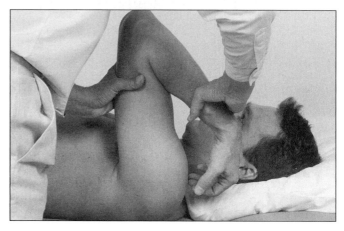

Figure 4-37 End position: triceps on stretch.

FUNCTIONAL APPLICATION

Joint Function

The function of the elbow complex is to serve the hand (3,6,19). Movement at the elbow joint adjusts the overall functional length of the arm (16). Elbow extension moves the hand away from the body; elbow flexion moves the hand toward the body. Hand orientation in space and hand mobility are enhanced through supination and pronation of the forearm. The elbow complex, including the forearm, contributes to many skilled and forceful hand movements involved in daily self-care, leisure, and work functions. The elbow complex also provides the power necessary to perform lifting activities (20) and activities involving raising and lowering of the body using the hands (19).

The elbow and forearm do not function in isolation, but link with the shoulder and wrist to enhance hand function (3). When the elbow is extended, supination and pronation are functionally linked with shoulder external and internal rotation, respectively (19). These linked movements occur simultaneously during activity. However, when the elbow is flexed, forearm rotation can be isolated from shoulder rotation (19). This is illustrated in activities such as turning a door handle or using a screwdriver (Fig. 4-38).

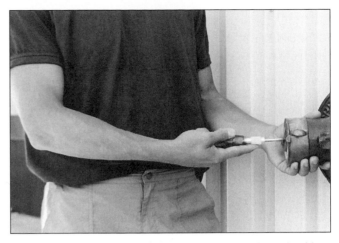

Figure 4-38 Elbow flexion isolates forearm rotation from shoulder rotation.

Functional Range of Motion

The normal AROM (12) at the elbow is from 0° of extension to 150° of flexion, 80° to 90° of forearm pronation, and 80° to 90° of forearm supination. However, many daily functions are performed with less than these ranges. The ROM required at the elbow and forearm for selected ADL is shown in Table 4-2, as adapted from the

TABLE 4-2 **Elbow and Forearm ROM Required for Selected ADL**[20-22]*						
Activity	Flexion ROM (°)		Supination ROM (°)		Pronation ROM (°)	
	Min	Max	Start	End	Start	End
Read a newspaper[20]	78	104	—	—	7	49
Rise from a chair[20]	20	95	—	—	10	34
Sit to stand to sit[22]	15	100	—	—	—	—
Cut with a knife[20]	89	107	—	—	27	42
Pour from a pitcher[20]	36	58	22	—	—	43
Drink from a cup[21]	72	129	3	31	—	—
Put glass to mouth[20]	45	130	13	—	—	10
Use a telephone[20]	43	136	23	—	—	41
Use a telephone[22]	75	140	—	—	—	—
Put fork to mouth[20]	85	128	—	52	10	—
Eat with a fork[21]	94	122	—	59	38	—
Eat with a spoon[21]	101	123	—	59	23	—
Eat with a spoon[22]	70	115	—	—	—	—
Open a door[20]	24	57	—	23	35	—

*Mean values from original sources (20,21) rounded to the nearest degree. Median values from original source (22).

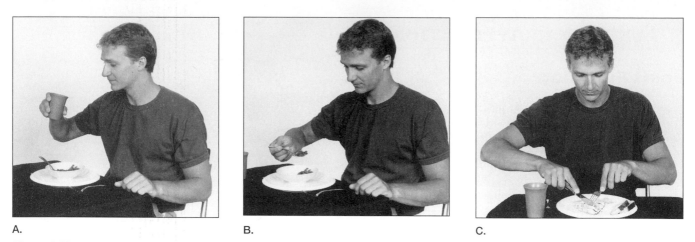

A.   B.   C.

Figure 4-39 Elbow range within the arc of movement from 45° to 136° of flexion and from 47° of pronation to 59° of supination. **A**. Drinking from a cup. **B**. Eating using a spoon. **C**. Eating using a knife and fork.

works of Morrey (20), Safaee-Rad (21), Packer (22), and their colleagues. Positions of the elbow and forearm required to touch different body parts for personal care and hygiene activities are shown in Table 4-3, as adapted from the work of Morrey and colleagues (20). The ROM requirements for ADL are influenced by the design of furniture, the placement of utensils, and the patient's posture. In part, these factors could account for the difference in ROM findings between studies for similar ADL shown in Table 4-2. Thus, the ROM values in Tables 4-2 and 4-3 should be used as a guide for ADL requirements.

Many self-care activities can be accomplished within the arc of movement from 30° to 130° of flexion and from 50° of pronation to 50° of supination (20). Writing, pour-

ing from a pitcher, reading a newspaper, and performing perineal hygiene are examples of activities performed within these ROMs. Feeding activities such as drinking from a cup, using a spoon or fork, and cutting with a knife (Fig. 4-39) may be performed within an arc of movement from about 45° to 136° of flexion and from about 47° pronation to 59° supination (20–23).

Daily functions that may involve extreme ranges of elbow motion include combing or washing the hair (flexion, pronation, and supination), reaching a back zipper at the neck level (flexion, pronation), using the telephone (135° to 140° flexion [20,22]), tying a shoe (16° flexion [20]), throwing a ball (extension), walking

TABLE 4-3	**Elbow and Forearm Positions* of Healthy Subjects, Measured During Personal Care and Hygiene Activities**[20]		
Hand to:	**Elbow Flexion (°)**	**Supination (°)**	**Pronation (°)**
Head-vertex	119	47	—
Head-occiput	144	2	—
Waist	100	12	—
Chest	120	29	—
Neck	135	41	—
Sacrum	70	56	—
Shoe	16	—	19

*Mean values from original source (20) rounded to the nearest degree.

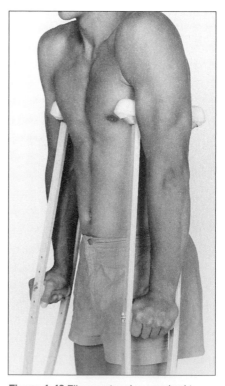

Figure 4-40 Elbow extension required to walk with axillary crutches.

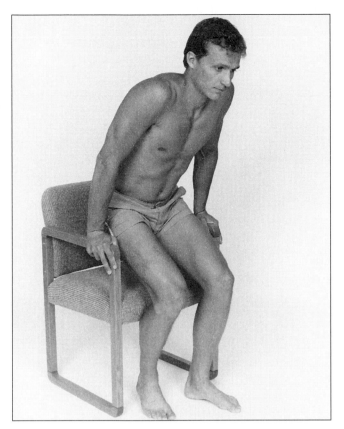

Figure 4-41 Elbow extension required to elevate the body when getting up from a chair.

with axillary crutches (extension) (Fig. 4-40), using the arms to elevate the body when getting up from a chair (15° flexion [22]) (Fig. 4-41), and playing tennis (extension).

Less elbow ROM is required to perform most upper extremity activities when elbow flexion and extension ROM is restricted and compensatory motions are allowed at normal adjacent joints. In this case, functional elbow ROM is from 75° to 120° flexion (24). These compensatory motions occur at the thoracic and lumbar spines, shoulder (primarily scapulothoracic and clavicular joints), and wrist (25). With the elbow in a fixed position of 90° flexion, although there are limitations in function, in most cases all personal care ADL (i.e., feeding and personal hygiene) can be performed (24,26).

With restriction of elbow ROM, loss of elbow flexion has a greater impact on loss of function than loss of elbow extension in a ratio of about 2:1 (27). Thus, the functional impact of a 5° loss of elbow flexion is approximately equivalent to a 10° loss of elbow extension ROM.

References

1. Standing S, ed. *Gray's Anatomy: The Anatomical Basis of Clinical Practice*. 39th ed. London: Elsevier Churchill Livingstone; 2005.
2. London JT. Kinematics of the elbow. *J Bone Joint Surg [Am]*. 1981;63(4):529–535.
3. Levangie PK, Norkin CC. *Joint Structure and Function: A Comprehensive Analysis*. 3rd ed. Philadelphia: FA Davis; 2001.
4. Steindler A. *Kinesiology of the Human Body Under Normal and Pathological Conditions*. Springfield: Charles C Thomas; 1955.
5. Nakamura T, Yabe Y, Horiuchi Y, Yamazaki N. In vivo motion analysis of forearm rotation utilizing magnetic resonance imaging. *Clin Biomechanics*. 1999;14:315–320.
6. Kapandji IA. *The Physiology of the Joints*. Vol. 1. 5th ed. New York: Churchill Livingstone; 1982.
7. Norkin CC, White DJ. *Measurement of Joint Motion: A Guide to Goniometry*. 3rd ed. Philadelphia: FA Davis; 2003.
8. Nordin M, Frankel VH. *Basic Biomechanics of the Musculoskeletal System*. 3rd ed. Philadelphia: Lippincott Williams & Wilkins; 2001.
9. Gabl M, et al. The interosseous membrane and its influence on the distal radioulnar joint. An anatomical investigation of the distal tract. *J Hand Surg [Br]*. 1998;23(2):179–182.
10. Cyriax J. *Textbook of Orthopaedic Medicine. Vol 1. Diagnosis of Soft Tissue Lesions*. 8th ed. London: Bailliere Tindall; 1982.
11. Magee DJ. *Orthopaedic Physical Assessment*. 4th ed. Philadelphia: WB Saunders; 2002.
12. American Academy of Orthopaedic Surgeons. *Joint Motion: Method of Measuring and Recording*. Chicago: AAOS; 1965.
13. Berryman Reese N, Bandy WD. *Joint Range of Motion and Muscle Length Testing*. Philadelphia: WB Saunders; 2002.
14. Hoppenfeld S. *Physical Examination of the Spine and Extremities*. New York: Appleton-Century-Crofts; 1976.
15. Kaltenborn FM. *Mobilization of the Extremity Joints*. 3rd ed. Oslo: Olaf Norlis Bokhandel; 1985.
16. Neumann DA. *Kinesiology of the Musculoskeletal System: Foundations for Physical Rehabilitation*. Philadelphia: Mosby; 2002.
17. Karagiannopoulos C, Sitler M, Michlovitz S. Reliability of 2 functional goniometric methods for measuring forearm pronation and supination active range of motion. *J Orthop Sports Phys Ther*. 2003;33(9):523–531.
18. Gajdosik RL. Comparison and reliability of three goniometric methods for measuring forearm supination and pronation. *Perceptual Motor Skills*. 2001;93:353–355.
19. Smith LK, Lawrence Weiss EL, Lehmkuhl LD. *Brunnstrom's Clinical Kinesiology*. 5th ed. Philadelphia: FA Davis; 1996.
20. Morrey BF, Askew LJ, An KN, Chao EY. A biomechanical study of normal functional elbow motion. *J Bone Joint Surg [Am]*. 1981;63:872–876.
21. Safaee-Rad R, Shwedyk E, Quanbury AO, Cooper JE. Normal functional range of motion of upper limb joints during performance of three feeding activities. *Arch Phys Med Rehabil*. 1990;71:505–509.
22. Packer TL, Peat M, Wyss U, Sorbie C. Examining the elbow during functional activities. *OTJR*. 1990;10:323–333.
23. Cooper JE, Shwedyk E, Quanbury AO, et al. Elbow joint restriction: effect on functional upper limb motion during performance of three feeding activities. *Arch Phys Med Rehabil*. 1993;74:805–809.
24. Vasen AP, Lacey SH, Keith MW, Shaffer JW. Functional range of motion of the elbow. *J Hand Surg [Am]*. 1995; 20:288–292.
25. O'Neill OR, Morrey BF, Tanaka S, An KN. Compensatory motion in the upper extremity after elbow arthrodesis. *Clin Orthop*. 1992;281:89–96.
26. Nagy SM, Szabo RM, Sharkey NA. Unilateral elbow arthrodesis: the preferred position. *J Southern Orthop Assoc*. 1999; 8(2):80–85.
27. Morrey BF, An KN. Functional evaluation of the elbow. In: Morrey BF, ed. *The Elbow and Its Disorders*. 3rd ed. Philadelphia: WB Saunders; 2000.

EXERCISES AND QUESTIONS

See the Answer Guide in Appendix F for suggested answers to the following exercises and questions.

1. PALPATION

A. Identify the anatomical reference points a therapist would use to align the universal goniometer axis and stationary and moveable arms when measuring the ROM at the elbow and forearm.

   i. Elbow flexion/extension:

   Goniometer axis _____

   Stationary arm _____

   Moveable arm _____

   ii. Forearm supination/pronation:

   Goniometer axis _____

   Stationary arm _____

   Moveable arm _____

B. Palpate the anatomical reference points used to align the goniometer when measuring elbow and forearm ROM on a skeleton and on a partner.

2. ASSESSMENT PROCESS

List the 10 main components of the assessment process performed by the therapist to assess pathology located at the elbow and forearm.

3. ASSESSMENT OF AROM AT THE ELBOW AND FOREARM ARTICULATIONS

A. Identify and describe the shape of the articular components that make up the elbow articulation and forearm articulations.

B. Demonstrate, define, and describe (i.e., identify the axis/plane of movement) all,

   i. Elbow joint movements.

   ii. Forearm movements with,

   a) your elbow in 90° flexion

   b) your elbow in the anatomical position (i.e., 0°), and identify the movements at the shoulder joint that augment each of the forearm movements.

C. For each of the movements listed below,

   • Assume the start position for the assessment and measurement of the ROM

   • Move the forearm through half of the full AROM, and hold the joint in this position to mimic a decreased AROM

   • Without allowing further movement of the forearm, try to give the appearance of further movement or a greater than available AROM

   • Identify the substitute movements used to give the appearance of a greater than available AROM for the movement being assessed. A patient may use the same substitute movement(s) to augment restricted AROM.

Elbow and Forearm AROM	Substitute Movement(s)
i. Forearm supination	_____
ii. Elbow extension	_____
iii. Elbow flexion	_____
iv. Forearm pronation	_____

D. The therapist assesses a patient's elbow AROM and PROM in sitting and measures 80° AROM and 130° PROM. Identify possible reasons why the AROM would be less than the PROM.

4. ASSESSMENT AND MEASUREMENT OF PROM AT THE ELBOW AND FOREARM

For each of the movements listed below, demonstrate the assessment and measurement of PROM on a partner and answer the questions that follow. Have a third partner evaluate your performance using the appropriate practical test form in Appendix E. Record your findings on the PROM Recording Form below.

Elbow Flexion

  i.   What normal end feel(s) is/are expected when assessing elbow flexion?
 ii.   Only one end feel can be identified for each joint motion assessed. True or false?
iii.   What elbow flexion end feel did you identify on your partner?
 iv.   Identify the normal limiting factor(s) that could have resulted in the end feel identified on your partner.

Elbow Extension/Hyperextension

  i.   Identify the two-joint muscle that crosses the shoulder and elbow joints and if placed on stretch could restrict elbow extension ROM. The muscle is placed on stretch during the assessment of elbow extension ROM if the shoulder is in _____ and the forearm is _____. Therefore, the therapist ensures the forearm is _____ and the shoulder is in the _____ position to avoid passive insufficiency of the two-joint muscle from restricting elbow extension ROM.
 ii.   A patient presents with decreased elbow extension PROM caused by decreased movement at the humeroulnar and humeroradial articulations. Identify the direction of the decreased glide of the trochlea of the ulna and the radial head that would cause the decreased elbow extension PROM.
iii.   Explain how a therapist would determine the direction(s) of decreased glide in ii above.

Forearm Supination

  i.   Assume a patient presents with decreased forearm supination PROM. Identify the joint(s) where motion could be decreased.
 ii.   Identify the motion that occurs between the radial head and the capitulum when the forearm is supinated.
iii.   In the presence of decreased forearm supination ROM, identify the direction of glide of the radial notch that could be limited and cause the decreased ROM.
 iv.   Explain how a therapist would determine the direction of decreased glide in iii above.
  v.   In full supination, the radius lies _____ to the ulna.

Forearm Pronation

  i.   What end feel was present when you assessed your partner's forearm pronation PROM?
 ii.   What normal end feel(s) can be expected when assessing forearm pronation?
iii.   List the normal limiting factors that would create the normal end feel(s) for forearm pronation.
 iv.   Moving from a position of full supination to one of full pronation, the radius _____ around the relatively _____ ulna.

PROM RECORDING FORM

Patient's Name _____ Therapist _____

				Left Side / Right Side				
*		*		**Date of Measurement**	*		*	
				Elbow and Forearm				
				Flexion (0–150°)				
				Supination (0–80°)				
				Pronation (0–80°)				
				Hypermobility:				
				Comments:				

5. MUSCLE LENGTH ASSESSMENT AND MEASUREMENT

Demonstrate the assessment and measurement of muscle length of the biceps brachii and triceps on a partner and answer the questions below that pertain to the tricep muscle. Have a third partner evaluate your performance using the appropriate practical test form in Appendix E.

Triceps

i.   Identify the origin and insertion of the triceps muscle.

ii. Identify the movements of the upper extremity that would place the origin and insertion of the triceps muscle farther apart and thus place the triceps on stretch.

iii. A therapist would identify a _____ end feel at the limit of _____ PROM when assessing triceps muscle length in the presence of an abnormally shortened triceps muscle.

6. FUNCTIONAL ROM AT THE ELBOW AND FOREARM

A. i. With your dominant elbow fixed in 0° extension, identify the regions/parts of your body you would be unable to contact with your dominant hand if you were:

(a) standing and

(b) sitting.

ii. List personal care ADL that would be impossible to perform using your dominant hand with the elbow fixed in 0° extension.

B. i. With your dominant elbow fixed in 90° flexion, identify the regions/parts of your body you would be unable to contact with your dominant hand if you were:

(a) standing and

(b) sitting.

ii. List personal care ADL that would be impossible to perform using your dominant hand with the elbow fixed in 90° flexion.

C. Have a partner perform or simulate the following functional activities. Use a universal goniometer and measure the maximum elbow flexion ROM required to successfully complete each of the following activities:

i. drinking from a cup;

ii. holding the telephone to the ear;

iii. tying a shoe lace;

iv. combing the hair on the back of the head;

v. reaching for a wallet in a back pocket.

D. Identify the forearm position(s) required to perform the following activities:

i. picking up a small object from a table top;

ii. receiving change in the palm of the hand;

iii. eating with a fork;

iv. reaching for a wallet in a back pocket;

v. combing the hair on the vertex of the head.

E. According to the findings of Morrey et al. (1), many self-care activities can be accomplished within the arc of movement from _____° to _____° flexion and from _____° of pronation to _____° of supination.

Reference

1. Morrey BF, Askew LJ, An KN, Chao EY. A biomechanical study of normal functional elbow motion. *J Bone Joint Surg [Am]*. 1981;63:872–876.

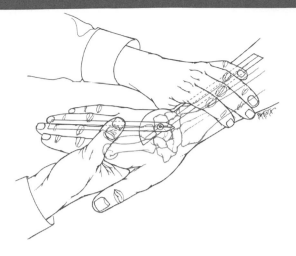

Wrist and Hand 5

ARTICULATIONS AND MOVEMENTS

The articulations of the wrist and hand are illustrated in Figures 5-1 and 5-2. The movements of the wrist and hand are described in Tables 5-1, 5-2, and 5-3.

Located between the forearm and hand, the wrist is made up of eight small bones. These bones are arranged in a proximal row (the scaphoid, lunate, triquetrum, and pisiform) and a distal row (the hamate, capitate, trapezoid, and trapezium). The proximal surface of the proximal row of carpal bones (excluding the pisiform, which articulates solely with the triquetrum) is convex. This convex surface articulates with the concave surface of the distal aspect of the radius and the articular disc of the inferior radioulnar joint to form the ellipsoidal, radiocarpal joint (2).

The midcarpal joint is a compound articulation (2) formed between the proximal and distal row of carpal bones. The proximal aspect of the distal row of carpal bones has a concave surface laterally (formed by the trapezoid and trapezium) and a convex surface medially (formed by the hamate and capitate). These surfaces articulate with the corresponding convex (formed by the scaphoid) and concave (formed by the scaphoid, lunate, and triquetrum) surfaces, respectively, on the distal aspect of the proximal row of carpal bones.

In the clinical setting, it is not possible to independently measure the motion at the radiocarpal joint and at the midcarpal joint. Thus, wrist range of motion (ROM) measurements include the combined motion of both joints. Movement at the radiocarpal and midcarpal joints produce the wrist movements of flexion, extension, radial deviation, and ulnar deviation. From the anatomical position, wrist flexion and extension occur in the sagittal plane around a frontal axis (Fig. 5-3). Wrist radial deviation

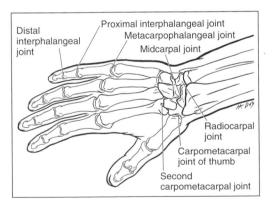

Figure 5-1 Wrist, finger, and thumb articulations.

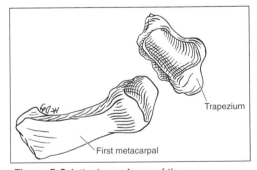

Figure 5-2 Articular surfaces of the carpometacarpal joint of the thumb.

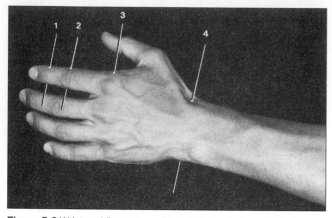

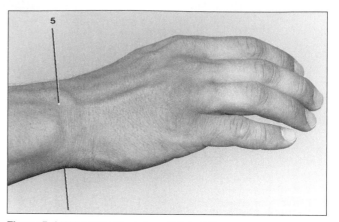

Figure 5-3 Wrist and finger axes: (1) distal interphalangeal flexion-extension, (2) proximal interphalangeal flexion-extension, (3) metacarpophalangeal flexion-extension, and (4) wrist flexion-extension.

Figure 5-4 Wrist axis: (5) ulnar-radial deviation.

and ulnar deviation occur in the frontal plane about a sagittal axis (Fig. 5-4).

Movement at the carpometacarpal (CM) joints (formed between the distal aspect of the distal row of carpal bones and the bases of the metacarpal bones) is essential for normal hand function. CM movement contributes to the flattening of the palm when the hand is opened fully, and the guttering of the palm when gripping or manipulating objects. The mobile peripheral metacarpals of the ring and little fingers and thumb move around the fixed metacarpals of the index and middle fingers. In the clinical setting, it is not possible to directly measure movements at the CM joints of the second through fifth metacarpals, but it is possible to measure movement at the CM joint of the thumb. The CM joint of the thumb (see Fig. 5-2) is a saddle joint formed by the distal surface of the trapezium, which is concave anteroposteriorly and convex mediolaterally and articulates with the corresponding reciprocal surface of the base of the first metacarpal. The movements at the first CM joint include flexion, extension, abduction, adduction, rotation, and opposition. Flexion and extension occur in an oblique frontal plane about an oblique sagittal axis (Fig. 5-5), and abduction and adduction occur in an oblique

sagittal plane around an oblique frontal axis. Opposition is a sequential movement incorporating abduction, flexion, and adduction of the first metacarpal, with simultaneous rotation (10).

The metacarpophalangeal (MCP) joints of the hand are classified as ellipsoid joints (2), each formed proximally by the convex head of the metatarsal articulating with the concave base of the adjacent proximal phalanx. The movements at the MCP articulations include flexion, extension, abduction, adduction, and rotation. The movements that are measured in the clinical setting are flexion and extension, which occur in the sagittal plane around a frontal axis (see Fig. 5-3), and abduction and adduction, which occur in the frontal plane around a sagittal axis. It is not possible to measure rotation at the MCP joints in the clinical setting.

The interphalangeal (IP) joints of the thumb and fingers are classified as hinge joints, formed by the convex head of the proximal phalanx articulating with the concave base of the adjacent distal phalanx. The IP joints allow flexion and extension movements of the fingers that occur in the sagittal plane around a frontal axis (see Figs. 5-3 and 5-5).

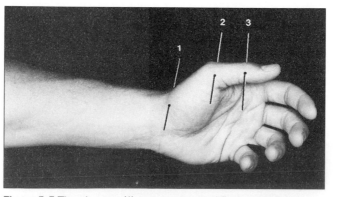

Figure 5-5 Thumb axes: (1) carpometacarpal flexion-extension, (2) metacarpophalangeal flexion-extension, and (3) interphalangeal flexion-extension.

TABLE 5-1 Joint Structure: Wrist Movements

	Flexion	Extension	Radial Deviation	Ulnar Deviation
Articulation[1,2]	Radiocarpal Midcarpal	Midcarpal Radiocarpal	Midcarpal Radiocarpal	Radiocarpal (predominant) Midcarpal
Plane	Sagittal	Sagittal	Frontal	Frontal
Axis	Frontal	Frontal	Sagittal	Sagittal
Normal limiting factors[1,3,4]* (See Figs. 5-6 and 5-7)	Tension in the posterior radiocarpal ligament and posterior joint capsule	Tension in the anterior radiocarpal ligament and anterior joint capsule; contact between the radius and the carpal bones	Tension in the ulnar collateral ligament, ulnocarpal ligament, and ulnar portion of the joint capsule; contact between the radial styloid process and the scaphoid bone	Tension in the radial collateral ligament and radial portion of the joint capsule
Normal end feel[3,5]	Firm	Firm/hard	Firm/hard	Firm
Normal AROM† (AROM[7])	0–80° (0–80°)	0–70° (0–70°)	0–20° (0–20°)	0–30° (0–30°)
Capsular pattern[5,8]	Flexion and extension are equally restricted			

*Note: There is a paucity of definitive research that identifies the normal limiting factors (NLF) of joint motion. The NLF and end feels listed here are based on a knowledge of anatomy, clinical experience, and available references.
†AROM, active range of motion.

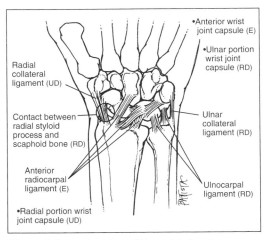

Figure 5-6 Anterior view of the wrist showing noncontractile structures that normally limit motion at the wrist.*

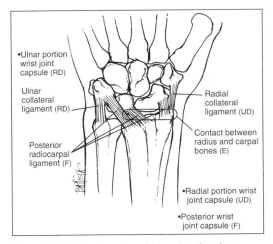

Figure 5-7 Posterior view of the wrist showing noncontractile structures that normally limit motion at the wrist.*

*Motion limited by structures is identified in brackets, using the following abbreviations: F, flexion; E, extension; UD, ulnar deviation; RD, radial deviation. Muscles normally limiting motion are not illustrated.

TABLE 5-2   Joint Structure: Finger Movements

	Flexion	Extension	Abduction	Adduction
Articulation[1,2]	Metacarpophalangeal (MCP) Proximal interphalangeal (PIP) Distal interphalangeal (DIP)	MCP PIP DIP	MCP	MCP
Plane	Sagittal	Sagittal	Frontal	Frontal
Axis	Frontal	Frontal	Sagittal	Sagittal
Normal limiting factors [1,3,4]* (See Fig. 5-8)	MCP: tension in the posterior joint capsule, collateral ligaments; contact between the proximal phalanx and the metacarpal; tension in extensor digitorum communis and extensor indicis (when the wrist is flexed)[9] PIP: contact between the middle and proximal phalanx; soft tissue apposition of the middle and proximal phalanges; tension in the posterior joint capsule, and collateral ligaments DIP: tension in the posterior joint capsule, collateral ligaments, and oblique retinacular ligament	MCP: Tension in the anterior joint capsule, palmar fibrocartilagenous plate (palmar ligament); tension in flexor digitorum profundus and flexor digitorum superficialis (when the wrist is extended)[9] PIP: tension in the anterior joint capsule, palmar ligament DIP: tension in the anterior joint capsule, palmar ligament	Tension in the collateral ligaments, fascia, and skin of the web spaces	Contact between adjacent fingers
Normal end feel[3,5]	MCP: firm/hard PIP: hard/soft/firm DIP: firm	MCP: firm PIP: firm DIP: firm	Firm	
Normal AROM[6] (AROM[7])	MCP: 0–90° (0–90°) PIP: 0–100° (0–100°) DIP: 0–90° (0–70°)	MCP: 0–45° (0–20°) PIP: 0° (0°) DIP: 0° (0°)		
Capsular pattern[5,8]	Metacarpophalangeal and interphalangeal joints: flexion, extension			

*Note: There is a paucity of definitive research that identifies the normal limiting factors (NLF) of joint motion. The NLF and end feels listed here are based on a knowledge of anatomy, clinical experience, and available references.

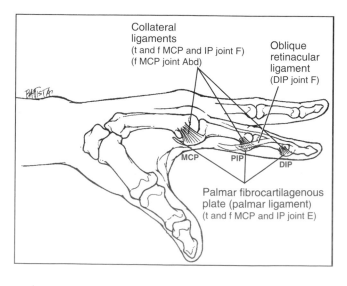

Collateral ligaments (t and f MCP and IP joint F) (f MCP joint Abd)

Oblique retinacular ligament (DIP joint F)

MCP   PIP   DIP

Palmar fibrocartilagenous plate (palmar ligament) (t and f MCP and IP joint E)

Figure 5-8 Lateral view of the wrist and hand showing noncontractile structures that normally limit motion at the MCP and IP joints of the fingers (f) and thumb (t). Other noncontractile structures that normally limit motion at the MCP and IP joints and first CM joint are listed in Table 5-2. Motion limited by structures is identified in brackets, using the following abbreviations: F, flexion; E, extension; Abd, abduction. Muscles normally limiting motion are not illustrated.

TABLE 5-3   Joint Structure: Thumb Movements

	Flexion	Extension	Palmar Abduction	Adduction
Articulation[1,2]	Carpometacarpal (CM) Metacarpophalangeal (MCP) Interphalangeal (IP)	CM MCP IP	CM MCP	CM MCP
Plane	CM: oblique frontal MCP: frontal IP: frontal	CM: oblique frontal MCP: frontal IP: frontal	CM: oblique sagittal	CM: oblique sagittal
Axis	CM: oblique sagittal MCP: sagittal IP: sagittal	CM: oblique sagittal MCP: sagittal IP: sagittal	CM: oblique frontal	CM: oblique frontal
Normal limiting factors[1,3,4]* (See Fig. 5-8)	CM: soft tissue apposition between the thenar eminence and the palm; tension in the posterior joint capsule, extensor pollicis brevis, and abductor pollicis brevis MCP: contact between the first metacarpal and the proximal phalanx; tension in the posterior joint capsule, collateral ligaments, and extensor pollicis brevis IP: tension in the collateral ligaments, and posterior joint capsule; contact between the distal phalanx, fibrocartilagenous plate and the proximal phalanx	CM: tension in the anterior joint capsule, flexor pollicis brevis, and first dorsal interosseous MCP: tension in the anterior joint capsule, palmar ligament, and flexor pollicis brevis IP: tension in the anterior joint capsule, palmar ligament	Tension in the fascia and skin of the first web space, first dorsal interosseous, and adductor pollicis	Soft tissue apposition between the thumb and index finger
Normal end feel[3,5,8]	CM: soft/firm MCP: hard/firm IP: hard/firm	CM: firm MCP: firm IP: firm	Firm	Soft
Normal AROM[6] (AROM[7])	CM: 0–15° (0–15°) MCP: 0–50° (0–50°) IP: 0–80° (0–65°)	CM: 0–20° (0–20°) MCP: 0° (0°) IP: 0–20° (0–10 to 20°)	0–70° (0–70°)	0° (0°)
Capsular pattern[5,8]	CM joint: abduction, extension MCP and IP joints: flexion, extension			

*Note: There is a paucity of definitive research that identifies the normal limiting factors (NLF) of joint motion. The NLF and end feels listed here are based on a knowledge of anatomy, clinical experience, and available references.

SURFACE ANATOMY

(Figs. 5-9 through 5-11)

Structure	Location
1. Styloid process of the ulna	Bony prominence on the posteromedial aspect of the forearm at the distal end of the ulna.
2. Styloid process of the radius	Bony prominence on the lateral aspect of the forearm at the distal end of the radius.
3. Metacarpal bones	The bases and shafts are felt through the extensor tendons on the posterior surface of the wrist and hand. The heads are the bony prominences at the bases of the digits.
4. Capitate bone	In the small depression proximal to the base of the third metacarpal bone.
5. Pisiform bone	Medial bone of the proximal row of carpal bones; proximal to the base of the hypothenar eminence.
6. Thumb web space	The web of skin connecting the thumb to the hand.
7. Distal palmar crease	Transverse crease commencing on the medial side of the palm and extending laterally to the web between the index and middle fingers.
8. Proximal palmar crease	Transverse crease commencing on the lateral side of the palm, extending medially and fading out on the hypothenar eminence.
9. Thenar eminence	The pad on the palm of the hand at the base of the thumb; bound medially and distally by the longitudinal palmar crease.
10. Hypothenar eminence	The pad on the medial side of the base of the palm.
11. First CM joint	At the distal aspect of the anatomical snuffbox, the articulation between the base of the first metacarpal and the trapezium. (*Anatomical snuffbox:* with the thumb held in extension, the triangular area on the posterolateral aspect of the wrist and hand outlined by the tendons of the extensor pollicis longus laterally and the extensor pollicis brevis medially.)

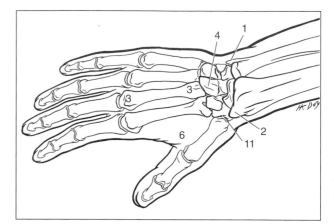

Figure 5-9 Bony anatomy, posterior aspect of the wrist and hand.

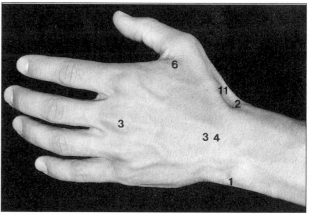

Figure 5-10 Posterior aspect of the wrist and hand.

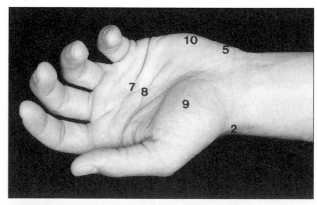

Figure 5-11 Anterior aspect of the wrist and hand.

RANGE OF MOTION ASSESSMENT AND MEASUREMENT

General Scan: Wrist and Hand Active Range of Motion

The AROM of the wrist and hand is scanned (not shown) to provide a general indication of the available ROM and/or muscle strength at the wrist and hand before proceeding with a detailed assessment of the region. First instruct the patient to make a fist. Observe the AROM of finger flexion, thumb flexion and adduction, and wrist extension. Then instruct the patient to open the hand and spread the fingers as far apart as possible. Observe the AROM for finger extension and abduction, thumb extension, and wrist flexion.

Wrist Flexion-Extension

AROM Assessment

Substitute Movement. Wrist ulnar or radial deviation.

PROM Assessment

Start Position. The patient is sitting. The elbow is flexed, the forearm is resting on a table in pronation, the wrist is in neutral position, the hand is over the end of the table, and the fingers are relaxed (Fig. 5-12).

Stabilization. The therapist stabilizes the forearm.

Therapist's Distal Hand Placement. The therapist grasps the metacarpals.

End Position. The therapist applies slight traction to and moves the hand anteriorly to the limit of motion to assess wrist flexion (Fig. 5-13). The therapist applies slight traction to and moves the hand posteriorly to the limit of motion for wrist extension (Fig. 5-14). The fingers should be relaxed when assessing the end feels.

End Feels. Wrist flexion—firm; wrist extension—firm or hard.

Joint Glides. *Flexion.* Radiocarpal joint: the convex surface of the proximal row of carpal bones glides posteriorly on the fixed concave surface of the distal radius and articular disc of the inferior radioulnar joint. Midcarpal joint: the concave surface formed by the trapezium and trapezoid glides in an anterior direction on the fixed convex surface of the scaphoid; the convex surface formed by the capitate and hamate glides in a posterior direction on the fixed

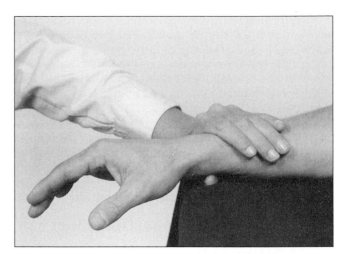
Figure 5-12 Start position for wrist flexion and extension.

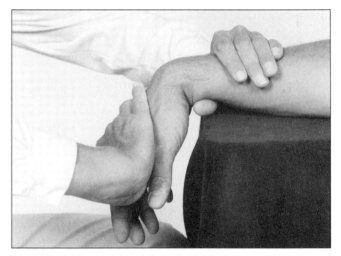
Figure 5-13 Firm end feel at limit of wrist flexion.

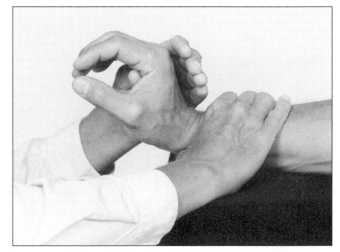
Figure 5-14 Firm or hard end feel at limit of wrist extension.

concave surface formed by the scaphoid, lunate, and triquetrum bones. *Extension.* Radiocarpal joint: the convex surface of the proximal row of carpal bones glides anteriorly on the fixed concave surface of the distal radius and articular disc of the inferior radioulnar joint. Midcarpal joint: the concave surface formed by the trapezium and trapezoid glides in a posterior direction on the fixed convex surface of the scaphoid; the convex surface formed by the capitate and hamate glides in an anterior direction on the fixed concave surface formed by the scaphoid, lunate, and triquetrum bones. The above represents a simplified explanation of wrist arthrokinematics with application of the concave–convex rule during wrist movement.

Measurement: Universal Goniometer

Start Position. The patient is sitting. The elbow is flexed, the forearm is resting on a table in pronation, the wrist is in a neutral position, and the fingers are slightly extended for measurement of flexion and slightly flexed for measurement of extension. The hand is over the end of the table (Fig. 5-15).

Stabilization. The therapist stabilizes the forearm.

Goniometer Axis. The axis is placed at the level of the ulnar styloid process (Fig. 5-16).

Stationary Arm. Parallel to the longitudinal axis of the ulna.

Movable Arm. Parallel to the longitudinal axis of the fifth metacarpal.

End Positions. Wrist flexion: the wrist is moved in an anterior direction (80°) (Figs. 5-16 and 5-17). Wrist extension: the wrist is moved in a posterior direction to the limit of motion of 70° (Fig. 5-18). For both movements, ensure that the mobile fourth and fifth metacarpals are not moved away from the start position throughout the assessment procedure, and ensure that no wrist deviation occurs if full range cannot be obtained.

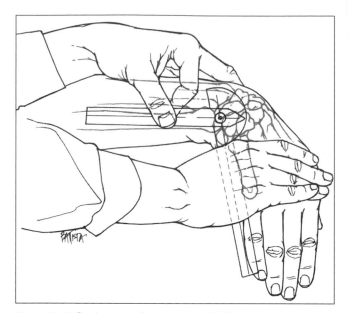

Figure 5-16 Goniometer alignment for wrist flexion and extension, illustrated at limit of wrist flexion.

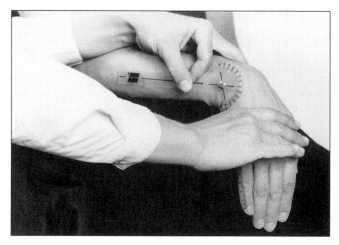

Figure 5-17 End position for wrist flexion.

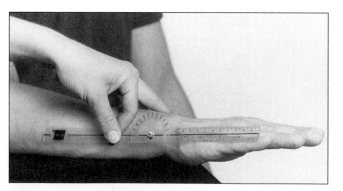

Figure 5-15 Start position for wrist flexion and extension.

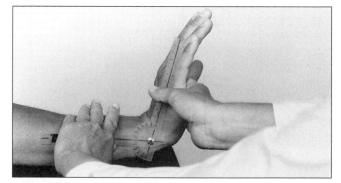

Figure 5-18 End position for wrist extension.

Wrist Ulnar and Radial Deviation

AROM Assessment

Substitute Movement. Ulnar or radial deviation of the fingers, wrist flexion, and wrist extension.

PROM Assessment

Start Position. The patient is sitting. The forearm is resting on a table in pronation, the wrist is in neutral position, the hand is over the end of the table, and the fingers are relaxed (see Fig. 5-12).

Stabilization. The therapist stabilizes the forearm.

Therapist's Distal Hand Placement. The therapist grasps the metacarpals from the radial aspect of the hand to assess wrist ulnar deviation. The therapist grasps the metacarpals from the ulnar aspect of the hand to assess wrist radial deviation.

End Positions. The therapist applies slight traction and moves the hand in an ulnar direction to the limit of motion to assess wrist ulnar deviation (Fig. 5-19). The therapist applies slight traction to and moves the hand in a radial direction to the limit of motion for wrist radial deviation (Fig. 5-20).

End Feels. Ulnar deviation—firm; radial deviation—firm or hard.

Joint Glides (11). *Ulnar deviation.* Radiocarpal joint: the convex surface of the proximal row of carpal bones glides laterally on the fixed concave surface of the distal radius and articular disc of the inferior radioulnar joint. Midcarpal joint: the convex surface formed by the capitate and hamate glides in a lateral direction on the fixed concave surface formed by the scaphoid, lunate, and triquetrum bones. *Radial deviation.* Radiocarpal joint: the convex surface of the proximal row of carpal bones glides medially on the fixed concave surface of the distal radius and articular disc of the inferior radioulnar joint. Midcarpal joint: the convex surface formed by the capitate and hamate glides in a medial direction on the fixed concave surface formed by the scaphoid, lunate, and triquetrum bones.

The above represents a simplified explanation of wrist arthrokinematics with application of the concave–convex rule during wrist movement.

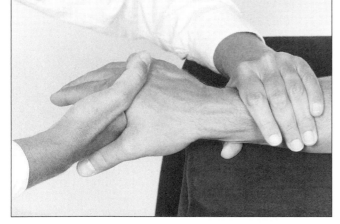

Figure 5-19 Firm end feel at limit of wrist ulnar deviation.

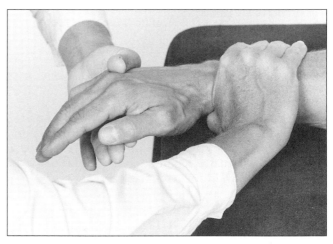

Figure 5-20 Firm or hard end feel at limit of wrist radial deviation.

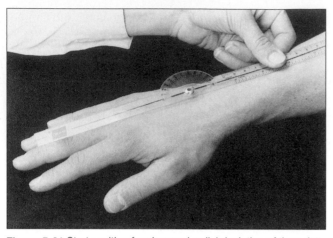

Figure 5-21 Start position for ulnar and radial deviation of the wrist.

Measurement: Universal Goniometer

Start Position. The patient is sitting. The elbow is flexed, the forearm is pronated, and the palmar surface of the hand is resting lightly on a table. The wrist remains in a neutral position and the fingers are relaxed (Fig. 5-21).

Stabilization. The therapist stabilizes the forearm.

Goniometer Axis. The axis is placed on the posterior aspect of the wrist joint over the capitate bone (Fig. 5-22).

Stationary Arm. Along the midline of the forearm.

Movable Arm. Parallel to the longitudinal axis of the shaft of the third metacarpal.

End Positions. Ulnar deviation (Figs. 5-22 and 5-23): the wrist is adducted to the ulnar side to the limit of motion (30°). Radial deviation (Fig. 5-24): the wrist is abducted to the radial side to the limit of motion (20°). Ensure that the wrist is not moved into flexion or extension.

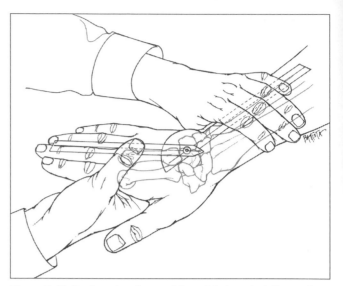

Figure 5-22 Goniometer alignment for wrist ulnar deviation and radial deviation, illustrated at limit of ulnar deviation.

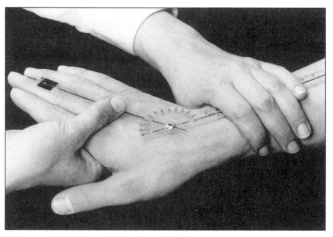

Figure 5-23 End position: ulnar deviation.

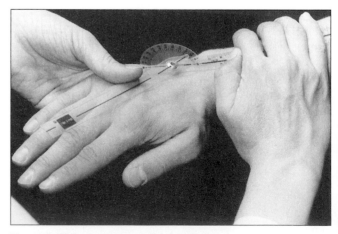

Figure 5-24 End position: radial deviation.

Finger MCP Flexion-Extension

PROM Assessment

Start Position. The patient is sitting. The forearm is resting on a table in midposition, the wrist is in neutral position, and the fingers are relaxed (Fig. 5-25).

Stabilization. The therapist stabilizes the metacarpal.

Therapist's Distal Hand Placement. The therapist grasps the proximal phalanx.

End Positions. The therapist applies slight traction to and moves the proximal phalanx in an anterior direction to the limit of motion to assess MCP joint flexion (Fig. 5-26). The therapist applies slight traction to and moves the proximal phalanx in a posterior direction to the limit of motion for MCP joint extension (Fig. 5-27).

End Feels. MCP joint flexion—firm or hard; MCP joint extension—firm.

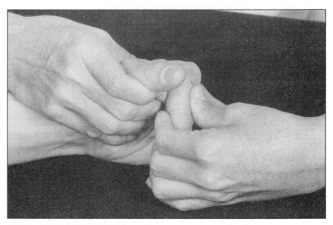

Figure 5-26 Firm or hard end feel at the limit of MCP flexion.

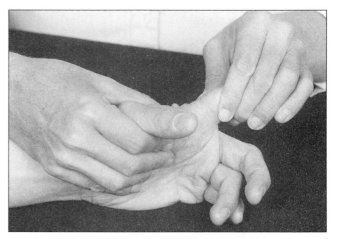

Figure 5-27 Firm end feel at the limit of MCP extension.

Joint Glides. *MCP joint flexion*—the concave base of the proximal phalanx glides in an anterior direction on the fixed convex head of the adjacent metacarpal. *MCP joint extension*—the concave base of the proximal phalanx glides in a posterior direction on the fixed convex head of the adjacent metacarpal.

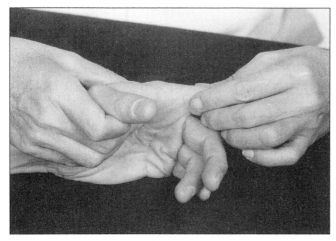

Figure 5-25 Start position: MCP joint flexion and extension.

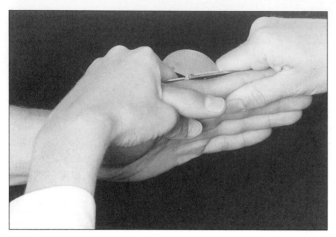

Figure 5-28 Start position for MCP flexion.

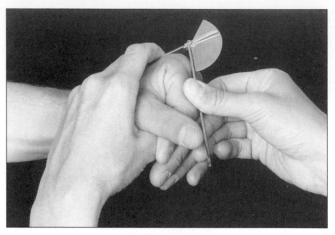

Figure 5-29 End position: MCP flexion.

Measurement: Universal Goniometer

Finger MCP Flexion

Start Position. The patient is sitting. The forearm is resting on a table, the elbow is flexed, the wrist is slightly extended, and the MCP joint of the finger being measured is in 0° of extension (Fig. 5-28).

Stabilization. The therapist stabilizes the metacarpal.

Goniometer Axis. The axis is placed on the posterior aspect of the MCP joint being measured.

Stationary Arm. Parallel to the longitudinal axis of the shaft of the metacarpal.

Movable Arm. Parallel to the longitudinal axis of the proximal phalanx.

End Position. All fingers are moved toward the palm to the limit of motion of 90° (Fig. 5-29). Range increases progressively from the index to the fifth finger (1). The IP joints are allowed to extend so that flexion at the MCP joint is not restricted due to tension of the long finger extensor tendons.

Alternate Goniometer Placement. The index and fifth MCP joints may be measured on the lateral aspect of the joint (Figs. 5-30 and 5-31). Should joint enlargement prevent measurement on the posterior aspect, the index and fifth fingers may be measured and the range estimated for the middle and fourth fingers (12).

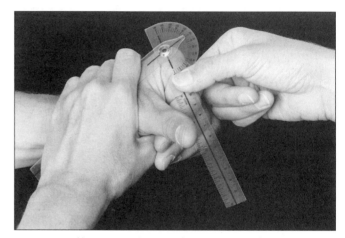

Figure 5-30 Alternate goniometer placement for MCP flexion.

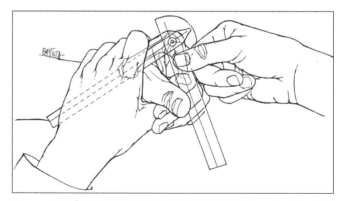

Figure 5-31 Goniometer alignment on the lateral aspect of the joint for MCP joint flexion and extension, illustrated with the MCP joint in flexion.

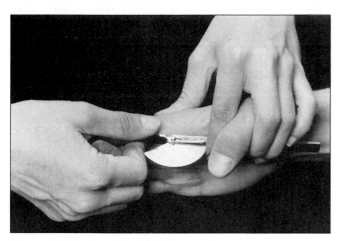

Figure 5-32 Start position for MCP extension.

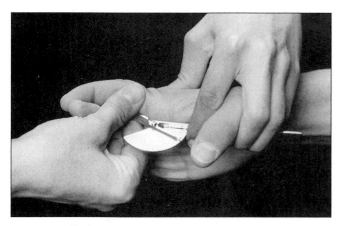

Figure 5-33 End position: MCP extension.

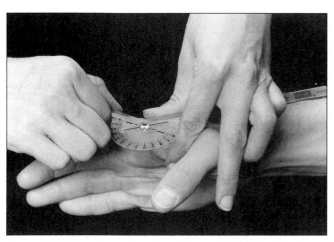

Figure 5-34 Alternate goniometer placement for MCP extension.

Measurement: Universal Goniometer

Finger MCP Extension

Start Position. The patient is sitting. The forearm is resting on a table, the elbow is flexed, the wrist is slightly flexed, and the MCP joint of the finger being measured is in 0° of extension (Fig. 5-32).

Stabilization. The therapist stabilizes the metacarpal.

Goniometer Axis. The axis is placed on the anterior surface of the MCP joint being measured.

Stationary Arm. Parallel to the longitudinal axis of the shaft of the metacarpal.

Movable Arm. Parallel to the longitudinal axis of the proximal phalanx.

End Position. The finger is moved in a posterior direction to the limit of motion of 45° (Fig. 5-33). The IP joints are allowed to flex so that extension at the MCP joint is not restricted due to tension of the long finger flexor tendons.

Alternate Goniometer Placement. The index and fifth MCP joints may be measured on the lateral aspect of the MCP joint (Fig. 5-34).

Finger MCP Abduction-Adduction

AROM Assessment

MCP Abduction

To gain a composite measure of finger spread and thumb web stretch, finger abduction and thumb extension can be measured in centimeters. A sheet of paper is placed under the patient's hand. The therapist stabilizes the wrist and metacarpals. The patient spreads all fingers and thumb and the therapist traces the contour of the hand (Fig. 5-35). The patient's hand is removed, and a linear measure of the distances between the midpoint of the tip of each finger and the index finger and thumb is recorded in centimeters (Fig. 5-36). *Note*: The ROM at the IP, MCP, and CM joints of the thumb influence the measurement of thumb extension ROM using this method.

PROM Assessment

MCP Abduction (not shown)

Start Position. The patient is sitting. The forearm is resting on a table, the wrist is in neutral position, and the fingers are in the anatomical position.

Stabilization. The therapist stabilizes the metacarpal.

Therapist's Distal Hand Placement. The therapist grasps the sides of the proximal phalanx.

End Position. The therapist applies slight traction to and moves the proximal phalanx to the limit of motion to assess MCP joint abduction.

End Feel. MCP joint abduction—firm.

Joint Glides. *MCP joint abduction*—the concave base of the proximal phalanx moves on the fixed convex head of the

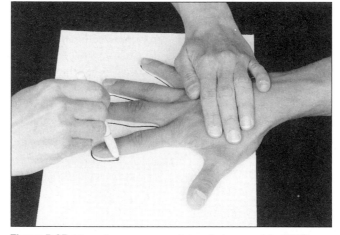

Figure 5-35 Alternate measurement: hand placement for MCP abduction and thumb extension.

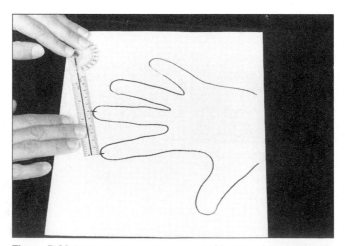

Figure 5-36 Ruler measurement: finger MCP abduction and thumb extension.

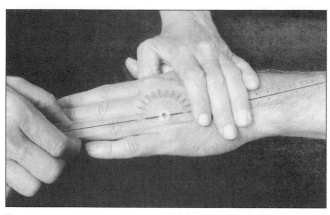

Figure 5-37 Start position: MCP abduction and adduction.

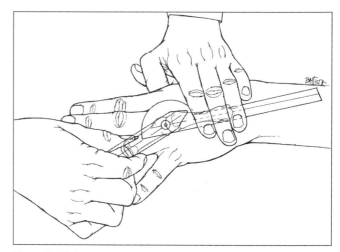

Figure 5-38 Goniometer alignment for MCP joint abduction/adduction, shown with the ring finger in abduction.

corresponding metacarpal in the same direction of movement as the shaft of the proximal phalanx. *MCP joint adduction*—the concave base of the proximal phalanx moves on the fixed convex head of the corresponding metacarpal in the same direction of movement as the shaft of the proximal phalanx.

Measurement: Universal Goniometer

Start Position. The patient is sitting. The elbow is flexed to 90°, the forearm is pronated and resting on a table, the wrist is in neutral position, and the fingers are in the anatomical position (Fig. 5-37).

Stabilization. The therapist stabilizes the metacarpal bones.

Goniometer Axis. The axis is placed on the posterior surface of the MCP joint being measured (Fig. 5-38).

Stationary Arm. Parallel to the longitudinal axis of the shaft of the metacarpal.

Movable Arm. Parallel to the longitudinal axis of the proximal phalanx.

End Position. The finger is moved away from the midline of the hand to the limit of motion in abduction (Fig. 5-39). The finger is moved toward the midline of the hand to the limit of motion in adduction (Fig. 5-40). The remaining fingers are moved to allow full adduction.

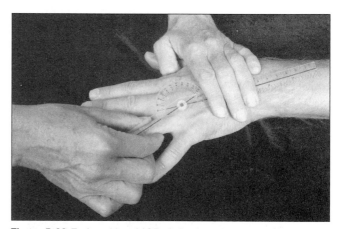

Figure 5-39 End position: MCP abduction of the fourth finger.

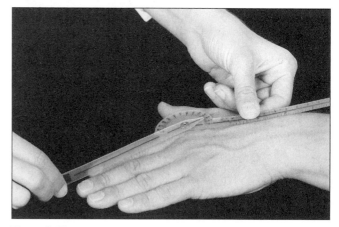

Figure 5-40 End position: MCP adduction of the index finger.

Finger IP Flexion-Extension

PROM Assessment

Start Position. The patient is sitting. The forearm is resting on a table, the wrist is in neutral position, and the fingers are relaxed.

Stabilization. The therapist stabilizes the proximal phalanx for assessment of the proximal interphalangeal (PIP) joint and the middle phalanx for the distal interphalangeal (DIP) joint.

Therapist's Distal Hand Placement. The therapist grasps the middle phalanx to assess the PIP joint and the distal phalanx to assess the DIP joint.

End Positions. The therapist applies slight traction to and moves the middle or distal phalanx in an anterior direction to the limit of motion to assess PIP (not shown) or DIP joint flexion (Fig. 5-41), respectively. The therapist applies slight traction to and moves the middle or distal phalanx in a posterior direction to the limit of motion for PIP joint (not shown) or DIP joint extension (Fig. 5-42), respectively.

End Feels. PIP joint flexion—hard, soft, or firm; DIP joint flexion—firm; PIP joint extension—firm; DIP joint extension—firm.

Joint Glides. *IP joint flexion*—the concave base of the distal phalanx glides in an anterior direction on the fixed convex head of the adjacent proximal phalanx. *IP joint extension*—the concave base of the distal phalanx glides in a posterior direction on the fixed convex head of the adjacent proximal phalanx.

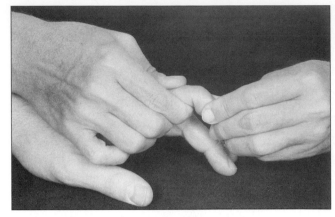

Figure 5-41 Firm end feel at limit of DIP joint flexion.

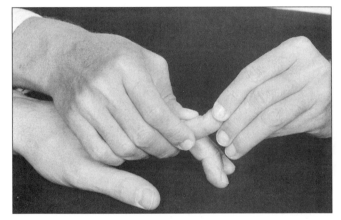

Figure 5-42 Firm end feel at limit of DIP joint extension.

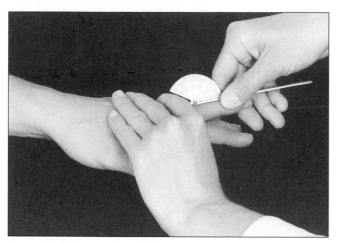

Figure 5-43 Start position: PIP joint flexion.

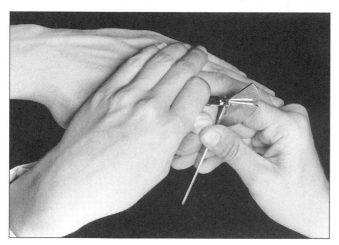

Figure 5-44 End position: PIP joint flexion.

Measurement: Universal Goniometer

Start Position. The patient is sitting. The forearm is resting on a table in either midposition or pronation. The wrist and fingers are in the anatomical position (0° extension at the MCP and IP joints).

Stabilization. The therapist stabilizes the proximal phalanx for measurement of the PIP joint and the middle phalanx for the DIP joint.

Goniometer Axis. To measure IP joint flexion, the axis is placed over the posterior surface of the PIP (Figs. 5-43 and 5-44) or DIP joint being measured. To measure IP joint extension, the axis is placed over the anterior surface of the PIP or DIP joint being measured.

Stationary Arm. PIP joint: parallel to the longitudinal axis of the proximal phalanx. DIP joint: parallel to the longitudinal axis of the middle phalanx.

Movable Arm. PIP joint: parallel to the longitudinal axis of the middle phalanx. DIP joint: parallel to the longitudinal axis of the distal phalanx.

End Positions. The PIP joint (Figs. 5-44 and 5-45) or DIP joint (not shown) is flexed to the limit of motion (100° or 90°, respectively). The PIP joint (Fig. 5-46) or DIP joint (not shown) is extended to the limit of motion (0°).

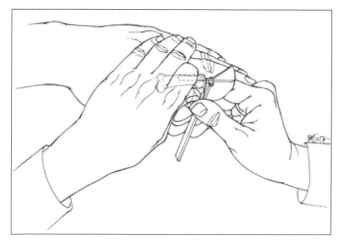

Figure 5-45 Goniometer alignment over posterior surface of PIP joint to assess flexion.

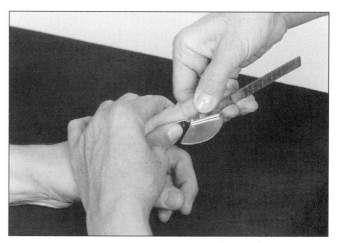

Figure 5-46 End position: PIP joint extension.

Finger MCP and IP Flexion

When evaluating impairment of hand function, a linear measurement of finger flexion should be used in conjunction with goniometry. This measure is particularly relevant in evaluating the extent of impairment (13) associated with grasp. The patient is sitting. The elbow is flexed and the forearm is resting on a table in supination. Two measurements are taken. First, the patient flexes the

IP joints while maintaining 0° of extension at the MCP joints (Fig. 5-47). A ruler measurement is taken from the pulp or tip of the middle finger to the distal palmar crease. Then the patient flexes the MCP and IP joints (Fig. 5-48), and a ruler measurement is taken from the pulp of the finger to the proximal palmar crease. *Note:* Long fingernails limit the flexion ROM at the finger joints (MCP joint flexion being the most affected) when the fingernails contact the palm (14).

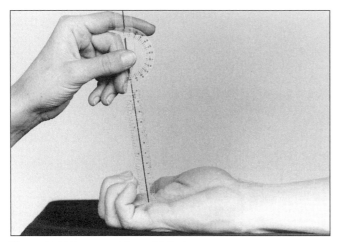

Figure 5-47 Decreased finger IP flexion.

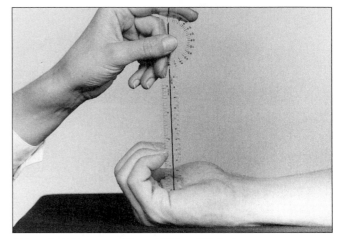

Figure 5-48 Decreased finger MCP and IP flexion.

Thumb CM Flexion-Extension

PROM Assessment

Start Position. The patient is sitting. The elbow is flexed with the forearm in midposition and resting on a table. The wrist is in neutral position, the fingers are relaxed, and the thumb is in the anatomical position (Fig. 5-49).

Stabilization. The therapist stabilizes the trapezium, wrist, and forearm (see Fig. 5-49).

Therapist's Distal Hand Placement. The therapist grasps the first metacarpal (Fig. 5-50).

End Positions. The therapist applies slight traction to and moves the first metacarpal in an ulnar direction to the limit of motion to assess thumb CM joint flexion (Fig. 5-51). The therapist applies slight traction to and moves the first metacarpal in a radial direction to the limit of motion for thumb CM joint extension (Fig. 5-52).

End Feels. Thumb CM joint flexion—soft or firm; thumb CM joint extension—firm.

Joint Glides (11). *Thumb CM joint flexion*—the concave surface of the base of the first metacarpal glides in a medial direction (i.e., in the same direction to the movement of the shaft of the first metacarpal) on the convex surface of the trapezium. *Thumb CM joint extension*—the concave surface of the base of the first metacarpal glides in a lateral direction (i.e., in the same direction to the movement of the shaft of the first metacarpal) on the convex surface of the trapezium.

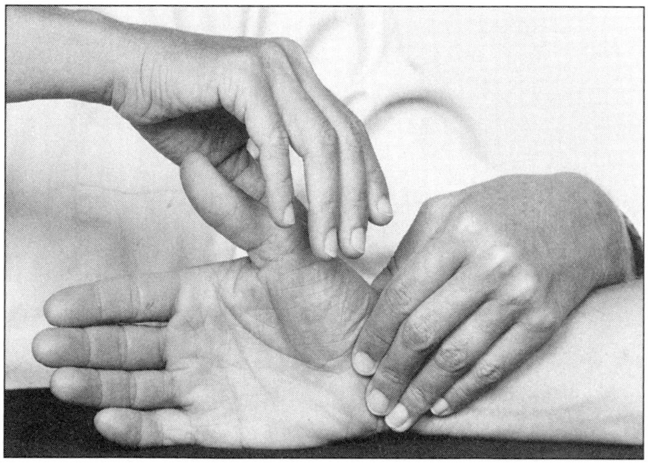

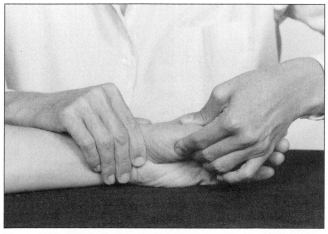

Figure 5-49 Start position: thumb CM flexion and extension. The therapist stabilizes the trapezium between the left thumb and index finger.

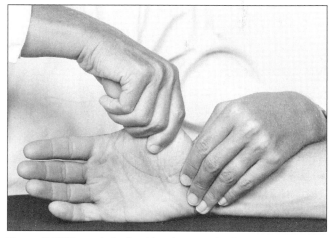

Figure 5-50 Therapist's distal hand grasps the first metacarpal.

Figure 5-51 Soft or firm end feel at the limit of thumb CM flexion.

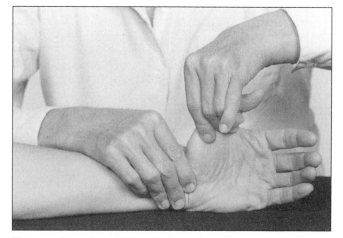

Figure 5-52 Firm end feel at the limit of thumb CM extension.

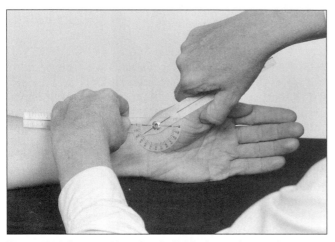

Figure 5-53 Start position: thumb CM flexion and extension.

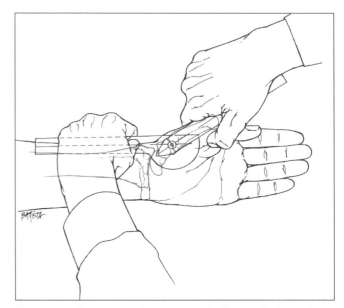

Figure 5-54 Goniometer alignment thumb CM joint flexion and extension.

Measurement: Universal Goniometer

Start Position. The patient is sitting. The elbow is flexed with the forearm in midposition and resting on a table. The wrist is in slight ulnar deviation, the fingers assume the anatomical position, and the thumb maintains contact with the metacarpal and proximal phalanx of the index finger (Fig. 5-53).

Stabilization. The therapist stabilizes the trapezium, wrist, and forearm.

Goniometer Axis. The axis is placed over the CM joint (Fig. 5-54).

Stationary Arm. Parallel to the longitudinal axis of the radius.

Movable Arm. Parallel to the longitudinal axis of the thumb metacarpal. *Note:* Although the goniometer arms are not aligned at 0° in this start position, this position is recorded as the 0° start position. The number of degrees the metacarpal is moved away from this 0° start position is recorded as the ROM for the movement. For example, if the goniometer read 30° at the start position for CM joint flexion/extension (see Fig. 5-53) and 15° at the end position for CM joint flexion (see Fig. 5-55), the CM joint flexion ROM would be 15°.

End Positions. Flexion (Fig. 5-55): the thumb is flexed across the palm to the limit of motion (15°). Extension (Fig. 5-56): the thumb is extended away from the palm to the limit of motion (20°).

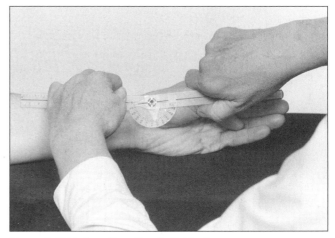

Figure 5-55 End position: thumb CM flexion.

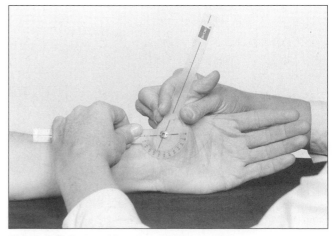

Figure 5-56 End position: thumb CM extension.

Thumb MCP and IP Flexion-Extension

PROM Assessment

Start Position. The patient is sitting. The elbow is flexed and the forearm is resting on a table in midposition. The wrist is in the neutral position and the fingers are relaxed. The MCP and IP joints of the thumb are in extension (0°).

Stabilization. First MCP joint: the therapist stabilizes the first metacarpal. IP joint: the therapist stabilizes the proximal phalanx.

Therapist's Distal Hand Placement. First MCP joint: the therapist grasps the proximal phalanx. IP joint: the therapist grasps the distal phalansx.

End Positions. The therapist applies slight traction to and moves the proximal phalanx across the palm to the limit of motion to assess thumb MCP flexion (Fig. 5-57), and to the limit of motion in a radial direction for thumb MCP extension (Fig. 5-58). The therapist applies slight traction to and moves the distal phalanx in an anterior (Fig. 5-59) or a posterior (Fig. 5-60) direction to the limit of motion for thumb IP flexion or extension, respectively.

End Feels. *Thumb MCP flexion*—hard or firm; thumb IP flexion—hard or firm; thumb MCP and IP extension—firm.

Joint Glides. *Thumb MCP flexion*—the concave base of the proximal phalanx moves in an anterior direction on the fixed convex head of the first metacarpal. *Thumb IP joint flexion*—the concave base of the distal phalanx glides in an anterior direction on the fixed convex head of the proximal phalanx. *Thumb MCP extension*—the concave base of the proximal phalanx moves in a posterior direction on the fixed convex head of the first metacarpal. *Thumb IP joint extension*—the concave base of the distal phalanx glides in a posterior direction on the fixed convex head of the proximal phalanx.

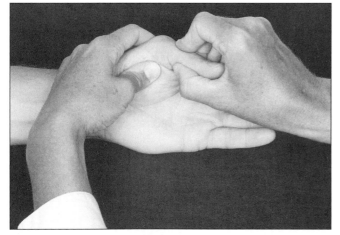

Figure 5-57 Hard or firm end feel at the limit of thumb MCP flexion.

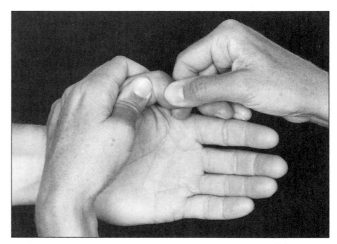

Figure 5-59 Hard or firm end feel at the limit of thumb IP flexion.

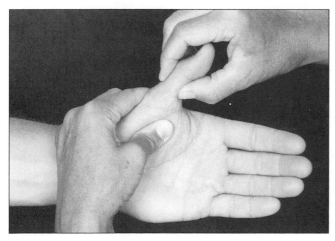

Figure 5-58 Firm end feel at the limit of thumb MCP extension.

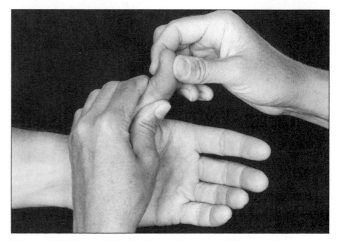

Figure 5-60 Firm end feel at the limit of thumb IP extension.

Measurement: Universal Goniometer

Start Position. The patient is sitting. The elbow is flexed and the forearm is resting on a table in midposition. The wrist and fingers are in the anatomical position. The MCP and IP joints are in extension (0°).

Stabilization. MCP joint: the therapist stabilizes the first metacarpal. IP joint: the therapist stabilizes the proximal phalanx.

Goniometer Axis. The axis is placed over the posterior or lateral aspect of the MCP joint (Fig. 5-61) or IP joint (Fig. 5-62) of the thumb.

Stationary Arm. MCP joint: parallel to the longitudinal axis of the shaft of the thumb metacarpal. IP joint: parallel to the longitudinal axis of the proximal phalanx.

Movable Arm. MCP joint: parallel to the longitudinal axis of the proximal phalanx. IP joint: parallel to the longitudinal axis of the distal phalanx.

End Positions. The MCP joint is flexed so that the thumb moves across the palm to the limit of MCP flexion (50°) (Fig. 5-63). The IP joint is flexed to the limit of motion (80°) (Fig. 5-64). The goniometer is positioned on the lateral or anterior surface of the thumb to assess MCP and IP joint extension. The MCP joint is extended to the limit of extension (0°).

Hyperextension. Hyperextension of the IP joint of the thumb (see Fig. 5-60) occurs beyond 0° of extension. The IP joint can actively be hyperextended to 10° and passively to 30° (1).

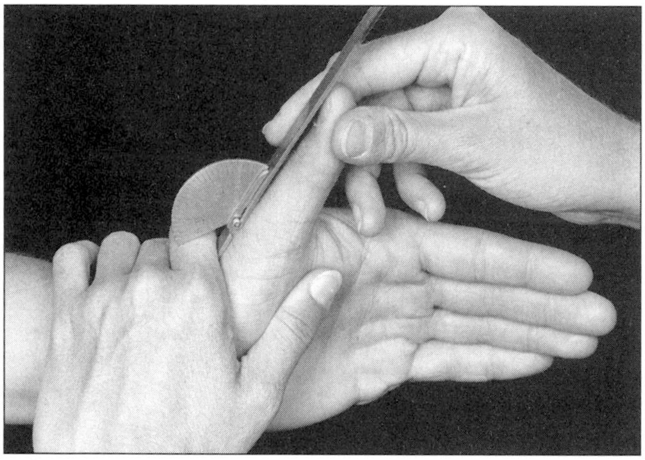

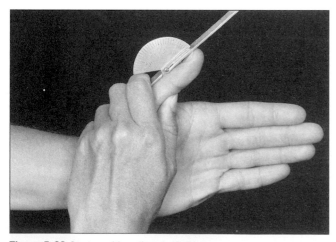

Figure 5-61 Start position: thumb MCP flexion.

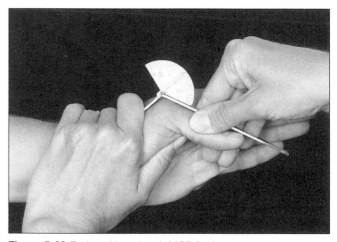

Figure 5-63 End position: thumb MCP flexion.

Figure 5-62 Start position: thumb IP flexion.

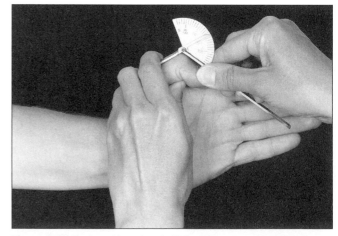

Figure 5-64 End position: thumb IP flexion.

Thumb CM Abduction

PROM Assessment (not shown)

Start Position. The patient is sitting. The forearm is in midposition resting on a table, the wrist is in neutral position, and the fingers and thumb are relaxed.

Stabilization. The therapist stabilizes the second metacarpal.

Therapist's Distal Hand Placement. The therapist grasps the first metacarpal.

End Position. The therapist applies slight traction to and moves the first metacarpal away from the second metacarpal in an anterior direction perpendicular to the plane of the palm to the limit of motion to assess CM joint abduction.

End Feel. CM joint abduction—firm.

Joint Glide (11). *CM joint abduction*—the convex surface of the base of the first metacarpal glides in a posterior direction (i.e., in the opposite direction as the shaft of the first metacarpal) on the fixed concave surface of the trapezium.

Measurement: Universal Goniometer

Start Position. The patient is sitting. The elbow is flexed and the forearm is resting on a table in midposition. The wrist and fingers are in the anatomical position. The thumb maintains contact with the metacarpal and proximal phalanx of the index finger (Fig. 5-65).

Stabilization. The therapist stabilizes the second metacarpal.

Goniometer Axis. The axis is placed at the junction of the bases of the first and second metacarpals (Fig. 5-66).

Stationary Arm. Parallel to the longitudinal axis of the second metacarpal.

Movable Arm. Parallel to the longitudinal axis of the first metacarpal. In the start position described, the goniometer will indicate 15° to 20°. This is recorded as 0° (12). For example, if the goniometer read 15° at the start position for CM joint abduction (see Fig. 5-65) and 60° at the end position for CM joint abduction (Fig. 5-67), the first CM joint abduction ROM would be 45°.

End Position. The thumb is abducted to the limit of motion (70°) so that the thumb column moves in the plane perpendicular to the palm (see Fig. 5-67).

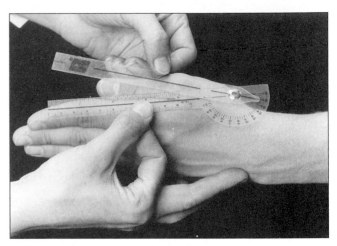

Figure 5-65 Start position: thumb abduction.

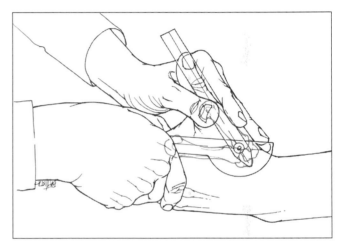

Figure 5-66 Goniometer alignment for end position thumb CM joint abduction.

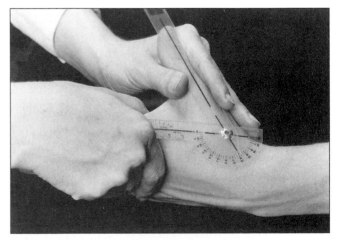

Figure 5-67 End position: thumb abduction.

Measurement: Ruler

As an alternate measurement to goniometry, thumb abduction may be measured by using a ruler or tape measure. With the thumb in the abducted position, a ruler measurement is taken from the lateral aspect of the midpoint of the MCP joint of the index finger to the posterior aspect of the midpoint of the MCP joint of the thumb (Fig. 5-68).

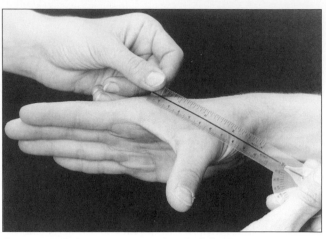

Figure 5-68 Ruler measurement: thumb abduction.

Thumb Opposition

Measurement: Ruler

On completion of full range of opposition between the thumb and fifth finger (Fig. 5-69), it is normally possible to place the pads of the thumb and fifth finger in the same plane (15). An evaluation of a deficit in opposition (Fig. 5-70) can be obtained by taking a linear measurement between the center of the tip of the thumb pad and the center of the tip of the fifth finger pad.

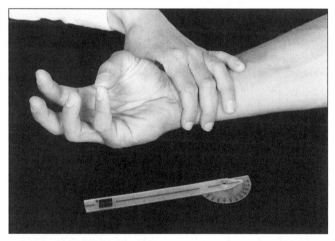

Figure 5-69 Full opposition ROM.

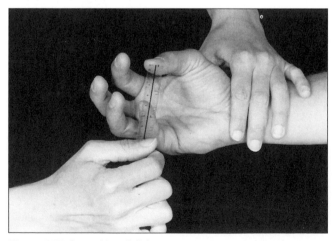

Figure 5-70 Opposition deficit.

MUSCLE LENGTH ASSESSMENT AND MEASUREMENT

Flexor Digitorum Superficialis, Flexor Digitorum Profundus, Flexor Digiti Minimi, and Palmaris Longus

Start Position. The patient is in supine or sitting with the elbow in extension, the forearm supinated, wrist in neutral position, and the fingers extended (Fig. 5-71).

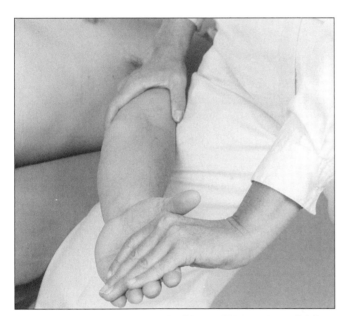

Figure 5-71 Start position: length of flexor digitorum superficialis, flexor digitorum profundus, and flexor digiti minimi.

Origin (2)	Insertion (2)
Flexor Digitorum Superficialis	
a. Humeroulnar head: common flexor origin on the medial epicondyle of the humerus, the anterior band of the ulnar collateral ligament, and the medial aspect to the coronoid process. b. Radial head: anterior border of the radius from the radial tuberosity to the insertion of pronator teres.	Anterior surface of the middle phalanges of the index, middle, ring, and little fingers.
Flexor Digitorum Profundus	
Upper three fourths of the anterior and medial aspects of the ulna; medial aspect of the coronoid process; by an aponeurosis on the upper three fourths of the posterior border of the ulna; anterior surface of the medial half of the interosseous membrane.	Palmar aspect of the bases of the distal phalanges of the index, middle, ring, and little fingers.
Flexor Digiti Minimi	
Hook of hamate; flexor retinaculum.	Ulnar aspect of the base of the proximal phalanx of the little finger.
Palmaris Longus (vestigial)	
Common flexor origin on the medial epicondyle of the humerus.	Palmar aspect of the flexor retinaculum; the palmar aponeurosis.

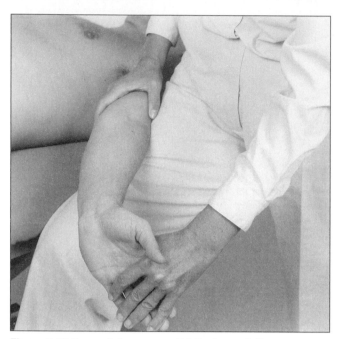

Figure 5-72 Flexor digitorum superficialis, flexor digitorum profundus, and flexor digiti minimi on stretch.

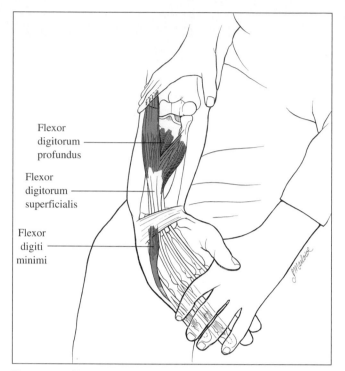

Flexor
digitorum
profundus

Flexor
digitorum
superficialis

Flexor
digiti
minimi

Figure 5-73 Flexor digitorum superficialis, flexor digitorum profundus, and flexor digiti minimi on stretch.

Stabilization. The therapist manually stabilizes the humerus. The radius and ulna are stabilized against the therapist's thigh.

End Position. The therapist maintains the fingers in extension and applies slight traction to and extends the wrist to the limit of motion so that the long finger flexors are put on full stretch (Figs. 5-72 and 5-73).

Assessment and Measurement. If the finger flexors are shortened, wrist extension ROM will be restricted proportional to the decrease in muscle length. The therapist either observes the available PROM or uses a goniometer to measure and record the available wrist extension PROM.

End Feel. Finger flexors on stretch—firm.

Extensor Digitorum Communis, Extensor Indicis Proprius, and Extensor Digiti MInimi

Origin (2)	Insertion (2)
Extensor Digitorum Communis	
Common extensor origin on the lateral epicondyle of the humerus.	Posterior surfaces of the bases of the distal and middle phalanges of the index, middle, ring, and little fingers.
Extensor Indicis Proprius	
Posterior surface of the ulna distal to the origin of extensor pollicis longus; posterior aspect of the interosseous membrane.	Ulnar side of the extensor digitorum tendon to the index finger at the level of the second metacarpal head.
Extensor Digiti Minimi	
Common extensor origin on the lateral epicondyle of the humerus.	Dorsal digital expansion of the fifth digit.

Start Position. The patient is in supine or sitting. The elbow is extended, the forearm is pronated, the wrist is in the neutral position, and the fingers are flexed (Fig. 5-74).

Stabilization. The therapist stabilizes the radius and ulna.

End Position. The therapist applies slight traction to and flexes the wrist to the limit of motion so that the long finger extensors are fully stretched (Figs. 5-75 and 5-76).

Assessment and Measurement. If the finger extensors are shortened, wrist flexion PROM will be restricted proportional to the degree of muscle shortening. The therapist either observes the available PROM or uses a goniometer to measure and record the available wrist flexion PROM.

End Feel. Long finger extensors on stretch—firm.

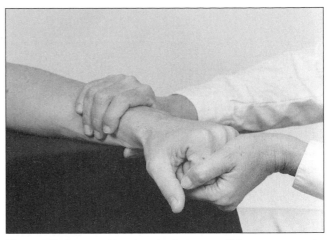

Figure 5-74 Start position: length of extensor digitorum communis, extensor indicis proprius, and extensor digiti minimi.

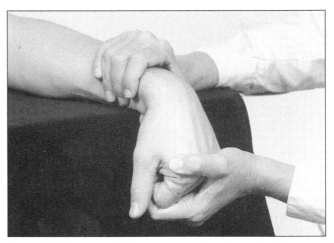

Figure 5-75 Extensor digitorum communis, extensor indicis proprius, and extensor digiti minimi on stretch.

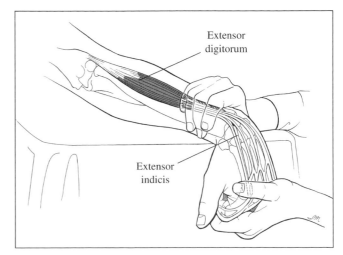

Extensor digitorum

Extensor indicis

Figure 5-76 Long finger extensors on stretch.

Lumbricales

Origin (2)	Insertion (2)
Lumbricales	
Tendons of flexor digitorum profundus: a. First and second lumbricales: radial sides and palmar surfaces of the tendons of the index and middle fingers. b. Third: adjacent sides of the tendons of the middle and ring fingers. c. Fourth: adjacent sides of the tendons of the ring and little fingers.	Radial aspect of the dorsal digital expansion of the corresponding index, middle, ring, and little fingers.

Start Position. The patient is in sitting or supine with the elbow flexed, forearm in midposition or supination, and the wrist in extension. The IP joints of the fingers are flexed (Fig. 5-77).

Stabilization. The therapist stabilizes the metacarpals.

End Position. The therapist simultaneously applies overpressure to flex the IP joints and extend the MCP joints of the fingers to the limit of motion so that lumbricales are put on full stretch (Figs. 5-78 and 5-79). The lumbricales may be stretched as a group or individually.

Assessment and Measurement. If the lumbricales are shortened, MCP joint extension ROM will be restricted proportional to the degree of muscle shortness. The therapist either observes the available PROM or uses a goniometer to measure and record the available MCP joint extension PROM.

End Feel. Lumbricales on stretch—firm.

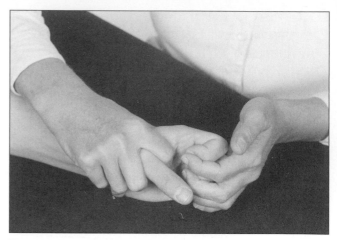

Figure 5-77 Start position: length of lumbricales.

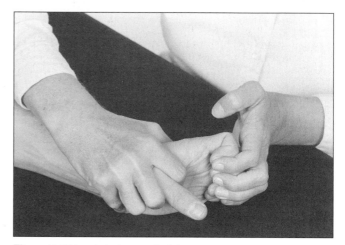

Figure 5-78 Lumbricales on stretch.

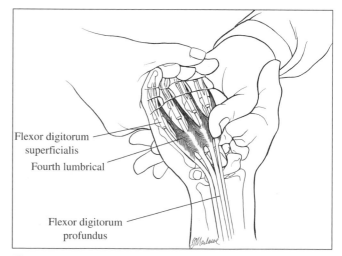

Flexor digitorum superficialis

Fourth lumbrical

Flexor digitorum profundus

Figure 5-79 Wrist extension, MCP joint extension, and IP joint flexion to place lumbricales on stretch.

FUNCTIONAL APPLICATION

Joint Function: Wrist

The wrist optimizes the function of the hand to touch, grasp, or manipulate objects. Wrist motion positions the hand in space relative to the forearm and serves to transmit load between the hand and forearm (16). Because of wrist motion and static positioning, the wrist serves to control the length–tension relations of the extrinsic muscles of the hand.

Functional Range of Motion: Wrist

Wrist extension and ulnar deviation are the most important positions or movements (17) for activities of daily living (ADL). In most daily activities, the wrist usually assumes a position of extension for the purposes of stabilization of the hand and flexion of the distal joints (Fig. 5-80). However, in the performance of perineal hygiene activities and dressing activities at the back (Fig. 5-81), the wrist assumes a flexed posture. Two approaches have been used to determine the wrist ROM required to successfully perform ADL.

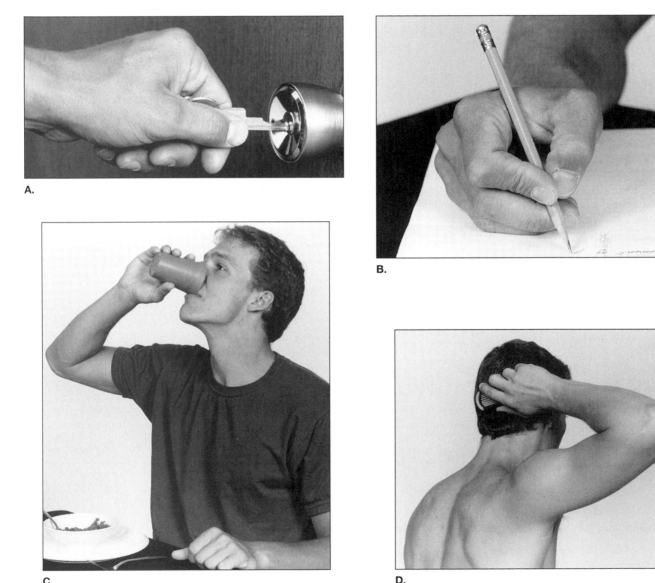

A.

B.

C.

D.

Figure 5-80 In most ADL the wrist assumes a position of extension: **A.** unlocking a door with a key, **B.** writing, **C.** drinking from a cup, and **D.** brushing one's hair.

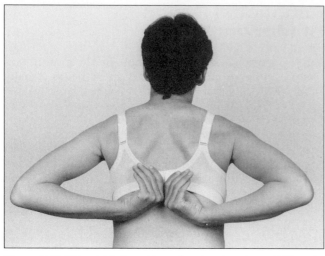

Figure 5-81 The wrist is flexed in performing dressing activities at the back.

In one approach, the wrist ROM was assessed as normal subjects performed ADL. Brumfield and Champoux (18) evaluated 15 ADL and found the normal functional range of wrist motion for most activities was between 10° flexion and 35° extension. Palmer and coworkers (19), evaluating 52 standardized tasks, found comparable required ranges of 5° flexion and 30° extension. Normal functional range for radial deviation was 10° and ulnar deviation 15° (19).

Higher values (54° flexion, 60° extension, 40° ulnar deviation, and 17° radial deviation) for the maximum wrist motion required for ADL were reported by Ryu and colleagues (17) in evaluating 31 activities. The authors suggested differing methods of data analysis and the design and application of the goniometer as possible reasons for these values being higher compared to other studies.

More specific ROM requirements for feeding activities (i.e., drinking from a cup or glass, eating using a fork or spoon, and cutting using a knife) are from approximately 3° wrist flexion to 35° wrist extension (18,20) and from 20° ulnar deviation to 5° radial deviation (20).

Using another approach, wrist ROM was artificially restricted and the ability to complete ADL was assessed. Nelson (21) evaluated the ability to perform 125 ADL (activities of work or recreation were not included) with the wrist splinted to allow for only 5° flexion, 6° extension, 7° radial deviation, and 6° ulnar deviation. With the wrist splinted in this manner, 123 ADL could be completed. Therefore, marked loss of wrist ROM may not significantly hinder a patient's ability to carry out ADL.

Joint Function: Hand

The hand has multiple functions associated with ADL. The primary functions are to grasp, communicate, manipulate objects, and receive sensory information from the environment.

Functional Range of Motion: Hand

Hume and coworkers (22) reported the IP and MCP joint ROM needed to perform many ADL. No significant differences in the functional positions of the individual fingers were found; therefore, the finger positions were reported as one. The ROM at the MCP joints of the fingers and thumb were 33° to 73° flexion and 10° to 32° flexion, respectively. The PIP and DIP joint ROM of the fingers was 36° to 86° flexion and 20° to 61° flexion, respectively. The ROM of the IP joint of the thumb was 2° to 43° flexion.

Full opening of the hand is not required for grasping tasks in daily self-care activities but may be required for grasp in leisure or occupational tasks. When grasping an object, the shape, size, and weight of the object influence the degree of finger flexion, the area of palmar contact, and thumb position (Fig. 5-82). The thumb may or may not be included in the grip (10) (see Fig. 5-82A and B). When grasping different-sized cylinders, the DIP joint angle remains constant and the fingers adjust to the new cylinder size through changes in the joint angles at the MCP and PIP joints (23).

Arches of the Hand

The arches of the hand are described in Table 5-4. The arches are observed with the forearm supinated and the

TABLE 5-4   Arches of the Hand

Arch	Location	Keystone	Mobility
Carpal arch	Distal row of carpal bones	Capitate	Fixed
	Proximal row of carpal bones	–	Mobile
Metacarpal arch	Level of metacarpal heads	Third metacarpal head	Mobile
Longitudinal arches	Carpals and each of the five rays*	MCP joints	Mobile; fixed (index and middle metacarpal)

*Ray: the metacarpal and phalanges of one finger or the thumb.
Adapted from Tubiana R, Thomine JM, Macklin E. *Examination of the Hand and Wrist*. 2nd ed. St. Louis: Mosby; 1996.

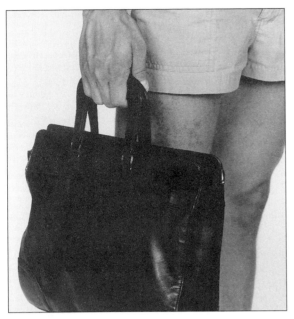

A.

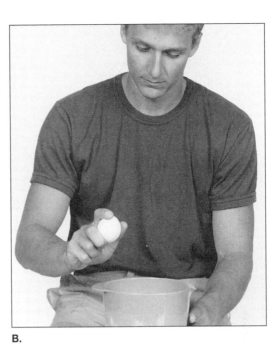

B.

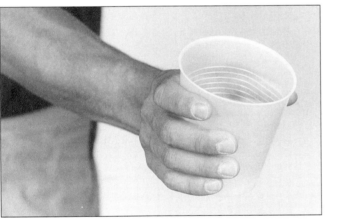

C.

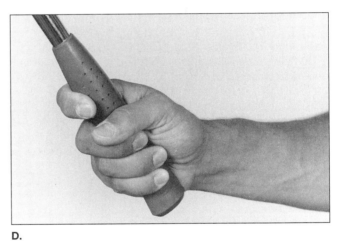

D.

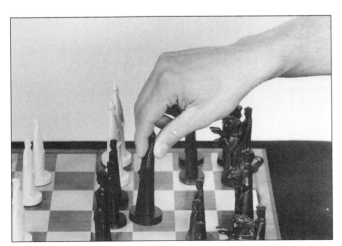

E.

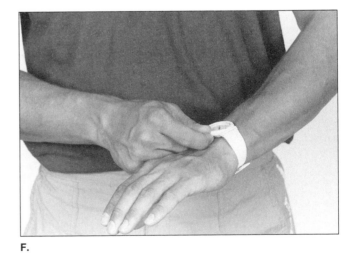

F.

Figure 5-82 When grasping an object, the shape, size, and/or weight of the object influence the degree of finger flexion, the area of palmar contact, and thumb position, as observed when **A.** carrying a briefcase, **B.** cracking an egg, **C.** holding a large cup, **D.** gripping the handle of a hammer, **E.** moving a chess piece, and **F.** winding a watch.

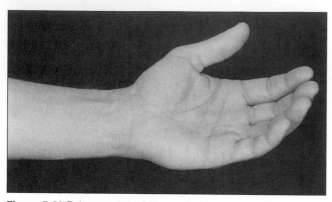

Figure 5-83 Palmar arches. Observe the transverse palmar concavities at the levels of the distal row of carpal bones and the metacarpal bones and the longitudinal concavities along the rays of each finger.

hand resting on a table (Fig. 5-83). The carpal arch, a relatively fixed segment, is covered by the flexor retinaculum. In the relaxed position of the hand, a gently cupped concavity is normally observed. When gripping or manipulating objects, the palmar concavity becomes deeper and more gutter-shaped. When the hand is opened fully, the palm flattens. The guttering and flattening of the palm results from the mobility available at the rays of the ring and little fingers and thumb. Each ray consists of the metacarpal and phalanges of a finger or the thumb. These rays flex, rotate, and move toward the center of the palm so the pads of the fingers and thumb are positioned to meet. This motion occurs at the CM joints so that the mobile peripheral rays move around the fixed metacarpals of the index and middle fingers.

References

1. Kapandji IA. *The Physiology of the Joints.* Vol 1. 5th ed. New York: Churchill Livingstone; 1982.
2. Standring S, ed. *Gray's Anatomy: The Anatomical Basis of Clinical Practice.* London: Elsevier Churchill Livingstone; 2005.
3. Norkin CC, White DJ. *Measurement of Joint Motion: A Guide to Goniometry.* 3rd ed. Philadelphia: FA Davis; 2003.
4. Daniels L, Worthingham C. *Muscle Testing: Techniques of Manual Examination.* 5th ed. Philadelphia: WB Saunders; 1986.
5. Magee DJ. *Orthopaedic Physical Assessment.* 4th ed. Philadelphia: WB Saunders; 2002.
6. American Academy of Orthopaedic Surgeons. *Joint Motion: Method of Measuring and Recording.* Chicago: AAOS; 1965.
7. Berryman Reese N, Bandy WD. *Joint Range of Motion and Muscle Length Testing.* Philadelphia: WB Saunders; 2002.
8. Cyriax J. *Textbook of Orthopaedic Medicine, Vol 1. Diagnosis of Soft Tissue Lesions.* 8th ed. London: Bailliere Tindall; 1982.
9. Knutson JS, Kilgore KL, Mansour JM, Crago PE. Intrinsic and extrinsic contributions to the passive movement at the metacarpophalangeal joint. *J Biomech.* 2000; 33:1675–1681.
10. Levangie PK, Norkin CC. *Joint Structure and Function: A Comprehensive Analysis.* 3rd ed. Philadelphia: FA Davis; 2001.
11. Neumann DA. *Kinesiology of the Musculoskeletal System: Foundations for Physical Rehabilitation.* Philadelphia: Mosby; 2002
12. Scott AD, Trombly CA. Evaluation. In: Trombly CA. *Occupational Therapy for Physical Dysfunction.* 2nd ed. Baltimore: Williams & Wilkins; 1983.
13. Swanson AB, Goran-Hagert C, DeGroot Swanson G. Evaluation of impairment of hand function. In: Hunter JM, Schneider LH, Mackin EJ, Bell JA. *Rehabilitation of the Hand.* St. Louis: CV Mosby; 1978.
14. Stegink Jansen CW, Patterson R, Viegas SF. Effects of fingernail length on finger and hand performance. *J Hand Therapy.* 2000;13:211–217.
15. Tubiana R, Thomine JM, Macklin E. *Examination of the Hand and Wrist.* 2nd ed. St. Louis: Mosby; 1996.
16. Nordin M, Frankel VH. *Basic Biomechanics of the Musculoskeletal System.* 3rd ed. Philadelphia: Lippincott Williams & Wilkins; 2001.
17. Ryu J, Cooney WP, Askew LJ, et al. Functional ranges of motion of the wrist joint. *J Hand Surg [Am].* 1991;16:409–419.
18. Brumfield RH, Champoux JA. A biomechanical study of normal functional wrist motion. *Clin Orthop.* 1984;187:23–25.
19. Palmer AK, Werner FW, Murphy DM, Glisson R. Functional wrist motion: a biomechanical study. *J Hand Surg [Am].* 1985;10:39–46.
20. Safaee-Rad R, Shwedyk E, Quanbury AO, Cooper JE. Normal functional range of motion of upper limb joints during performance of three feeding activities. *Arch Phys Med Rehabil.* 1990;71:505–509.
21. Nelson DL. Functional wrist motion. *Hand Clin.* 1997;13: 83–92.
22. Hume MC, Gellman H, McKellop H, Brumfield RH. Functional range of motion of the joints of the hand. *J Hand Surg [Am].* 1990;15:240–243.
23. Lee JW, Rim K. Measurement of finger joint angles and maximum finger forces during cylinder grip activity. *J Biomed Eng.* 1991;13:152–162.

EXERCISES AND QUESTIONS

See the Answer Guide in Appendix F for suggested answers to the following exercises and questions.

1. PALPATION

On a skeleton, and next on a partner, palpate the following anatomical structures and then identify the ranges of motion of the wrist and hand that can be measured using the structure to align the universal goniometer.

  i.   Styloid process of the ulna. _____

  ii. Distal palmar crease. _____

  iii. Third metacarpal bone. _____

  iv. First carpometacarpal joint. _____

  v.   Capitate bone. _____

  vi. Lateral aspect of the PIP joint line. _____

2. ASSESSMENT PROCESS

Are the following statements true or false?

  i.   AROM is normally assessed prior to assessing PROM at a joint.

  ii. End feels are determined when assessing AROM at a joint.

  iii. It is important to note the presence or absence of pain when assessing AROM and PROM at a joint.

  iv. A goniometer can be used only to measure PROM when assessing a joint.

3. ASSESSMENT OF AROM AT THE WRIST AND HAND ARTICULATIONS

A. Demonstrate the two movement patterns a therapist would have a patient perform when conducting a general scan of the active movements available at the wrist and hand. Identify the ROM the therapist would observe when performing the scan.

B. Identify and describe the shape of the articular components that make up the:

  i.   Wrist

  ii. CM joint of the thumb

  iii. MCP and IP joints of the thumb and fingers

C. Demonstrate, define, and describe* the following movements:

  i.   Wrist extension

  ii. Thumb abduction

  iii. Thumb extension at the CM joint

  iv. Finger abduction

  v.   Finger flexion at the PIP joint

  *Identify the axis/plane of movement.

D. When assessing wrist ulnar deviation, what substitute movements may give the appearance of greater ulnar deviation ROM than is actually present?

4. ASSESSMENT AND MEASUREMENT OF PROM AT THE WRIST AND HAND

For each of the movements listed below, demonstrate the assessment and measurement of PROM on a partner and answer the questions that follow. Have a third partner evaluate your performance using the appropriate practical test form in Appendix E. Record your findings on the PROM Recording Form on pages 137 and 138.

Wrist Ulnar Deviation

i.   What normal end feel(s) would be expected when assessing wrist ulnar deviation?

ii. List the normal limiting factor(s) that create the normal end feel(s) for wrist ulnar deviation.

iii. Assess the end feel for wrist ulnar deviation on your partner. Is the end feel normal?

iv. Identify the anatomical structure the axis of the goniometer is aligned with when measuring wrist ulnar deviation ROM.

v.   When measuring wrist ulnar deviation, the movable arm of the goniometer is aligned with the longitudinal axis of the third finger. True or false? Explain.

Wrist Extension

Assume a patient presents with decreased wrist extension PROM.

i.   What glide of the proximal row of carpal bones could be limited at the radiocarpal joint?

ii. Explain the reason for the glide being decreased in the direction indicated in i.

iii. The goniometer alignment for wrist extension is also used to assess wrist _____ ROM and muscle length for the _____ and the _____.

iv. What position should the fingers be in when assessing wrist extension PROM? Why?

MCP Joint Extension of the Fingers and Thumb

i.   A therapist assesses MCP joint extension PROM and notes decreased PROM and a firm end feel. Would the firm end feel be considered a normal end feel? Justify your answer.

ii. A patient has decreased passive thumb MCP joint extension ROM. What glide of the base of the proximal phalanx of the thumb would be decreased in this case? Explain the reason for the glide being decreased in the direction indicated.

iii. Identify the pattern of movement restriction at the MCP joints in the presence of a capsular pattern.

iv. When measuring PROM for finger MCP joint extension, why is the wrist positioned in slight flexion during the procedure?

Finger MCP Joint Abduction

i.   What normal end feel(s) would be expected when assessing MCP joint abduction?

ii. List the normal limiting factor(s) that create the normal end feel(s) for MCP joint abduction.

Thumb CM Joint ROM

i.   Identify the movements that occur at this joint that can be measured using a universal goniometer.

ii. When assessing the PROM at the CM joint of the thumb, identify the segment(s) proximal to the joint that must be stabilized to ensure movement is localized at the CM joint.

Ring Finger PIP Joint Flexion

i.   What normal end feel(s) would be expected when assessing ring finger PIP joint flexion?

ii. List the normal limiting factor(s) that create the normal end feel(s) for ring finger PIP joint flexion.

Thumb Opposition

If your partner has full opposition ROM, have your partner simulate a deficit in opposition so that you can demonstrate the measurement of thumb opposition.

i.   Opposition is a sequential movement that incorporates _____, _____, and _____ of the first metacarpal, with simultaneous _____.

ii. If mobility at the _____ joint is restricted, the motion of the first metacarpal and therefore thumb opposition would not be possible.

PROM RECORDING FORM

Patient's Name _____   Therapist _____

	Left Side			Date of Measurement		Right Side		
	*		*		*		*	
				Wrist				
				Flexion (0–80°)				
				Extension (0–70°)				
				Ulnar deviation (0–30°)				
				Radial deviation (0–20°)				
				Hypermobility:				
				Comments:				
				Thumb				
				CM flexion (0–15°)				
				CM extension (0–20°)				
				abduction (0–70°)				
				MCP flexion (0–50°)				
				IP flexion (0–80°)				
				Opposition				
				Hypermobility:				
				Comments:				
				Fingers				
				MCP digit 2 flexion (0–90°)				
				extension (0–45°)				
				abduction				
				adduction				
				MCP digit 3 flexion (0–90°)				
				extension (0–45°)				
				abduction (radial)				
				adduction (ulnar)				
				MCP digit 4 flexion (0–90°)				
				extension (0–45°)				

PROM RECORDING FORM

Patient's Name _____   Therapist _____

Left Side					Right Side			
*		*	**Date of Measurement**		*		*	
			Fingers (con't)					
			abduction					
			adduction					
			MCP digit 5 flexion (0–90°)					
			extension (0–45°)					
			abduction					
			adduction					
			PIP digit 2 flexion (0–100°)					
			3 flexion (0–100°)					
			4 flexion (0–100°)					
			5 flexion (0–100°)					
			DIP digit 2 flexion (0–90°)					
			3 flexion (0–90°)					
			4 flexion (0–90°)					
			5 flexion (0–90°)					
			Composite finger abduction/thumb extension—Distance between:					
			Thumb—digit 2					
			Digit 2—digit 3					
			Digit 3—digit 4					
			Digit 4—digit 5					
			Composite flexion—Distance between:					
			Finger pulp—distal palmar crease					
			Finger pulp—proximal palmar crease					
			Hypermobility:					
			Comments:					

5. MUSCLE LENGTH ASSESSMENT AND MEASUREMENT

For the muscles listed below, demonstrate the assessment and measurement of muscle length on a partner and answer the questions. Have a third partner evaluate your performance using the appropriate practical test form in Appendix E.

Flexor Digitorum Superficialis, Flexor Digitorum Profundus, Flexor Digiti Minimi, and Palmaris Longus
   i. What position is the elbow in to assess the muscle length of the flexor muscles listed above? Why is the elbow held in this position?
   ii. If the length of the finger flexors is decreased, with the elbow extended, the forearm supinated, and the fingers _____, wrist _____ PROM will be restricted proportional to the decrease in muscle length. To assess this PROM restriction using a universal goniometer, the goniometer axis is placed at the _____, the stationary arm is aligned parallel to the _____, and the movable arm is aligned parallel to the _____. The therapist will note a _____ end feel at the end of the restricted wrist PROM.

Lumbricales
   i. Explain why the wrist would be positioned in extension to assess the length of the lumbricales.
   ii. If the length of the lumbricales is decreased, with the wrist in extension and the fingers _____, MCP joint _____ PROM will be restricted proportional to the degree of muscle shortness.

Extensor Digitorum Communis, Extensor Indicis Proprius, and Extensor Digiti Minimi
   i. If the length of the long finger extensors is decreased, with the elbow _____, forearm pronated, and fingers _____, wrist _____ PROM will be restricted proportional to the degree of muscle shortness.

6. FUNCTIONAL ROM AT THE WRIST AND HAND

A. What two wrist positions have been identified as the most important positions or movements for ADL?
B. For feeding activities (i.e., drinking from a cup or glass, eating using a fork or spoon, and cutting using a knife) the ROM requirements are approximately ____° wrist flexion to ____° wrist extension and from ____° ulnar deviation to ____° of radial deviation.
C. What are the primary functions of the wrist?
D. What are the primary functions of the hand?
E. Motion at the _____ joints of the ring finger, little finger, and thumb results in the guttering of the palm for gripping and manipulating objects, and the flattening of the palm. Explain how the ROM of these joints is measured in the clinic.
F. For each of the following wrist and hand movements, identify two ADL that require the specified movement:
   i.   wrist flexion,
   ii. wrist extension,
   iii. wrist radial deviation,
   iv. wrist ulnar deviation,
   v.   finger flexion,
   vi. finger extension,
   vii. thumb opposition.
G. With the wrist splinted to allow for only 5° flexion, 6° extension, 7° radial deviation, and 6° ulnar deviation, Nelson (1) evaluated the ability to perform 125 ADL and found that 123 ADL could be completed. From these findings, what conclusion was made regarding wrist ROM and the ability to carry out ADL?

Reference

1. Nelson DL. Functional wrist motion. *Hand Clin.* 1997; 13:83–92.

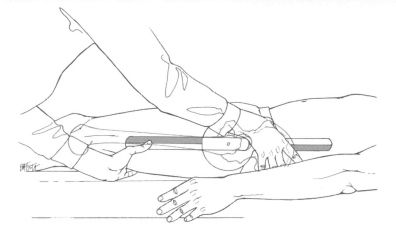

ARTICULATIONS AND MOVEMENTS

The hip joint is a ball-and-socket joint (Fig. 6-1) formed proximally by the cup-shaped, concave surface of the acetabulum and distally by the ball-shaped, convex head of the femur. From the anatomical position, the hip joint may be flexed and extended in the sagittal plane, with movement occurring around a frontal axis, and abducted and adducted in the frontal plane about a sagittal axis (Fig. 6-2). With the hip positioned in 90° of flexion, hip internal and external rotation occurs in the frontal plane about a sagittal axis (Fig. 6-3). Hip rotation can also be performed in the anatomical position, with movement occurring in the transverse plane about a longitudinal (vertical) axis. The movements of the hip joint are described in Table 6-1.

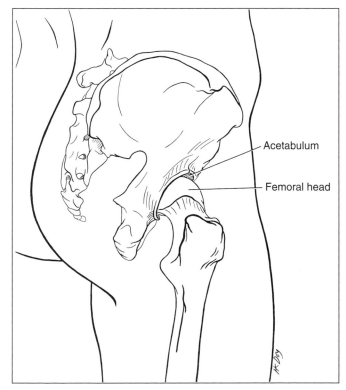

Acetabulum

Femoral head

Figure 6-1 Hip joint: the convex head of the femur articulates with the concave surface of the acetabulum.

TABLE 6-1 Joint Structure: Hip Movements

	Flexion	Extension	Abduction	Adduction	Internal Rotation	External Rotation
Articulation[1,2]	Hip	Hip	Hip	Hip	Hip	Hip
Plane	Sagittal	Sagittal	Frontal	Frontal	Horizontal	Horizontal
Axis	Frontal	Frontal	Sagittal	Sagittal	Longitudinal	Longitudinal
Normal limiting factors[1,3–6]* (See Figs. 6-4 and 6-5)	Soft tissue apposition of the anterior thigh and the abdomen (knee is flexed); tension in the posterior hip joint capsule and gluteus maximus	Tension in the anterior joint capsule, the iliofemoral, ischiofemoral, and pubofemoral ligaments and iliopsoas	Tension in pubofemoral and ischiofemoral ligaments, the inferior band of the iliofemoral ligament, the inferior joint capsule, and hip adductor muscles	Soft tissue appositon of the thighs With the contralateral leg in abduction or flexion: tension in the iliotibial band, the superior joint capsule, superior band of the iliofemoral ligament, the ischiofemoral ligament, and hip abductor muscles	Tension in the ischiofemoral ligament, the posterior joint capsule, and the external rotator muscles	Tension in the iliofemoral and pubofemoral ligaments, the anterior joint capsule, and the medial rotator muscles
Normal end feel[3,7]	Soft/firm	Firm	Firm	Soft/firm	Firm	Firm
Normal AROM[8]† (AROM[9])	0–120° (0–120°)	0–30° (0–20°)	0–45° (0–40° to 45°)	0–30° (0–20° to 25°)	0–45° (0–25° to 30°)	0–45° (0–35° to 40°)
Capsular pattern[7,10]	The order of restriction may vary: flexion, abduction, and internal rotation					

*Note: There is a paucity of definitive research that identifies the normal limiting factors (NLF) of joint range of motion. The NLF and end feels listed here are based on a knowledge of anatomy, clinical experience, and available references.
†AROM, active range of motion

Note: Normal hip extension range of motion (ROM) varies between sources, ranging from 10° to 30°.[4,8,9,11–13]

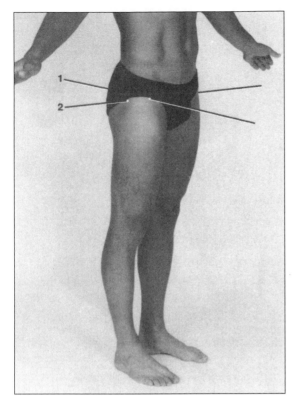

Figure 6-2 Hip joint axes: (1) abduction-adduction and (2) flexion-extension.

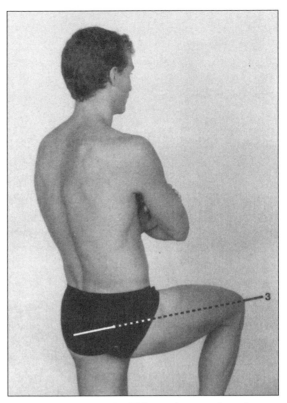

Figure 6-3 Hip joint axis: (3) internal-external rotation.

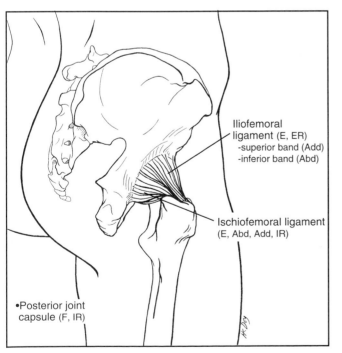

Iliofemoral ligament (E, ER)
-superior band (Add)
-inferior band (Abd)

Ischiofemoral ligament (E, Abd, Add, IR)

•Posterior joint capsule (F, IR)

Figure 6-4 Posterolateral view of the hip joint showing noncontractile structures that normally limit motion.*

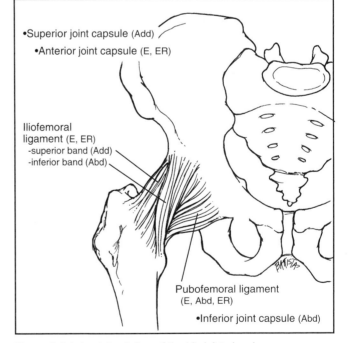

•Superior joint capsule (Add)

•Anterior joint capsule (E, ER)

Iliofemoral ligament (E, ER)
-superior band (Add)
-inferior band (Abd)

Pubofemoral ligament (E, Abd, ER)

•Inferior joint capsule (Abd)

Figure 6-5 Anterolateral view of the hip joint showing noncontractile structures that normally limit motion.*

*Motion limited by structure is identified in brackets, using the following abbreviations: F, flexion; E, extension; Abd, abduction; Add, adduction; ER, external rotation; IR, internal rotation. Muscles normally limiting motion are not illustrated.

SURFACE ANATOMY

(Figs. 6-6 through 6-10)

Structure	Location
1. Iliac crest	A convex bony ridge on the upper border of the ilium; the top of the iliac crest is level with the space between the spinous processes of L4 and L5.
2. Anterior superior iliac spine (ASIS)	Round bony prominence at the anterior end of the iliac crest.
3. Tubercle of the ilium	Approximately 5 cm above and lateral to the ASIS along the lateral lip of the iliac crest.
4. Posterior superior iliac spine (PSIS)	Round bony prominence at the posterior end of the iliac crest, felt subcutaneously at the bottom of the dimples on the proximal aspect of the buttocks; the spines are at the level of the spinous process of S2.
5. Ischial tuberosity	With the hip passively flexed, this bony prominence is lateral to the midline of the body and just proximal to the gluteal fold (the deep transverse groove between the buttock and the posterior aspect of the thigh).
6. Greater trochanter	With the tip of the thumb on the lateral aspect of the iliac crest, the tip of the third digit placed distally on the lateral aspect of the thigh locates the upper border of the greater trochanter.
7. Adductor tubercle	Medial projection at the distal end of the femur at the proximal aspect of the medial epicondyle.
8. Lateral epicondyle of the femur	Small bony prominence on the lateral condyle of the femur.
9. Patella	Large triangular sesamoid bone on the anterior aspect of the knee. The base is proximal and the apex distal.
10. Anterior border of the tibia	Subcutaneous bony ridge along the anterior aspect of the leg.

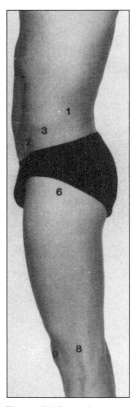

Figure 6-6 Lateral aspect of the trunk and thigh.

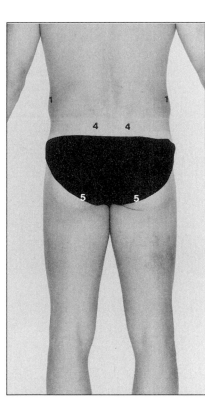

Figure 6-7 Posterior aspect of the trunk and thigh.

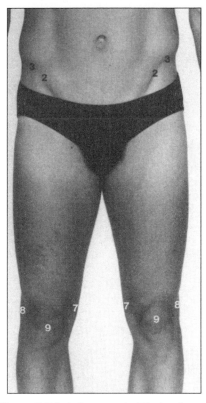

Figure 6-8 Anterior aspect of the trunk and thigh.

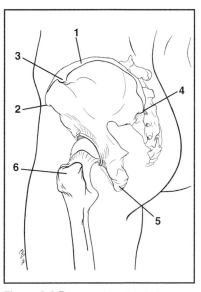

Figure 6-9 Bony anatomy, postero-lateral aspect of the pelvis and thigh.

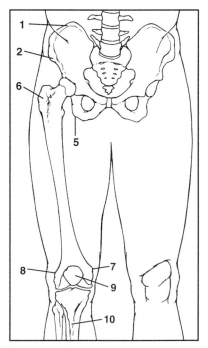

Figure 6-10 Bony anatomy, anterior aspect of the pelvis, thigh, and knee.

RANGE OF MOTION ASSESSMENT AND MEASUREMENT

General Scan: Lower Extremity Active Range of Motion

Active range of motion (AROM) of the lower extremity joints is scanned with the patient either non-weight-bearing or weight-bearing, as follows:

A. Non-weight-bearing. The patient is in the supine position with the legs in the anatomical position. In supine-lying position, the patient extends the toes, dorsiflexes the ankle, and brings the heel toward the contralateral hip (Fig. 6-11). The therapist observes the AROM of hip flexion, abduction, external rotation, knee flexion, ankle dorsiflexion, and toe extension. As the patient attempts to touch the contralateral hip, the level reached by the heel may be used as a guide of AROM of the hip and knee joints.

The patient flexes the toes, plantarflexes the ankle, extends the knee, and adducts, internally rotates, and extends the hip to move the great toe toward the corner on the other side of the plinth (Fig. 6-12). The therapist observes the AROM of hip adduction, internal rotation, knee extension, ankle plantarflexion, and toe flexion.

B. Weight-bearing. The patient squats (Fig. 6-13). The therapist observes bilateral hip flexion, knee flexion, ankle dorsiflexion, and toe extension ROM. Standing, the patient rises onto the toes (Fig. 6-14), while the therapist observes hip extension, knee extension, ankle plantarflexion, and toe extension ROM bilaterally.

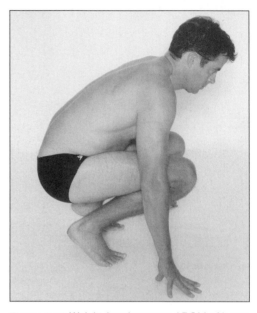

Figure 6-13 Weight-bearing scan: AROM of lower extremity.

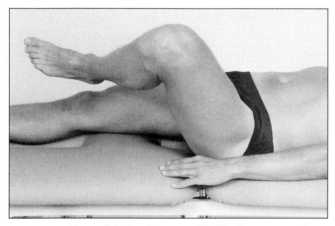

Figure 6-11 Non-weight-bearing scan: AROM of lower extremity.

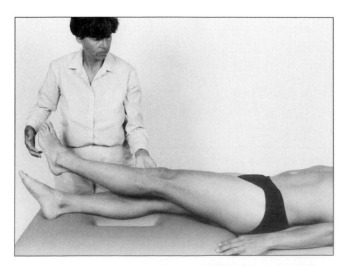

Figure 6-12 Non-weight-bearing scan: AROM of lower extremity.

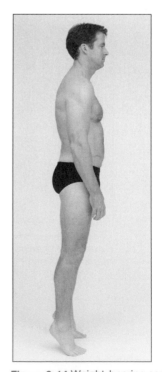

Figure 6-14 Weight-bearing scan: AROM of lower extremity.

Hip Flexion

AROM Assessment

Substitute Movement. Posterior pelvic tilt and flexion of the lumbar spine.

PROM Assessment

Start Position. The patient is supine. The hip and knee on the test side are in the neutral position. The other hip may be flexed or extended (Fig. 6-15). The pelvis is in the neutral position; that is, the ASISs and the symphysis pubis are in the same frontal plane and the right and left ASISs are in the same transverse plane (11,14).

Stabilization. The therapist stabilizes the ipsilateral pelvis at the ASIS and iliac crest to maintain a neutral position. The trunk is stabilized through body positioning.

Therapist's Distal Hand Placement. The therapist raises the lower extremity off the plinth and grasps the posterior aspect of the distal femur.

End Position. While maintaining pelvic stabilization, the therapist applies slight traction to move the femur anteriorly to the limit of hip flexion (Fig. 6-16).

End Feel. Hip flexion—soft or firm.

Joint Spin (15). *Hip flexion*—the convex femoral head spins in the fixed concave acetabulum.

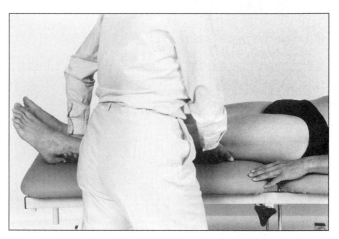

Figure 6-15 Start position: hip flexion.

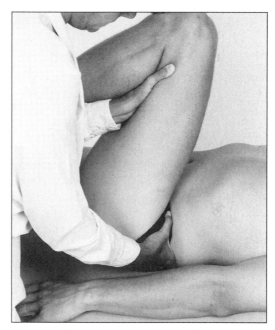

Figure 6-16 Soft or firm end feel at limit of hip flexion.

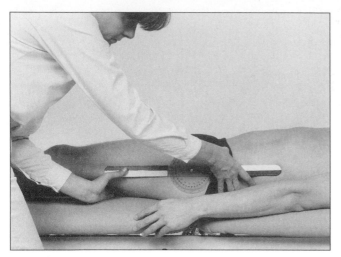

Figure 6-17 Start position: hip flexion.

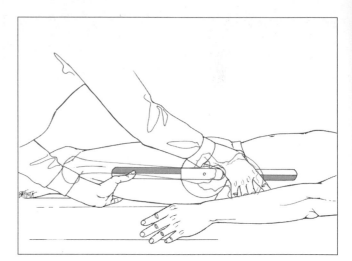

Figure 6-18 Goniometer alignment: hip flexion and extension.

Measurement: Universal Goniometer

Start Position. The patient is supine. The hip and knee on the test side are in the neutral position. The contralateral hip may be flexed or extended (Fig. 6-17). The pelvis is in the neutral position.

Stabilization. The trunk is stabilized through body positioning and the therapist stabilizes the ipsilateral pelvis.

Goniometer Axis. The axis is placed over the greater trochanter of the femur (Fig. 6-18).

Stationary Arm. Parallel to the midaxillary line of the trunk.

Movable Arm. Parallel to the longitudinal axis of the femur, pointing toward the lateral epicondyle.

End Position. The hip is flexed to the limit of motion (120°) while flexing the knee (Fig. 6-19).

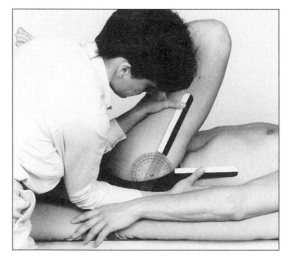

Figure 6-19 End position: hip flexion.

Hip Internal and External Rotation

AROM Assessment

Substitute Movement. Lateral tilting of the pelvis. In sitting, the patient shifts body weight to raise the pelvis and lift the buttocks off the sitting surface.

PROM Assessment

Start Position. The patient is sitting or supine with the hip and knee flexed to 90° (Fig. 6-32).

Stabilization. The pelvis is stabilized through body positioning. The therapist maintains the position of the femur, without restricting movement.

Therapist's Distal Hand Placement. The therapist grasps the distal tibia and fibula.

End Position. The therapist applies slight traction to the distal femur, then moves the tibia and fibula in a lateral direction to the limit of hip internal rotation (Fig. 6-33) and in a medial direction to the limit of hip external rotation (Fig. 6-34).

End Feels. Hip internal rotation—firm; hip external rotation—firm.

Joint Glides. *Hip internal rotation*—the convex femoral head glides on the fixed concave acetabulum in a posterior direction with the hip in anatomical position, and in an inferior direction with the hip in a position of 90° flexion. *Hip external rotation*—the convex femoral head glides on the fixed concave acetabulum in an anterior direction with the hip in anatomical position, and in a superior direction with the hip in a position of 90° flexion.

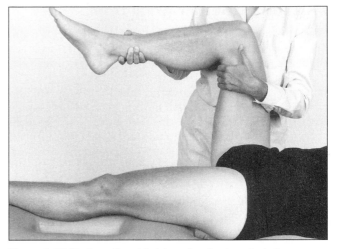

Figure 6-32 Start position: hip internal and external rotation.

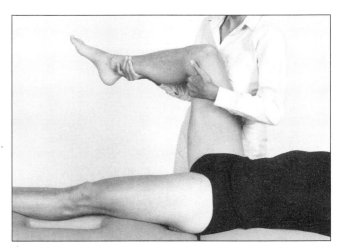

Figure 6-33 Firm end feel at the limit of hip internal rotation.

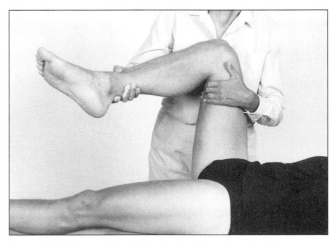

Figure 6-34 Firm end feel at the limit of hip external rotation.

Measurement: Universal Goniometer

Start Position. The patient is sitting. In sitting, the hip being measured is in 90° of flexion and neutral rotation with the knee flexed to 90°. A pad is placed under the distal thigh to keep the thigh in a horizontal position. The contralateral hip is abducted and the foot is supported on a stool (Fig. 6-35). Alternative starting positions are supine with the lower extremities in anatomical position (not shown), supine with the hip and knee flexed to 90° (see Fig. 6-32), sit-lying (i.e., supine with the knees flexed 90° over the end of the plinth; not shown), or prone with the knee flexed 90° (see Fig. 6-40). In prone, the pelvis is stabilized through strapping. Hip rotation PROM is greater when measured with the patient in prone than when measured in sitting (16). Therefore, the position used to measure hip rotation PROM should be noted on the chart (16) and the same position used when subsequently measuring the PROM to evaluate patient progress.

Stabilization. In sitting, the pelvis is stabilized through body positioning and the patient grasps the edge of the plinth. The therapist maintains the position of the femur without restricting movement.

Goniometer Axis. The axis is placed over the midpoint of the patella (Figs. 6-36 and 6-37).

Stationary Arm. Perpendicular to the floor.

Movable Arm. Parallel to the anterior midline of the tibia.

End Positions. Internal rotation (Figs. 6-37 and 6-38): The hip is internally rotated to the limit of motion (45°) to move the leg and foot in a lateral direction.

External rotation (Figs. 6-39 and 6-40): The hip is externally rotated to the limit of motion (45°) to move the leg and foot in a medial direction.

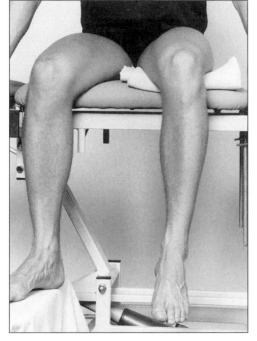

Figure 6-35 Start position: hip internal and external rotation.

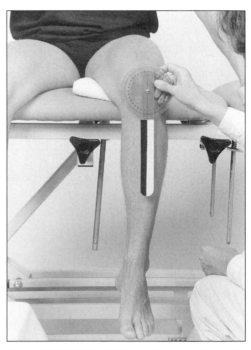

Figure 6-36 Start position: goniometer placement for hip internal and external rotation.

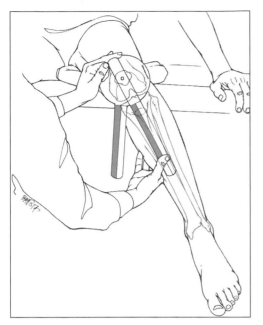

Figure 6-37 Goniometer alignment: hip internal rotation and external rotation. Illustrated with the hip in internal rotation.

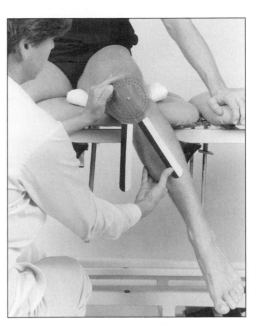

Figure 6-38 End position: internal rotation.

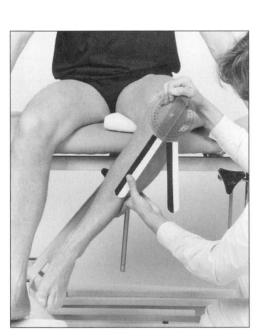

Figure 6-39 End position: external rotation.

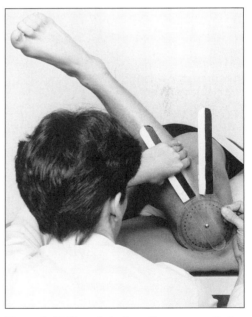

Figure 6-40 Alternate test position: prone with the knee flexed 90° and the hip in external rotation.

MUSCLE LENGTH ASSESSMENT AND MEASUREMENT

Hamstrings (Semitendinosus, Semimembranous, Biceps Femoris)

Origins (2)	Insertions (2)
Semitendinosus	
Inferomedial impression on the superior aspect of the ischial tuberosity	Proximal part of the medial surface of the tibia.
Semimembranosus	
Superolateral aspect of the ischial tuberosity	Tubercle on the posterior aspect of the medial tibial condyle.
Biceps Femoris	
a. Long head: inferomedial impression of the superior aspect of the ischial tuberosity; lower portion of the sacrotuberous ligament	Head of the fibula; slip to the lateral condyle of the tibia; slip to the lateral collateral ligament.
b. Short head: lateral lip of the linea aspera and lateral supracondylar line	

Passive Straight Leg Raise (SLR)

Start Position. The patient is supine with the lower extremities in the anatomical position (Fig. 6-41). The low back and sacrum should be flat on the plinth (11). Since ankle dorsiflexion limits the ROM of SLR (17), the test is performed with the ankle relaxed in plantarflexion.

Stabilization. It is difficult to stabilize the pelvis when performing passive SLR, and pelvic rotation is not eliminated from the movement (18). However, the therapist must ensure that excessive anterior or posterior pelvic tilt is avoided through use of a precise start position, adequate stabilization, and observation of pelvic motion. To stabilize the pelvis, the patient's nontest thigh is held on the plinth with the use of a strap (see Fig. 6-41), or the therapist's knee is placed over the distal aspect of the anterior surface of the patient's nontest thigh (not shown).

End Position. The hip is flexed to the limit of motion while maintaining knee extension so that the biceps femoris, semitendinosus, and semimembranosus are put on full stretch (Figs. 6-42 and 6-43). The ankle is relaxed in plantarflexion during the test.

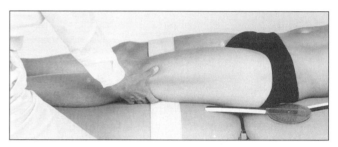

Figure 6-41 Start position: length of hamstrings.

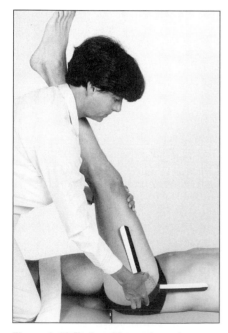

Figure 6-42 End position: universal goniometer measurement of hamstrings length.

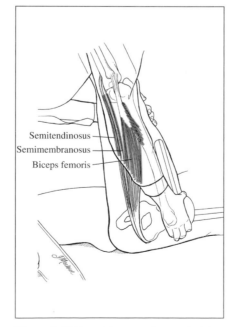

Semitendinosus
Semimembranosus
Biceps femoris

Figure 6-43 Hamstring muscles on stretch.

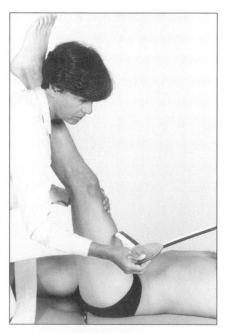

Figure 6-44 Reading goniometer: hamstrings length.

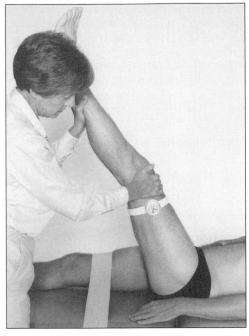

Figure 6-45 End position: OB goniometer measurement of hamstrings length.

End Feel. Hamstrings on stretch—firm.

Measurement. The therapist uses a goniometer to measure and record the available hip flexion PROM (Figs. 6-42, 6-43, and 6-44).

Universal Goniometer Placement. The goniometer is placed the same as for hip flexion. A second therapist may assist to align and read the goniometer. Normal ROM and hamstring length is about 80° hip flexion (11). A restriction of less than 80° for SLR in normal subjects is generally imposed by lack of extensibility of hamstrings (19). When interpreting test results, consider that changes in passive SLR might also result from changes in the degree of pelvic rotation (20).

OB Goniometer Placement. This measurement procedure allows the therapist to easily assess SLR ROM without assistance. The strap is placed around the distal thigh

and the dial is placed on the lateral aspect of the thigh (Fig. 6-45).

Alternate Measurement: Passive Knee Extension (PKE) Supine (21)

Start Position. The patient is supine. The hip is flexed to 90°. The patient supports the thigh in this position by placing both hands around the distal thigh. If the patient cannot hold this position, the therapist stabilizes the thigh. The knee is flexed, and the ankle is relaxed in plantarflexion (Fig. 6-46).

Stabilization. The patient or the therapist stabilizes the femur to maintain the hip in 90° flexion. Posterior tilt of the pelvis is avoided through use of a precise start position, observation of pelvic motion, and if necessary use of a strap placed over the anterior aspect of the distal thigh on the nontest side (see Fig. 6-41).

End Position. While maintaining the hip in 90° flexion, the knee is extended to the limit of motion so that the hamstring muscles are put on full stretch (Fig. 6-47). The ankle is relaxed in plantarflexion during the test.

End Feel. Hamstrings on stretch—firm.

Measurement. The angle of knee flexion is used to indicate the hamstring muscle length. Hamstring tightness is indicated if the knee cannot be extended beyond 20° knee flexion (22).

Universal Goniometer Placement. The goniometer is placed the same as for knee flexion. Should the therapist stabilize the thigh, a second therapist may be required to assist with the alignment and reading of the universal goniometer.

Alternate Measurement: Sitting

See page 182 for an alternate test to evaluate hamstring muscle length.

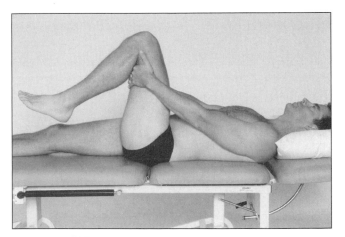

Figure 6-46 PKE: hamstrings length.

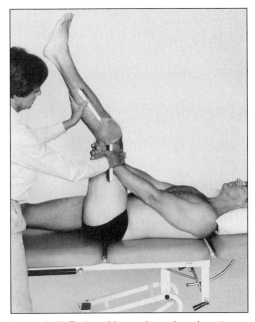

Figure 6-47 End position: universal goniometer measurement of knee flexion for hamstrings length.

Hip Flexors (11) (Iliacus, Psoas Major, Tensor Fascia Latae, Sartorius, Rectus Femoris)- Thomas Test

Origins (2)	Insertions (2)
Iliacus	
Superior two thirds of the iliac fossa, inner lip of the iliac crest; ventral sacroiliac and iliolumbar ligaments; and the upper surface of the lateral aspect of the sacrum.	Lateral side of the tendon of psoas major; and into the lesser trochanter.
Psoas Major	
Anterior aspects of the transverse processes of all of the lumbar vertebrae; sides of the bodies and intervertebral discs of T12 and all the lumbar vertebrae.	Lesser trochanter of the femur.
Tensor Fascia Latae	
Anterior aspect of the outer lip of the iliac crest; outer surface and notch below the ASIS; and the deep surface of the fascia latae.	Via the iliotibial tract onto the lateral condyle of the tibia.
Sartorius	
ASIS and the upper half of the notch below it.	Upper part of the medial surface of the tibia (anterior to gracilis and semitendinosus).
Rectus Femoris	
a. Straight head: anterior aspect of the anterior inferior iliac spine. b. Reflected head: groove above the acetabulum and the capsule of the hip joint.	Base of the patella, via the quadriceps tendon into the tibial tuberosity.

Start Position. The patient sits at the end of the plinth with the edge of the plinth at midthigh level. From this position, the patient is assisted into supine. Using both hands, the patient holds the hip of the nontest leg in flexion so that the sacrum and lumbar spine are flat on the plinth (Fig. 6-48). Care should be taken to avoid flexion of the lumbar spine due to excessive hip flexion ROM.

Stabilization. The patient's supine position and holding of the nontest hip in flexion stabilizes the pelvis and lumbar spine. The therapist observes the ASIS to ensure there is no pelvic tilting.

End Position. The test leg is allowed to fall toward the plinth into hip extension (Fig. 6-49). As the test leg falls toward

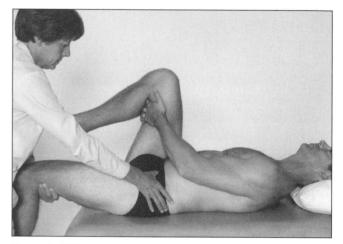

Figure 6-48 Start position: length of hip flexors.

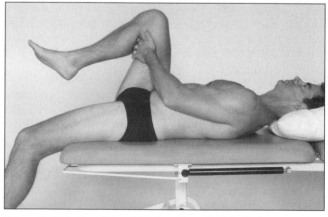

Figure 6-49 End position: thigh touching plinth indicates normal length of hip flexors.

the plinth, the therapist ensures the knee is free to move into extension (i.e., to avoid placing the rectus femoris on stretch and restrict hip extension ROM), and the thigh remains in neutral adduction/abduction and rotation. If the thigh does not touch the plinth, slight overpressure is applied on the anterior aspect of the thigh to passively move the femur posteriorly to the limit of movement (Fig. 6-50). The hip flexors (i.e., iliopsoas) are considered to be of normal length if the thigh touches the plinth (11) (see Fig. 6-49). Note that a flexion deformity at the hip can be obscured by an increased lumbar lordosis (23).

End Feel. Iliacus and psoas major on stretch—firm.

Measurement. With shortness of the hip flexors (i.e., iliopsoas), the angle between the midaxillary line of the trunk and the longitudinal axis of the femur represents the degree of hip flexion contracture (Figs. 6-50 and 6-51).

Universal Goniometer Placement. The same as for hip flexion-extension with the axis over the greater trochanter of the femur (Figs. 6–50 and 6–51). If a restriction of hip joint extension is present (i.e., the thigh does not rest on the plinth) with the knee joint in extension, shortness of the iliopsoas, sartorius, or tensor fascia latae muscles may contribute to the limited ROM. The muscle shortness causing the restriction can be determined using the following criteria (11):

A. Shortness of the *sartorius* should be suspected if the hip joint assumes a position of external rotation and abduction and/or the knee flexes at the restricted limit of hip extension.

B. Shortness of the *tensor fascia latae* may be suspected if the thigh is observed to abduct as the hip joint extends. If during testing the thigh is abducted as the hip is extended, and this results in increased hip extension, there is shortness of the tensor fascia latae. Specific length testing of tensor fascia latae should be performed to confirm this finding. Van Dillen and colleagues (24) suggest that abducting the hip may place the anterior fibers of the gluteus medius and minimus on slack and thus also contribute to the increase in hip extension. If hip abduction makes no difference to the restricted hip extension ROM, the *iliopsoas* muscle is shortened and preventing the full movement.

If the thigh is prevented from abducting during testing, a shortened tensor fascia latae may also produce hip internal rotation, lateral deviation of the patella, external rotation of the tibia, or knee extension.

C. With the hip abducted as the hip is extended to the limit of motion when testing hip flexor muscle length, the knee is flexed to the limit of motion to assess shortness of the *rectus femoris* (24) (see Figs. 7–26 through 7–28). If the rectus femoris is shortened, knee flexion PROM will be restricted proportional to the decrease in muscle length. Knee flexion of less than 80° indicates the degree of muscle shortening (11).

Note: In the presence of excessive hip flexor length, the patient's hips are positioned at the edge of the plinth to allow the full available ROM (11).

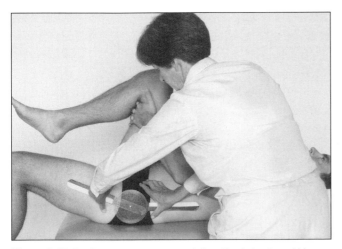

Figure 6-50 Goniometer measurement: length of shortened hip flexors.

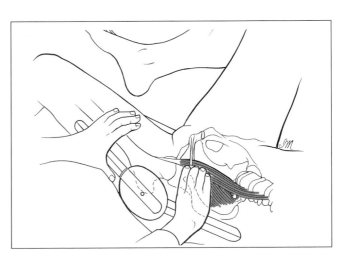

Figure 6-51 Hip flexors on stretch.

Hip Adductors (Adductor Longus, Adductor Brevis, Adductor Magnus, Pectineus, and Gracilis)

Start Position. The patient is supine with the lower extremity in the anatomical position. On the nontest side, the hip is abducted, the knee is flexed, and the foot rests on a stool beside the plinth (Fig. 6-52).

Stabilization. The therapist stabilizes the ipsilateral pelvis.

End Position. The hip is abducted to the limit of motion so that the hip adductor muscles are put on full stretch (Fig. 6-53).

End Feel. Hip adductors on stretch—firm.

Measurement. If the hip adductors are shortened, hip abduction PROM will be restricted proportional to the decrease in muscle length. The therapist uses a goniometer to measure and record the available hip abduction PROM (Figs. 6-54 and 6-55).

Universal Goniometer Placement. The goniometer is placed the same as for hip abduction (Fig. 6–55).

Origins (2)	Insertions (2)
Adductor Longus	
Front of the pubis in the angle between the crest and the symphysis.	Middle third of the linea aspera of the femur.
Adductor Brevis	
External surface of the inferior pubic ramus between gracilis and obturator externus.	Line between lesser trochanter and linea aspera; upper part of the linea aspera.
Adductor Magnus	
External surface of the inferior ramus of the pubis adjacent to the ischium; the external surface of the inferior ramus of the ischium; and the inferolateral aspect of the ischial tuberosity.	Medial margin of the gluteal tuberosity of the femur; medial lip of the linea aspera; medial supracondylar line; adductor tubercle.
Pectineus	
Pecten pubis between the iliopectineal eminence and the pubic tubercle.	Line between the lesser trochanter and the linea aspera.
Gracilis	
Lower half of the body of the pubis; the inferior ramus of the pubis and ischium.	Upper part of the medial surface of the tibia (between sartorius and semitendinosus).

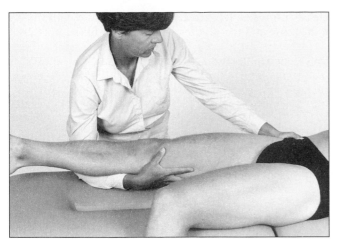

Figure 6-52 Start position: length of hip adductors.

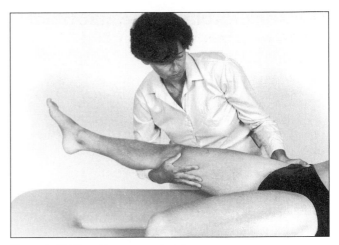

Figure 6-53 Hip adductors on stretch.

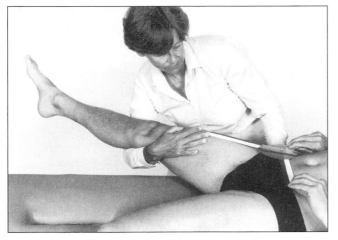

Figure 6-54 Goniometer measurement: length of hip adductors.

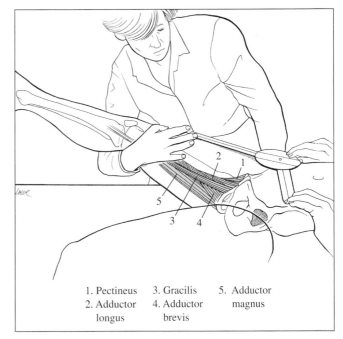

1. Pectineus 3. Gracilis 5. Adductor
2. Adductor 4. Adductor   magnus
   longus   brevis

Figure 6-55 Hip adductors on stretch.

Tensor Fascia Latae (Iliotibial Band)—Ober's Test (25)

Origin (2)	Insertion (2)
Tensor Fascia Latae	
Anterior aspect of the outer lip of the iliac crest; the outer surface and notch below the ASIS; and the deep surface of the fascia latae.	Via the iliotibial tract onto the antero lateral aspect of the lateral condyle of the tibia.

Start Position. The patient is in the side-lying position on the nontest side and holds the nontest leg in hip and knee flexion to flatten the lumbar spine. The therapist stands behind and against the patient's pelvis to maintain the side-lying position. The therapist positions the hip in abduction and then extension to stretch the iliotibial band over the greater trochanter. The hip is in neutral rotation and the knee is positioned in 90° flexion (Fig. 6-56).

Stabilization. The position of the nontest leg stabilizes the pelvis and lumbar spine; the therapist stabilizes the lateral pelvis at the superior aspect of the iliac crest.

End Position. The test leg is allowed to fall toward the plinth. The therapist may apply slight overpressure on the lateral aspect of the thigh to passively adduct the hip to the limit of movement (not shown). With shortness of the tensor fascia latae, the hip remains abducted (Figs. 6-57 and 6-58). If the leg cannot be passively adducted to the horizontal, there is maximal tightness; if the horizontal position is reached, there is moderate tightness; and if the leg falls below horizontal but does not completely reach the plinth, there is minimal tightness (26).

Note that tightness of the tensor fascia latae at the hip can be obscured by a downward lateral tilt of the pelvis on the test side that may be accompanied by trunk lateral flexion on the opposite side. The position of the test leg must be carefully maintained in hip extension and neutral or slight external rotation to perform an accurate test of tensor fascia latae tightness.

If the rectus femoris muscle is tight or there is a need to decrease stress in the region of the knee, the Ober's Test may be modified (Modified Ober's Test) and performed with the knee in extension (11) (not shown). The therapist should note that the degree of hip adduction ROM used to indicate the length of tensor fascia latae will be more restricted with the knee in flexion (Ober's Test) than with the knee in extension (Modified Ober's Test) (27,28). Therefore, these tests should not be used interchangeably (28) when assessing tensor fascia latae muscle length.

End Feel. Tensor fascia latae (iliotibial band) on stretch—firm.

Measurement. If the tensor fascia latae is shortened, hip adduction PROM will be restricted proportional to the de-crease in muscle length. The therapist uses a goniometer to measure and record the available hip adduction PROM.

Universal Goniometer Placement. The goniometer is placed the same as for hip abduction/adduction. A second therapist is required to assist with the alignment and reading of the goniometer.

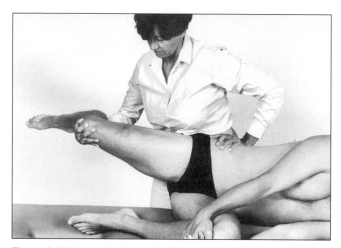
Figure 6-56 Ober's Test start position: length of tensor fascia latae.

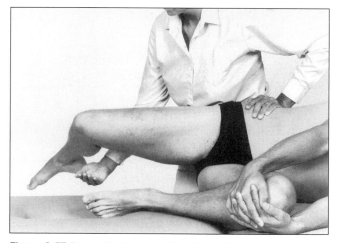
Figure 6-57 Ober's Test end position: tensor fascia latae on stretch.

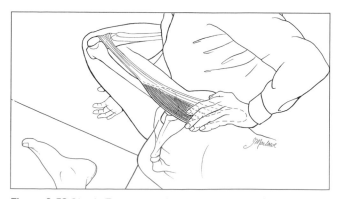
Figure 6-58 Ober's Test: tensor fascia latae on stretch.

Alternate Measurement: Ober's Test: Trunk Prone

Kendall and colleagues (11) describe the "Modified Ober Test: Trunk Prone" to assess tensor fascia latae muscle length. This test provides better stabilization than the Ober's Test and is described here. In this test and in the Ober's Test the knee is held in 90° flexion. To avoid confusion with the "Modified Ober's Test", in which the knee is held in extension, the test described here is referred as the "Ober's Test: Trunk Prone."

Start Position. The patient is standing at the end of the plinth and flexes the hips so the trunk is resting on the plinth (Fig. 6-59). The nontest leg is placed under the plinth with the hip and knee flexed. The patient positions the arms overhead and grasps the sides of the plinth. The therapist supports the test leg and, while maintaining the knee in 90° flexion and the hip in neutral rotation, moves the hip into full abduction, followed by full extension.

Stabilization. The therapist stabilizes the posterior aspect of the ipsilateral pelvis to prevent anterior pelvic tilt. It is also important that the therapist stabilize the lateral aspect of the contralateral pelvis to prevent elevation of the contralateral pelvis, and downward lateral tilt of the ipsilateral pelvis. The patient's arm position aids in preventing lateral pelvic tilt. The weight of the trunk offers stabilization.

End Position. With the hip maintained in full extension and neutral rotation, the hip is adducted to the limit of motion so that the tensor fascia latae is put on full stretch (Fig. 6-60). If the tensor fascia latae is shortened, hip adduction PROM, with the hip in extension, will be restricted proportional to the decrease in muscle length.

End Feel. Tensor fascia latae on stretch—firm.

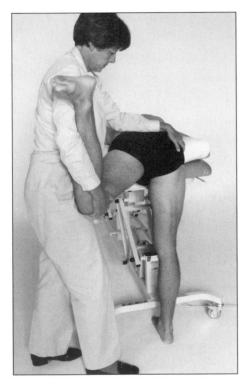

Figure 6-59 Ober's Test: Trunk Prone start position.

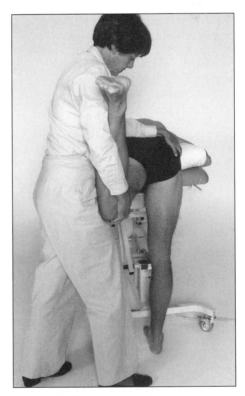

Figure 6-60 Ober's Test: Trunk Prone end position: tensor fascia latae on stretch.

FUNCTIONAL APPLICATION

Joint Function (29)

The hip joint transmits forces between the ground and the pelvis to support the body weight and acts as a fulcrum during single-leg stance. Through hip movement, the body may be moved closer to or farther away from the ground. The hip brings the foot closer to the trunk and positions the lower limb in space.

Functional Range of Motion

The hip joint may be flexed, extended, abducted, adducted, and internally and externally rotated. Common activities of daily living (ADL) can be accomplished in a normal manner with hip ROM of at least 120° flexion, 20° abduction, and 20° external rotation (30).

In performing functional activities, hip movements are accompanied at various points in the range of motion by lumbar-pelvic motions (31). These motions extend the functional range capabilities of the hip joint. The lumbar and pelvic motions are included in the following description of motion, with the purpose of explaining the interdependence of the components of the pelvic girdle and trunk throughout movement.

Hip Flexion and Extension

As in the shoulder joint, motions occurring at the more central joints augment movement at the hip joint. Hip movement "may result from movement of the pelvis on the

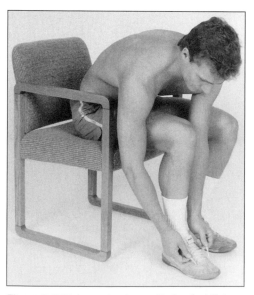

Figure 6-61 Tying a shoelace with the foot flat on the floor requires approximately 120° of hip flexion (27).

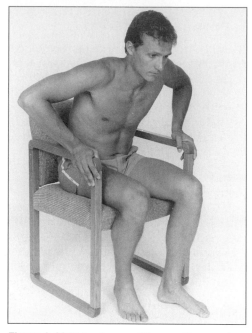

Figure 6-62 Rising from a sitting position requires at least 90° of hip flexion (27).

femur, from movement of the femur on the pelvis, or from a combination of pelvic and femoral motion" (5, p. 273). As the femur moves on the pelvis to produce hip flexion, hip range of motion is augmented by a posterior pelvic tilt (i.e., the ASIS moves superiorly and posteriorly) and flexion of the lumbar spine. In hip extension, the movement is increased by an anterior pelvic tilt (i.e., the ASIS moves inferiorly and anteriorly) and extension of the lumbar spine.

The normal AROM for hip flexion is 0° to 120° and extension is 0° to 30° (8). Full hip flexion and extension ranges of motion are required for many ADL. Standing requires 0° or slight hip extension (32). Using electrogoniometric measures, it has been found that without using compensatory movement patterns at other joints, activities such as squatting to pick up an object from the ground, tying a shoe lace with the foot on the ground (Fig. 6-61) or with the foot across the opposite thigh, and rising from a sitting position (Fig. 6-62) require an average of 110° to 120° of hip flexion (27).

Activities requiring less than 90° of hip flexion include ascending (Fig. 6-63) and descending stairs (30,33), sitting in a chair of standard height (30), and putting on a pair of trousers (Fig. 6-64). Ascending stairs requires an average of 67° hip flexion, descending an average of 36° hip flexion (30). A maximum of about 1° to 2° hip extension may be required to ascend and descend stairs (33).

The range required for sitting is determined by the height of the chair. To sit from standing requires an average of 104° hip flexion (30); to rise from sitting requires an average of 98° to 101° hip flexion ROM (34). About 84° of hip flexion is required for sitting in a standard chair (30). These ranges increase with decreased chair height and decrease with increased chair height.

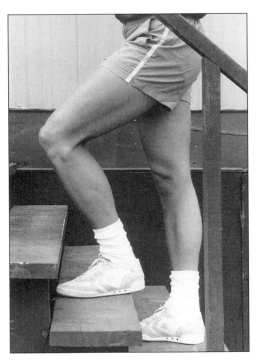

Figure 6-63 Ascending stairs.

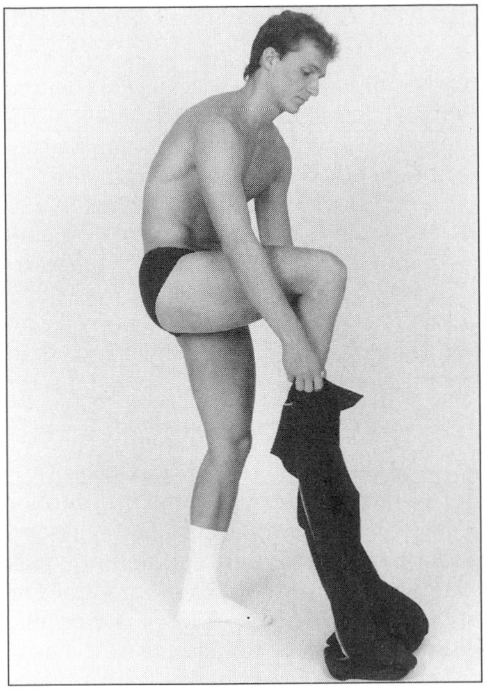

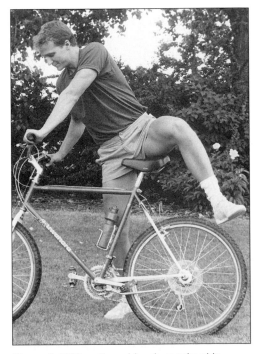

Figure 6-64 Putting on a pair of trousers.

Hip Abduction and Adduction

The normal AROM at the hip for abduction is 0° to 45°; for adduction, it is 0° to 30° (8). However, most daily functions do not require the full ranges of hip abduction and adduction. Many ADL can be performed within an arc of 0° to 20° of hip abduction (30). Squatting to pick up an object and sitting with the foot across the opposite thigh (Fig. 6-65) are examples of activities performed within this ROM. Mounting a men's bicycle (Fig. 6-66) may require the full range of hip abduction. Hip adduction in ADL is illustrated when sitting with the thighs crossed and when standing on one leg; the leg one stands on adducts as a result of the pelvis dropping on the contralateral side.

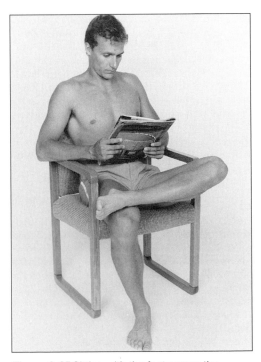

Figure 6-65 Sitting with the foot across the opposite thigh requires hip flexion, abduction, and external rotation.

Figure 6-66 Mounting a bicycle requires hip flexion, abduction, and external rotation.

Hip Internal and External Rotation

The AROM of hip internal and external rotation is 0° to 45° in both directions (8). The extremes of these rotational motions are seldom used in ADL. Ranges of 0° to 20° external rotation are required for most ADL (30). Mounting a bicycle (see Fig. 6-66), sitting on a chair with the foot across the opposite thigh to tie a shoelace, or visually observing the skin on the sole of the foot when performing foot hygiene activities illustrate the use of hip external rotation. Squatting to pick up an object from the floor is an example of a functional activity that requires 20° of hip internal rotation (30).

Gait

A normal walking pattern requires hip motion in the sagittal, frontal, and horizontal planes. In the sagittal plane, about 10° to 20° of hip extension is required at terminal stance and 30° of hip flexion is required at the end of swing phase and the beginning of stance phase as the limb is advanced forward to take the next step (from the Rancho Los Amigos gait analysis forms as cited in Levangie and Norkin [32]).

With the feet fixed on the ground, the femoral heads can act as fulcrums for the pelvis as it tilts anteriorly and posteriorly. The pelvis can also tilt laterally, causing the iliac crests to move either superiorly or inferiorly. Lateral tilting of the pelvis occurs when one leg is off the ground, the hip joint of the supporting leg acts as a fulcrum, and the tilting results in relative abduction and adduction at the hip joints (32). When walking, there is a lateral tilt of the pelvis inferiorly on the unsupported side during the swing phase of the gait cycle. This dropping of the pelvis on the unsupported side results in abduction at the hip on the same side. As the pelvis drops, the inferior aspect of the pelvis moves toward the femur of the stance leg, producing hip adduction on this side. About 7° of hip abduction is required at initial swing, and 5° of hip adduction is required at the end of the stance phase of the gait cycle (35).

Pelvic rotation occurs in the horizontal plane about a vertical axis. Rotations of the thigh occur relative to the pelvis. As the swinging leg advances during locomotion, the pelvis rotates forward on the same side. The fulcrum for this forward rotation of the pelvis is the head of the femur on the supporting leg. As the supporting or stance leg is fixed on the ground, the pelvis rotates around the femoral head, resulting in internal rotation at the hip joint. As the pelvis moves forward on the swing side, the swinging leg moves forward in the sagittal plane in the line of progression, resulting in external rotation of the hip during the swing phase of the gait cycle. During the normal gait cycle about 5° of internal rotation and 9° of external rotation are required at the hip joint (35). External rotation occurs at the end of the stance phase and through most of the swing phase, and internal rotation occurs at terminal swing before initial contact to the end of the stance phase (35). Refer to Appendix D for further description and illustrations of the positions and motions at the hip joint during gait.

Hip flexion and extension ROM requirements for slow-paced running (slower than an 8-minute mile) and fast-paced running (faster than a 7.5-minute mile) have been investigated and described by Pink and colleagues (36). Fast-paced running required averages of 31° maximum hip flexion at the end of middle swing and 11° maximum hip extension at toe off. Slower-paced running requires lower maximal ranges of hip flexion and extension than fast-paced running.

References

1. Kapandji IA. *The Physiology of the Joints.* Vol 2. 5th ed. New York: Churchill Livingstone; 1982.
2. Standring S, ed. *Gray's Anatomy: The Anatomical Basis of Clinical Practice.* 39th ed. London: Elsevier Churchill Livingstone, 2005.
3. Norkin CC, White DJ. *Measurement of Joint Motion: A Guide to Goniometry.* 3rd ed. Philadelphia: FA Davis; 2003.
4. Daniels L, Worthingham C. *Muscle Testing: Techniques of Manual Examination.* 5th ed. Philadelphia: WB Saunders; 1986.
5. Norkin CC, Levangie PK. *Joint Structure and Function: A Comprehensive Analysis.* Philadelphia: FA Davis; 1983.
6. Woodburne RT. *Essentials of Human Anatomy.* 5th ed. London: Oxford University Press; 1973.
7. Magee DJ. *Orthopaedic Physical Assessment.* 4th ed. Philadelphia: WB Saunders; 2002.
8. American Academy of Orthopaedic Surgeons. *Joint Motion: Method of Measuring and Recording.* Chicago: AAOS; 1965.
9. Berryman Reese N, Bandy WD. *Joint Range of Motion and Muscle Length Testing.* Philadelphia: WB Saunders; 2002.
10. Cyriax J. *Textbook of Orthopaedic Medicine. Vol 1. Diagnosis of Soft Tissue Lesions.* 8th ed. London: Bailliere Tindall; 1982.
11. Kendall FP, McCreary EK, Provance PG, et al. *Muscles Testing and Function with Posture and Pain.* 5th ed. Baltimore: Lippincott Williams & Wilkins; 2005.
12. Caillet R. *Soft Tissue Pain and Disability.* Philadelphia: FA Davis; 1977.
13. Boone DC, Azen SP. Normal range of motion of joints in male subjects. *J Bone Joint Surg [Am].* 1979;61:756–759.
14. Steindler A. *Kinesiology of the Human Body Under Normal and Pathological Conditions.* Springfield: Charles C Thomas; 1955.
15. Neumann DA. *Kinesiology of the Musculoskeletal System: Foundations for Physical Rehabilitation.* Philadelphia: Mosby; 2002.
16. Hollman JH, Burgess B, Bokermann JC. Passive hip rotation range of motion: effects of testing position and age in runners and non-runners. *Physiotherapy Theory and Practice.* 2003;19:77–86.
17. Gajdosik RL, LeVeau BF, Bohannon RW. Effects of ankle dorsiflexion on active and passive unilateral straight leg raising. *Phys Ther.* 1985;65:1478–1482.
18. Bohannon RW. Cinematographic analysis of the passive straight-leg-raising test for hamstring muscle length. *Phys Ther.* 1982;62:1269–1274.
19. Goeken LN, Nof AtL. Instrumental straight-leg raising. Results in healthy subjects. *Arch Phys Med Rehabil.* 1993;74:194–203.
20. Bohannon R, Gajdosik R, LeVeau BF. Contribution of pelvic and lower limb motion to increases in the angle of passive straight leg raising. *Phys Ther.* 1985;65:474–476.
21. Holt KS. *Assessment of Cerebral Palsy. I. Muscle Function, Locomotion and Hand Function.* London: Lloyd-Luke Medical Books; 1965.
22. Palmer ML, Epler ME. *Clinical Assessment Procedures in Physical Therapy.* Philadelphia: JB Lippincott; 1990.
23. Salter RB. *Textbook of Disorders and Injuries of the Musculoskeletal System.* 2nd ed. Baltimore: Williams & Wilkins; 1983.

24. Van Dillen LR, McDonnell MK, Fleming DA, Sahrmann SA. Effect of knee and hip position on hip extension range of motion in individuals with and without low back pain. *JOSPT*. 2000;30:307–316.

25. Ober FR. Back strain and sciatica. *JAMA*. 1935;104: 1580–1583.

26. Gose JC, Schweizer P. Iliotibial band tightness. *JOSPT*. 1989;10:399–407.

27. Gajdosik RL, Sandler MM, Marr HL. Influence of knee positions and gender on the Ober test for length of the iliotibial band. *Clin Biomechanics*. 2003;18:77–79.

28. Reese NB, Bandy WD. Use of an inclinometer to measure flexibility of the iliotibial band using the Ober test and the modified Ober test: differences in magnitude and reliability of measurements. *JOSPT*. 2003;33:326–330.

29. Smith LK, Weiss EL, Lehmkuhl LD. *Brunnstrom's Clinical Kinesiology*. 5th ed. Philadelphia: FA Davis; 1996.

30. Johnston RC, Smidt GL. Hip motion measurements for selected activities of daily living. *Clin Orthop Relat Res.* 1970;72: 205–215.

31. Cailliet R. *Low Back Pain Syndrome*. 2nd ed. Philadelphia: FA Davis; 1968.

32. Levangie PK, Norkin CC. *Joint Structure and Function. A Comprehensive Analysis*. 3rd ed. Philadelphia: FA Davis; 2001.

33. Livingston LA, Stevenson JM, Olney SJ. Stairclimbing kinematics on stairs of differing dimensions. *Arch Phys Med Rehabil*. 1991;72:398–402.

34. Ikeda ER, Schenkman ML, Riley PO, Hodge WA. Influence of age on dynamics of rising from a chair. *Phys Ther*. 1991; 71:473–481.

35. Johnston RC, Smidt GL. Measurement of hip-joint motion during walking. Evaluation of an electrogoniometric method. *J Bone Joint Surg [Am]*. 1969;51:1083–1094.

36. Pink M, Perry J, Houglum PA, Devine DJ. Lower extremity range of motion in the recreational sport runner. *Am J Sports Med*. 1994;22:541–549.

EXERCISES AND QUESTIONS

See the Answer Guide in Appendix F for suggested answers to the following exercises and questions.

1. PALPATION

A. Palpate the following anatomical structures on a skeleton and on a partner.

Iliac crest	Greater trochanter of the femur
Anterior superior iliac spine (ASIS)	Lateral epicondyle of the femur
Tubercle of the ilium	Adductor tubercle
Posterior superior iliac spine (PSIS)	Patella
Ischial tuberosity	Anterior border of the tibia

B. For each anatomical structure listed below, identify the hip joint ROM that would be measured using the structure to align the universal goniometer. Also identify the part of the goniometer (i.e., axis, stationary arm, or moveable arm) that would be aligned with the anatomical structure for the purpose of the measurement.

   i.   Greater trochanter of the femur. _____

   ii. Anterior border of the tibia. _____

   iii. Anterior superior iliac spines (ASISs). _____

   iv. Lateral epicondyle of the femur. _____

   v.   Patella. _____

C. Identify the muscle(s) that attach to the following structures:

   i.   Adductor tubercle. _____

   ii. Ischial tuberosity. _____

2. ASSESSMENT OF AROM AT THE HIP JOINT

A. Identify and describe the shape of the articular components that make up the hip articulation.

B. Demonstrate, define, and describe* the following movements of the hip joint and identify the reciprocal movement:

   i.   Hip extension.

   ii. Hip internal rotation.

   iii. Hip abduction.

   *Identify the plane and axis of movement.

C. Demonstrate a quick scan of the AROM for the lower extremities on a partner under the following conditions:

   i. Unable to weight-bear.

   ii. Able to weight-bear.

D. List the active movements a therapist would assess when evaluating the hip joint (i.e., include active movements for the appropriate joints proximal and distal to the hip joint).

E. Identify patient criteria that would have to be met for the therapist to safely assess hip joint AROM in standing.

F. For each of the movements listed below,

   • Assume the start position for the assessment and measurement of the ROM,

   • Move your hip through half of the full AROM, and hold the joint in this position to mimic a decreased AROM.

   • Without allowing further movement of the thigh, try to give the appearance of further movement or a greater than available AROM.

   • Identify the substitute movements used to give the appearance of a greater than available AROM for the movement being assessed. These should be the same substitute movement(s) a patient may use to augment a restricted AROM for each movement.

Hip AROM	Substitute Movement(s)
i. Hip flexion	_____
ii. Hip abduction	_____
iii. Hip internal rotation	_____

3. ASSESSMENT AND MEASUREMENT OF PROM AT THE HIP JOINT

A. For each of the movements listed below, demonstrate the assessment and measurement of PROM on a partner and answer the questions. Have a third partner evaluate your performance using the appropriate practical test form in Appendix E. Record your findings on the PROM Recording Form on page 170.

Hip Flexion

When you correctly assessed and measured the PROM for hip flexion,
i.   What position was the knee in on the test side?

ii. Why was the knee maintained in this position during the PROM assessment and measurement of hip flexion?

iii. Identify the normal end feel(s) expected when assessing hip flexion.

iv. What end feel did you identify on your partner for hip flexion?

v.   List the normal limiting factors that created the end feel identified on your partner.

Hip Extension

Having correctly assessed and measured the PROM for hip extension,
i.   What position was the knee in on the test side?

ii. Why was the knee maintained in this position during the PROM assessment and measurement of hip extension?

iii. If stabilization was inadequate when assessing the PROM for hip extension, the movements of _____ will result in erroneously large PROM values for hip extension.

iv. If a patient presents with decreased hip extension PROM, what arthrokinematic motion (i.e., glide/slide) of the femoral head could be decreased?

Hip Abduction

i.   The pelvis should be level when assessing hip abduction PROM. How does the therapist ensure that the pelvis is level?

ii. If a patient presents with decreased hip abduction PROM, what glide of the femoral head could be restricted in this case? Explain the reason for the glide being decreased in the direction indicated.

Hip Internal Rotation

i.   What end feel was present when you assessed your partner's hip internal PROM? Would this be considered a normal end feel?

ii. List the normal limiting factors that create a normal end feel for internal rotation.

iii. List the patient start position(s) that could be used to assess and measure the PROM for hip internal rotation. Assess and measure the PROM for hip internal rotation on your partner, using these alternate positions.

iv. If a patient presents with decreased hip internal PROM, what glide of the femoral head could be limited in this case? Explain the reason for the glide being decreased in the direction indicated.

B. A therapist evaluates the hip PROM and finds hip flexion to be the most restricted motion, followed by abduction and then internal rotation. This pattern of restricted motion could be a _____ pattern that would indicate to the therapist the presence of _____.

PROM RECORDING FORM

Patient's Name_____   Therapist_____

			Left Side ... Date of Measurement ... Right Side			
*		*	**Date of Measurement**	*		*	
			Hip				
			Flexion (0–120°)				
			Extension (0–30°)				
			Abduction (0–45°)				
			Adduction (0–30°)				
			Internal rotation (0–45°)				
			External rotation (0–45°)				
			Hypermobility: Comments:				

4. MUSCLE LENGTH ASSESSMENT AND MEASUREMENT

Demonstrate the assessment and measurement of the length of the following muscles on a partner and answer the questions below that pertain to the muscle(s) assessed. Have a third partner evaluate your performance using the appropriate practical test form in Appendix E.

Hamstrings
i.   When correctly assessing the hamstrings length using the SLR technique, the therapist must ensure the knee is maintained in full extension at the limit of motion and the pelvis is not moving into a _____ tilt position that would decrease the stretch on the hamstrings.

ii. When using the PKE test, hamstring tightness is indicated if the knee cannot be _____.

iii. Identify the end feel at the limit of the PROM when the hamstrings muscles are put on full stretch.

Hip Flexors
i.   Identify the muscles for which muscle length is being assessed when assessing hip flexor muscle shortness.

ii. When assessing the hip flexor muscle length, in what position is the nontest hip held, and why?

iii. An *increased* or *decreased* (choose one) lumbar lordosis can mask a hip flexion contracture; therefore, this position of the lumbar spine should be avoided when assessing the length of the hip flexors.

iv. When assessing the hip flexor muscle length, the hip is positioned in abduction to place the _____ on slack.

Tensor Fascia Latae
i.   If a skeleton is available, tape one end of a piece of string to the site of origin of the tensor fascia latae muscle and tape the other end of the string to the site of insertion of the iliotibial tract on the skeleton. If a skeleton is not available, hold the string at the sites of muscle origin and insertion on a partner. With the string in place, position the hip and knee articulations such that the muscle origin and insertion are as far apart as possible so as to maximally stretch the string (i.e., simulated muscle). Identify the positions of the hip and knee that place maximal stretch on the simulated tensor fascia latae.

ii. Perform both the Ober's Test and the Ober's Test: Trunk Prone on a partner. Identify the test that offers the optimal stability of the pelvis and lumbar spine.

5. FUNCTIONAL ROM AT THE HIP JOINT

A. Have a partner perform the following functional activities. For each activity, use a universal goniometer to measure the position of your partner's hip joint or the maximum hip ROM used for the movement indicated. Record your measurements.
   i.   Squatting to pick up an object on the ground—hip flexion.
   ii.   Sitting in a standard-height chair—hip flexion.
   iii. Sitting on a high stool—hip flexion.
   iv.   Rising from sitting—hip flexion.
   v.   Ascending a staircase—hip flexion.
   vi.   Descending a staircase—hip flexion.
   vii. Cutting one's toenails—hip flexion and hip abduction.
   viii. Walking—hip flexion and hip extension.

B. For each hip movement listed below, identify three daily activities that require the specified movement and demonstrate each activity:
   i.   Hip abduction ROM.
   ii.   Hip adduction ROM.
   iii. Hip internal rotation ROM.
   iv.   Hip external rotation ROM.

C. i. Identify the purposes served by the hip joint in performing ADL.

   ii. For each purpose the hip serves in performing ADL, identify an activity that illustrates the purpose.

   iii. According to Johnston and Smidt (1), common ADL can be accomplished in a normal manner with hip ROM of at least ____° flexion, ____° abduction, and ____° external rotation.

Reference

1. Johnston RC, Smidt GL. Hip motion measurements for selected activities of daily living. *Clin Orthop Relat Res.* 1970;72:205–215.

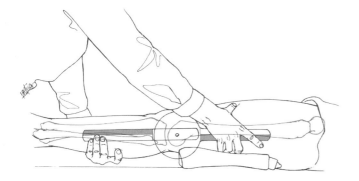

Knee

ARTICULATIONS AND MOVEMENTS

The knee is made up of the femorotibial and patellofemoral articulations (Fig. 7-1). The femorotibial articulation is a bicondylar joint formed proximally by the convex condyles of the femur and distally by the concave surfaces of the tibial condyles. The congruency of these surfaces is enhanced by the menisci located between the articulating surfaces (1). From the anatomical position, the femorotibial joint may be flexed and extended in the sagittal plane, with movement occurring around a frontal axis (Fig. 7-2). Rota-

tion also occurs at the femorotibial joint and is an essential component of normal range of motion (ROM) at the knee. Rotation occurs in the horizontal plane around a longitudinal axis (see Fig. 7-2). At the beginning of knee flexion, the tibia automatically rotates internally on the femur, and at the end of knee extension, the tibia automatically rotates externally. The external rotation at the end of knee extension locks the knee in full extension and is referred to as the "screw home mechanism." The greatest range of tibial rotation is available when the knee is flexed 90° (2). Knee movements are described in Table 7-1.

The patellofemoral articulation, an incongruous joint, is also contained within the capsule of the knee joint (see Fig. 7-1). The patellar articular surface, divided by a vertical

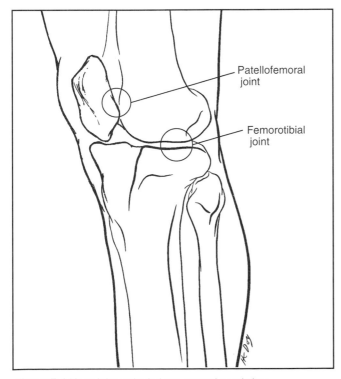

Figure 7-1 Knee joint articulations, anterolateral view.

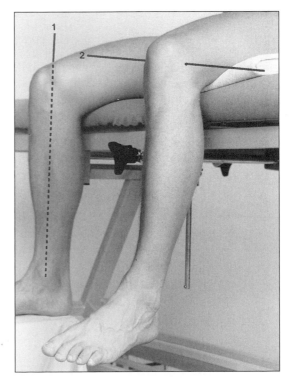

Figure 7-2 Knee joint axes: (*1*) tibial internal-external rotation; (*2*) flexion-extension.

TABLE 7-1   Joint Structure: Knee Movements

	Flexion	Extension	Internal Rotation	External Rotation
Articulation[1,3]	Femorotibial Patellofemoral	Femorotibial Patellofemoral	Femorotibial	Femorotibial
Plane	Sagittal	Sagittal	Horizontal	Horizontal
Axis	Frontal	Frontal	Longitudinal	Longitudinal
Normal limiting factors[2–6]* (See Figs. 7-3 and 7-4)	Tension in the rectus femoris (with the hip in extension); tension in the vasti muscles; soft tissue apposition of the posterior aspects of the calf and thigh or the heel and buttock	Tension in parts of both cruciate ligaments, the medial and lateral collateral ligaments, the posterior aspect of the capsule, and the oblique popliteal ligament	Tension in the cruciate ligaments	Tension in the collateral ligaments
Normal end feel[4,7]	Firm/soft	Firm	Firm	Firm
Normal AROM[8]† (AROM[9])	0–135° (0–140° to 145°)	135–0° (0°)	40°[11] to 58°[12] total active range at 90° knee flexion	
Capsular pattern[7,10]	Knee joint: flexion, extension			

*Note: There is a paucity of definitive research that identifies the normal limiting factors (NLF) of joint motion. The NLF and end feels listed here are based on knowledge of anatomy, clinical experience, and available references.
†AROM, active range of motion.

ridge, is flat or slightly convex mediolaterally and superoinferiorly (2) and articulates with the anterior surface of the femur, a surface that is divided by the intercondylar groove and is concave mediolaterally and convex superoinferiorly (1). The "motion of the patella relative to the femur or femoral groove in knee flexion and extension" is referred to as patellar tracking (13, p. 241). The gliding of the patella on the femur during knee flexion and extension is essential for normal motion at the knee. In full knee flexion, the patella slides distally and lies in the intercondylar notch (2). In full knee extension, the patella slides proximally and the lower portion of the patellar surface articulates with the anterior surface of the femur (1). In addition to proximal-distal glide, the patella glides medial-laterally during knee joint movement (14). At the beginning of knee flexion the patella shifts slightly medial, and as knee flexion increases, the patella gradually shifts laterally (13).

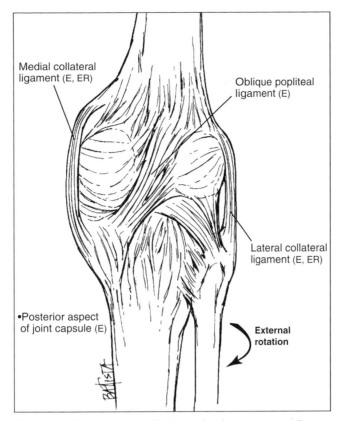

Medial collateral
ligament (E, ER)

Oblique popliteal
ligament (E)

Lateral collateral
ligament (E, ER)

•Posterior aspect
of joint capsule (E)

**External
rotation**

Figure 7-3 Posterior view of the knee showing noncontractile
structures that normally limit motion.*

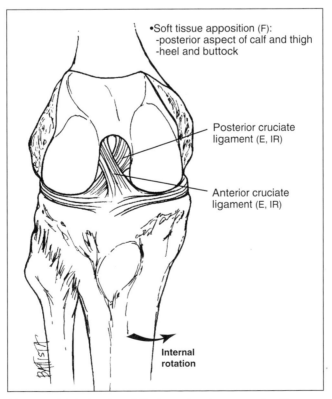

•Soft tissue apposition (F):
  -posterior aspect of calf and thigh
  -heel and buttock

Posterior cruciate
ligament (E, IR)

Anterior cruciate
ligament (E, IR)

**Internal
rotation**

Figure 7-4 Anterior view of the knee showing noncontractile
structures that normally limit motion.*

*Motion limited by structure is identified in brackets, using the following abbreviations: E, extension; ER, external rotation; IR, internal rotation. Muscles
normally limiting motion are not illustrated.

SURFACE ANATOMY

(Figs. 7-5 and 7-6)

Structure	Location
1. Greater trochanter	The superior border of the greater trochanter can be found with the tip of the thumb placed on the iliac crest at the midline and the tip of the third finger placed distally on the lateral aspect of the thigh.
2. Patella	Large triangular sesamoid bone on the anterior aspect of the knee. The base is proximal and the apex distal.
3. Ligamentum patellae (quadriceps tendon, patellar ligament, or patellar tendon)	Extends from the apex of the patella to the tibial tuberosity. As the patient attempts to extend the knee, the edges of the tendon are palpable.
4. Tibial tuberosity	Bony prominence at the proximal end of the anterior border of the tibia and the insertion of the ligamentum patellae.
5. Tibial plateaus	The upper edges of the medial and lateral tibial plateaus are located in the soft tissue depressions on either side of the ligamentum patellae. Follow the plateau medially and laterally to ascertain the knee joint line.
6. Head of the fibula	A round bony prominence on the lateral aspect of the leg on a level with the tibial tuberosity.
7. Lateral malleolus	The prominent distal end of the fibula on the lateral aspect of the ankle.
8. Lateral epicondyle of the femur	Small bony prominence on the lateral condyle of the femur.

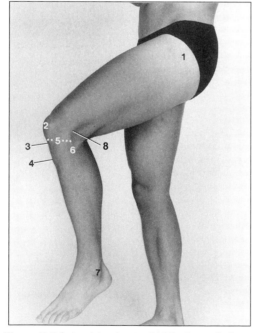

Figure 7-5 Anterolateral aspect of the lower limb.

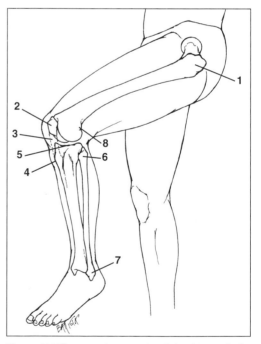

Figure 7-6 Bony anatomy, anterolateral aspect of the lower limb.

RANGE OF MOTION ASSESSMENT AND MEASUREMENT

Knee Flexion-Extension

AROM Assessment

PROM Assessment

Start Position. The patient is supine with the hip and knee in the anatomical position (Fig. 7-7). A towel is placed under the distal thigh.

Stabilization. The pelvis is stabilized by the weight of the patient's body. The therapist stabilizes the femur.

Therapist's Distal Hand Placement. The therapist grasps the distal tibia and fibula.

End Positions. The therapist applies slight traction and moves the lower leg to flex the hip and knee (Fig. 7-8). Slight overpressure is applied at the limit of knee flexion.

The therapist applies slight traction and extends the knee, applying slight overpressure at the limit of knee extension/hyperextension (Fig. 7-9).

End Feels. Flexion—firm/soft; extension/hyperextension—firm.

Joint Glides. *Flexion*—the concave tibial condyles glide posteriorly on the fixed convex femoral condyles. *Extension*—the concave tibial condyles glide anteriorly on the fixed convex femoral condyles.

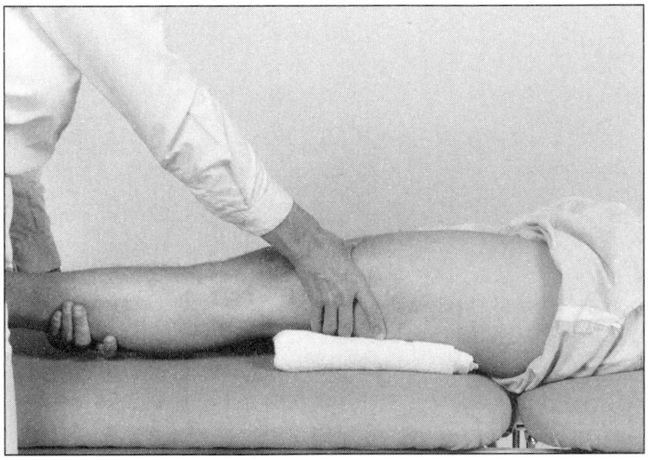

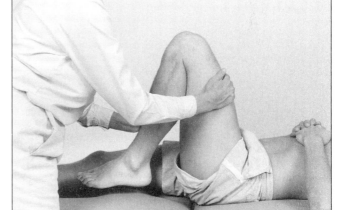

Figure 7-7 Start position: knee flexion and extension or hyperextension.

Figure 7-8 Firm or soft end feel at the limit of knee flexion.

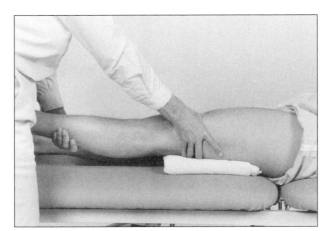

Figure 7-9 Firm end feel at the limit of knee extension or hyperextension.

Measurement: Universal Goniometer

Start Position. The patient is supine. The hip is in the anatomical position and the knee is in extension (0°) (Fig. 7-10). A towel is placed under the distal thigh.

Stabilization. The pelvis is stabilized by the weight of the patient's body. The therapist stabilizes the femur.

Goniometer Axis. The axis is placed over the lateral epicondyle of the femur (Fig. 7-11).

Stationary Arm. Parallel to the longitudinal axis of the femur, pointing toward the greater trochanter.

Movable Arm. Parallel to the longitudinal axis of the fibula, pointing toward the lateral malleolus.

End Position. From the start position of knee extension, the hip and knee are flexed (Fig. 7-12). The heel is moved toward the buttock to the limit of knee flexion (135°).

Hyperextension. The femur is stabilized, and the lower leg is moved in an anterior direction beyond 0° of extension (Fig. 7-13). Hyperextension from 0° to 10° may be present.

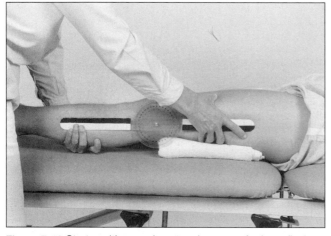

Figure 7-10 Start position: goniometer placement for knee flexion and extension/hyperextension.

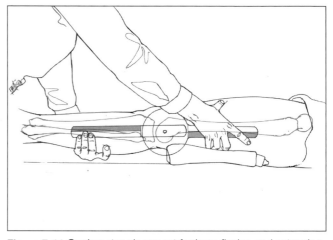

Figure 7-11 Goniometer placement for knee flexion and extension.

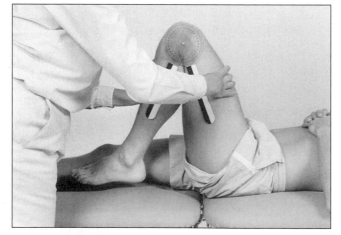

Figure 7-12 Knee flexion.

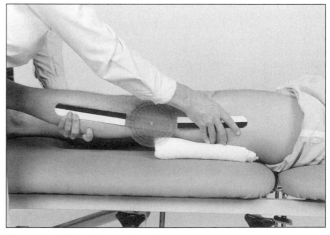

Figure 7-13 Knee hyperextension.

Patellar Mobility— Distal Glide

PROM Assessment

Start Position. The patient is supine; a roll supports the knee joint in slight flexion (Fig. 7-14).

Stabilization. The femur rests on the plinth.

Procedure (15). The heel of one hand is against the base of the patella, with the forearm lying along the thigh. The other hand is placed on top, and both hands move the patella in a distal direction to the end of the movement. Movement of the patella in a posterior direction compresses the patella against the femur and should be avoided. The therapist records whether the movement is full or restricted. The patella moves vertically a total of 8 cm from full flexion to full extension of the knee (16).

End Feel. Firm.

Patellar Mobility— Medial-Lateral Glide

PROM Assessment

Start Position. The patient is supine; a roll supports the knee joint in slight flexion (Fig. 7-15).

Stabilization. The therapist stabilizes the femur and tibia.

Procedure. The palmar aspects of the thumbs are placed on the lateral border of the patella. The pads of the index fingers are placed on the medial border of the patella. The thumbs move the patella medially, and the index fingers move the patella laterally in a side-to-side motion. With the knee in extension, passive movement of the patella should average 9.6 mm medially and 5.4 mm laterally (17). Excessive, normal, or restricted ROM is recorded.

End Feel. Firm.

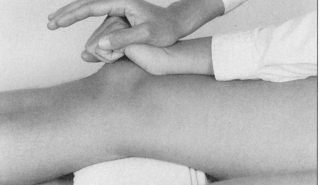

Figure 7-14 Distal glide of the patella.

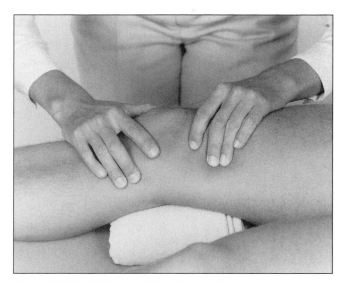

Figure 7-15 Medial-lateral glide of the patella.

Tibial Rotation

Tibial rotation is an essential component of normal ROM at the knee. Assessment of total rotation ROM is more reliable than assessment of internal and external tibial rotation because of the difficulty of defining the zero start position for the individual movements (18). The greatest range of tibial rotation is available when the knee is flexed 90° (2).

AROM Assessment

Substitute Movement. Tibial internal rotation—hip internal rotation, ankle dorsiflexion/plantarflexion, subtalar joint inversion, forefoot adduction. Tibial external rotation—hip external rotation, ankle dorsiflexion/plantarflexion, subtalar joint eversion, forefoot abduction.

PROM Assessment

Start Position. The patient is sitting with the knee in 90° flexion and the tibia in full internal rotation (Fig. 7-16A). A pad is placed under the distal thigh to maintain the thigh in a horizontal position.

Stabilization. The therapist stabilizes the femur.

Procedure. From full internal rotation, the therapist rotates the tibia externally through the full available ROM (Fig. 7-17A). The total range of tibial rotation is observed (average total active range, about 40° in women [11] and 58° in men [12]) and recorded as excessive, normal, or restricted.

End Feels. Internal rotation—firm; external rotation—firm.

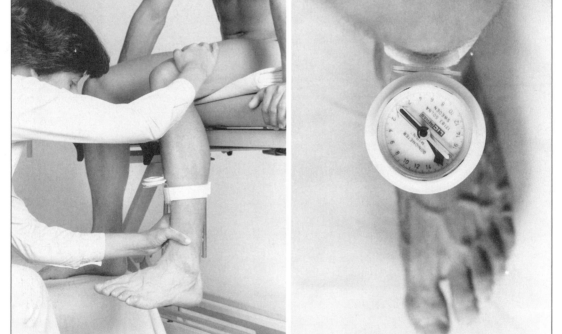

A.   B.

Figure 7-16 A. and B. Start position for total tibial rotation: tibial internal rotation.

Joint Spin. The proximal concave surface of the tibia spins on the convex condyles of the fixed femur. This spin occurs in conjunction with roll and glide of the articular surface during flexion and extension at the knee joint.

Measurement: OB Goniometer

Start Position. The patient is sitting with the knee in 90° flexion and the tibia in full internal rotation (see Fig. 7-16A). A pad is placed under the distal thigh to maintain the thigh in a horizontal position. In the start position the fluid-filled container of the goniometer is rotated until the 0° arrow lines up directly underneath the compass needle (see Fig. 7-16B).

Goniometer Placement. The strap is placed around the leg distal to the gastrocnemius muscle, and the dial is placed on the right-angle extension plate on the anterior aspect of the leg.

Stabilization. The therapist stabilizes the femur.

End Position. From full internal rotation, the therapist rotates the tibia externally through the full available PROM (see Fig. 7-17A). The number of degrees the compass needle moves away from the 0° arrow on the compass dial is recorded as the total range of tibial rotation (see Fig. 7-17B) (average total active range, about 40° in women [11] and 58° in men [12]).

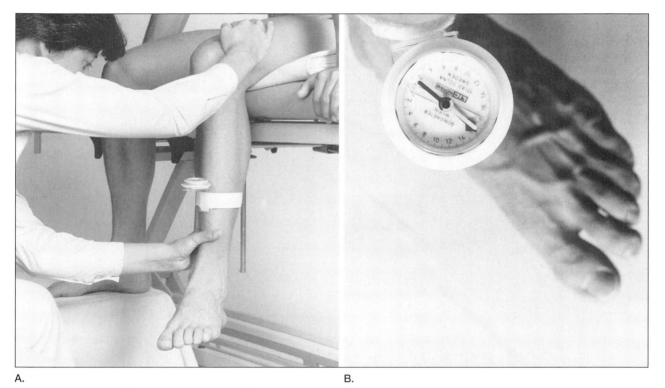

A.   B.

Figure 7-17 A. and B. End position for total tibial rotation: tibial external rotation.

MUSCLE LENGTH ASSESSMENT AND MEASUREMENT

Hamstrings (Semitendinosus, Semimembranosus, Biceps Femoris)

Origins (1)	Insertions (1)
Semitendinosus	
Inferomedial impression on the superior aspect of the ischial tuberosity.	Proximal part of the medial surface of the tibia.
Semimembranosus	
Superolateral aspect of the ischial tuberosity.	Tubercle on the posterior aspect of the medial tibial condyle.
Biceps Femoris	
a. Long head: inferomedial impression of the superior aspect of the ischial tuberosity; lower portion of the sacrotuberous ligament.	Head of the fibula; slip to the lateral condyle of the tibia; slip to the lateral collateral ligament.
b. Short head: lateral lip of the linea aspera and lateral supracondylar line.	

Start Position. The patient is sitting, grasps the edge of the plinth, and has the nontest foot supported on a stool (Fig. 7-18). A pad is placed under the distal thigh to maintain the thigh in a horizontal position. The ankle on the test side is relaxed in plantarflexion.

Stabilization. The therapist stabilizes the femur. The patient grasps the edge of the plinth and is instructed to maintain the upright sitting position.

Goniometer Placement. The goniometer is placed the same as for knee flexion-extension.

End Position. The therapist extends the knee to the limit of motion so that hamstrings are put on full stretch (Fig. 7-19). The ankle is relaxed in plantarflexion throughout the test movement to prevent gastrocnemius muscle tightness from limiting knee ROM.

End Feel. Hamstrings on stretch—firm.

Substitute Movement. The patient leans back to posteriorly tilt the pelvis, extending the hip joint to place the hamstrings on slack and thus allow increased knee extension (Fig. 7-20).

Alternate Test Positions. See pages 156 and 157 for alternate tests of hamstring muscle length.

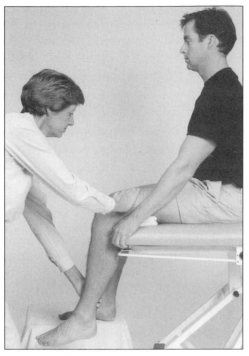

Figure 7-18 Start position: length of hamstrings.

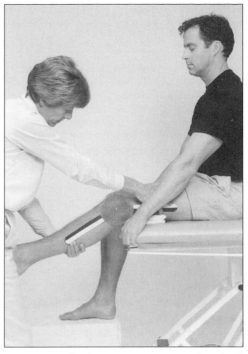

Figure 7-19 Goniometer measurement: length of hamstrings.

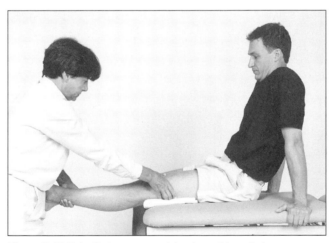

Figure 7-20 Substitute movement: backward lean during hamstrings length test.

Measurement of Muscle Length: Rectus Femoris

Origins (1)	Insertion (1)
Rectus Femoris	
a. Straight head: anterior inferior iliac spine.	Base of the patella, via the quadriceps tendon into the tibial tuberosity.
b. Reflected head: groove above the acetabulum and the capsule of the hip joint.	

Start Position. The patient is prone. To position the pelvis in a posterior tilt, the nontest leg is over the side of the plinth with the hip flexed and the foot on the floor (Fig. 7-21). This positioning of the nontest leg has been shown to effectively tilt the pelvis posteriorly and thus increase hip extension of the test leg to better ensure maximum stretch of the rectus femoris muscle (19). The test leg is in the anatomical position with the knee in extension (0°). A towel may be placed under the thigh to eliminate pressure on the patella.

Stabilization. The patient's prone position with the nontest leg over the side of the plinth with the hip flexed and the foot on the floor stabilizes the pelvis. A strap may also be placed over the buttocks to stabilize the pelvis. The therapist stabilizes the femur.

Goniometer Placement. The goniometer is placed the same as for knee flexion-extension.

End Position. The lower leg is moved in a posterior direction so that the heel approximates the buttock to the limit of knee flexion. Decreased length of the rectus femoris restricts the range of knee flexion when the patient is prone (Fig. 7-22).

End Feel. Rectus femoris on stretch—firm.

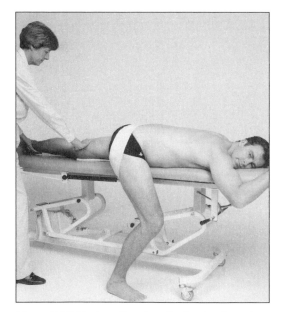

Figure 7-21 Start position: length of rectus femoris.

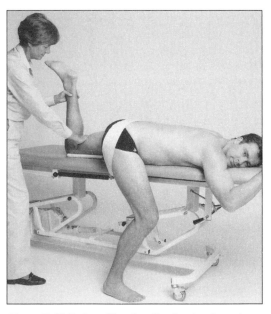

Figure 7-22 End position: length of rectus femoris.

Alternate Position

Start Position. The patient is prone. A towel may be placed under the thigh to eliminate pressure on the patella. The leg is in the anatomical position with the knee in extension (0°) (Fig. 7-23).

Stabilization. The patient's prone position stabilizes the pelvis. A strap may also be placed over the buttocks to stabilize the pelvis. The therapist observes the pelvis to ensure there is no tilting of the pelvis. The therapist stabilizes the femur.

Goniometer Placement. The goniometer is placed the same as for knee flexion-extension.

End Position. The lower leg is moved in a posterior direction so the heel approximates the buttock to the limit of knee flexion. Decreased length of the rectus femoris restricts the range of knee flexion when the patient is prone (Fig. 7-24).

Substitute Movement. The patient anteriorly tilts the pelvis and flexes the hip to place the rectus femoris on slack and thus allow increased knee flexion (Fig. 7-25).

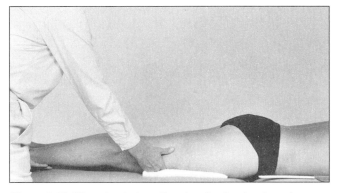

Figure 7-23 Alternate start position: length of rectus femoris.

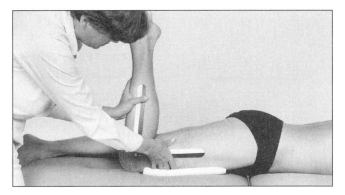

Figure 7-24 Goniometer measurement: length of rectus femoris.

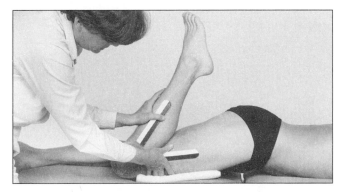

Figure 7-25 Substitute movement: anterior pelvic tilt and hip flexion placing rectus femoris on slack.

Alternate Position

Start Position. The patient sits at the end of the plinth with the edge of the plinth at midthigh level. From this position, the patient is assisted into supine. Using both hands, the patient holds the hip of the nontest leg in flexion so that the sacrum and lumbar spine are flat on the plinth. Care should be taken to avoid flexion of the lumbar spine due to excessive hip flexion ROM. The test leg is allowed to fall toward the plinth into hip extension and the knee is flexed (Fig. 7-26).

Stabilization. The patient's supine position and holding of the nontest hip in flexion stabilizes the pelvis and lumbar spine. The therapist observes the anterior superior iliac spine (ASIS) to ensure there is no pelvic tilting. The therapist stabilizes the femur.

Goniometer Placement. The goniometer is placed the same as for knee flexion-extension.

End Position. With the hip held in the extended position, the therapist flexes the knee to the limit of motion to put the rectus femoris on full stretch (Figs. 7-27 and 7-28).

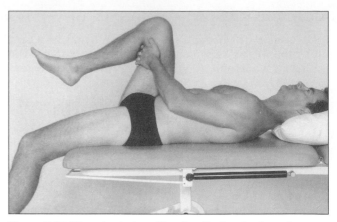

Figure 7-26 Alternate start position: length of rectus femoris.

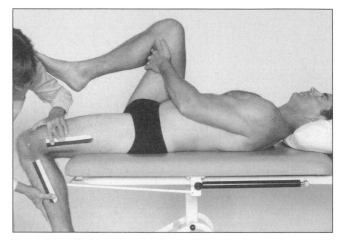

Figure 7-27 End position: length of rectus femoris.

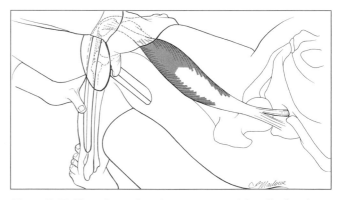

Figure 7-28 Alternate goniometer measurement: length of rectus femoris.

FUNCTIONAL APPLICATION

Joint Function

The knee joint functions to support the body weight and to shorten or lengthen the lower limb (2). Knee flexion with the foot planted lowers the body closer to the ground, while knee extension raises the body (20). With the foot off the ground, foot orientation in space is provided (2) by flexing or extending the knee or rotating the tibia. The rotational mobility of the knee joint makes twisting movements of the body possible when the foot is planted on the ground (20). In walking, the knee joint acts as a shock absorber, decreases the vertical displace-ment of the body, and through knee flexion shortens the lower limb to allow the toes to clear the ground during the swing phase of the gait cycle (21,22).

Functional Range of Motion

The normal AROM at the knee is from 0° of extension to 135° of flexion. Full extension is required for normal func-tion, but many daily activities require less than 135° of knee flexion.

The knee has to be fully extended to stand erect (Fig. 7-29). Full or near-full knee extension is required to reach a height (Fig. 7-30) or to contact a distant object or surface with the foot, such as depressing the brake pedal of a car or going downstairs (Fig. 7-31). When dressing, the knee

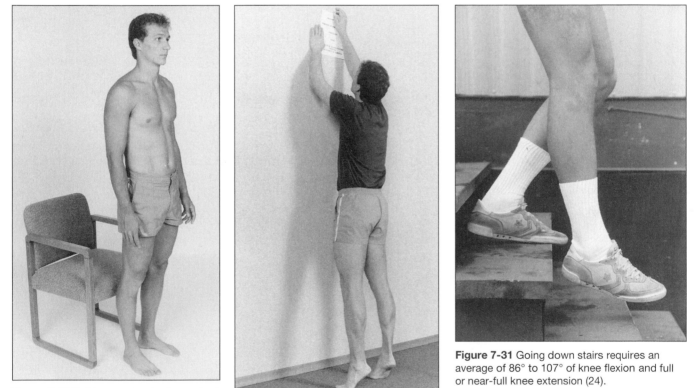

Figure 7-29 Full knee extension is required to stand erect.

Figure 7-30 To reach a height, full or near-full knee extension is required.

Figure 7-31 Going down stairs requires an average of 86° to 107° of knee flexion and full or near-full knee extension (24).

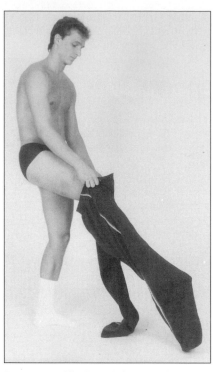

Figure 7-32 The knee is in extension to put on a pair of trousers.

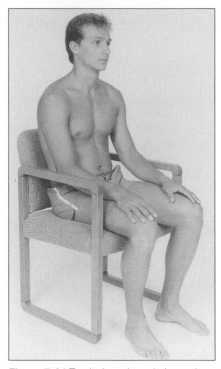

Figure 7-34 To sit down in a chair requires an average of 93° of knee flexion (23).

is extended to put on a pair of trousers (Fig. 7-32) or shorts. The fully extended position of the knee usually occurs in asymmetrical postures; for example, prolonged standing when one leg is used to support most of the body weight or when powerful thrusting motions (1) such as jumping are performed.

Daily activities involving ranges of knee motion up to an average of 117° of flexion include lifting an object off the floor (Fig. 7-33), sitting down in a chair (Fig. 7-34), ascending and descending stairs (Figs. 7-31 and 7-35), and tying a shoelace (23) or pulling on a sock (Fig. 7-36). The knee flexion ROM required for selected activities of daily

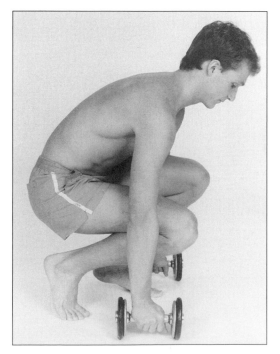

Figure 7-33 Lifting an object off the floor requires an average of 117° of knee flexion (23).

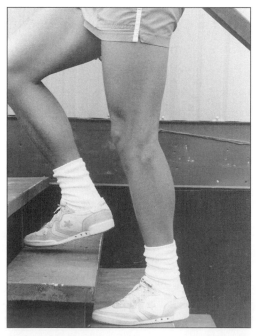

Figure 7-35 Climbing stairs requires an average of 83° to 105° of knee flexion and full or near-full knee extension (24).

TABLE 7-2   Knee Flexion ROM Average Values Required for ADL

Activity	Flexion
Tying shoe: sitting and bringing the foot up from the floor*	106°
Sitting: without touching the chair with the hands*	93°
Lifting object from floor*	
Bending at hips to reach down	71°
Back straight, bending knees	117°
Stairs[†]	
Ascending	83–105°
Descending	86–107°
Walking[‡]	60°
Fast-paced running[25] (faster than 7.5-minute mile)	103°

‡Data from the Rancho Los Amigos gait analysis forms as cited in Levangie and Norkin (2).
*Knee flexion ROM for 30 subjects were measured from the subject's normal stance position and not anatomical zero position (23).
†Knee flexion ROM for 15 subjects during ascent and descent of three stairs of different dimensions. Maximum knee flexion ROM requirements varied depending on the stair dimensions and subject height (24).

living (ADL) is shown in Table 7-2. Many of the daily functions previously mentioned require on average less than 25° of tibial rotation (23).

Livingston and coworkers (24) evaluated the knee flexion ROM required to ascend and descend three stairs of different dimensions. Depending on the stair dimensions and subject height, the maximum knee flexion ROM required ranged between averages of 83° and 105° to ascend and 86° and 107° to descend the stairs. Minimum knee flexion ROM averages of between 1° or 2° and 15° were required to ascend or descend stairs. It appears that changes of ROM at the knee joint, rather than the hip and ankle, are used to adjust to different stair dimensions (24).

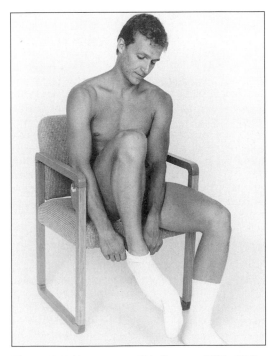

Figure 7-36 Knee range within the arc of 0° to 117° of flexion.

Gait

Walking requires an ROM from about 0° of knee extension as the leg advances forward to make initial contact with the ground (Fig. 7-37) to a maximum of about 60° of knee flexion at initial swing so that the foot clears the ground as the extremity is advanced forward (from the Rancho Los Amigos gait analysis forms, as cited in the work of Levangie and Norkin [2]). The tibia rotates internally on the femur at the end of the swing phase and maintains the position of internal rotation through the stance phase until preswing, when the tibia externally rotates through to midswing (26). An average of about 13° of tibial rotation is required for normal gait (27). For further description and illustrations of the positions and motions at the knee joint during gait, see Appendix D.

Pink and colleagues (25) investigated and described the ROM requirement at the knee for slow-paced running (slower than an 8-minute mile) and fast-paced running (faster than a 7.5-minute mile). Fast-paced running required a range of knee joint motion from an average of 11° flexion at terminal swing to an average 103° maximum knee flexion near the end of middle swing. Slower-paced running required less flexion throughout most of the swing phase compared to fast-paced running.

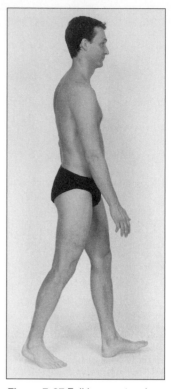

Figure 7-37 Full knee extension is required for normal gait.

References

1. Standring S, ed. *Gray's Anatomy: The Anatomical Basis of Clinical Practice*. 39th ed. London: Elsevier Churchill Livingstone; 2001.
2. Levangie PK, Norkin CC. *Joint Structure and Function. A Comprehensive Analysis*. 3rd ed. Philadelphia: FA Davis; 2001.
3. Kapandji IA. *The Physiology of the Joints*. Vol. 2. 2nd ed. New York: Churchill Livingstone; 1982.
4. Norkin CC, White DJ. *Measurement of Joint Motion: A Guide to Goniometry*. 3rd ed. Philadelphia: FA Davis; 2003.
5. Daniels L, Worthingham C. *Muscle Testing: Techniques of Manual Examination*. 5th ed. Philadelphia: WB Saunders; 1986.
6. Woodburne RT. *Essentials of Human Anatomy*. 5th ed. London: Oxford University Press; 1973.
7. Magee DJ. *Orthopedic Physical Assessment*. 4th ed. Philadelphia: WB Saunders; 2002.
8. American Academy of Orthopaedic Surgeons. *Joint Motion: Method of Measuring and Recording*. Chicago: AAOS; 1965.
9. Berryman Reese N, Bandy WD. *Joint Range of Motion and Muscle Length Testing*. Philadelphia: WB Saunders; 2002.
10. Cyriax J. *Textbook of Orthopaedic Medicine. Vol. 1. Diagnosis of Soft Tissue Lesions*. 8th ed. London: Bailliere Tindall; 1982.
11. Mossberg KA, Smith LK. Axial rotation of the knee in women. *JOSPT*. 1983;4(4):236–240.
12. Osternig LR, Bates BT, James SL. Patterns of tibial rotary torque in knees of healthy subjects. *Med Sci Sports Exerc*. 1980;12:195–199.
13. Katchburian MV, Bull AMJ, Shih Y-F, et al. Measurement of patellar tracking: assessment and analysis of the literature. *Clin Orthop Relat Res*. 2003;412:241–259.
14. Heegaard J, Leyvraz P-F, Van Kampen A, et al. Influence of soft structures on patellar three-dimensional tracking. *Clin Orthop Relat Res*. 1994;299:235–243.
15. Kaltenborn FM. *Mobilization of the Extremity Joints: Examination and Basic Treatment Techniques*. 3rd ed. Oslo: Olaf Norlis Bokhandel; 1985.
16. Soderberg GL. *Kinesiology: Application to Pathological Motion*. 2nd ed. Baltimore: Williams & Wilkins; 1997.
17. Skalley TC, Terry GC, Teitge RA. The quantitative measurement of normal passive medial and lateral patellar motion limits. *Am J Sports Med*. 1993;21:728–732.
18. Zarins B, Rowe CR, Harris BA, Watkins MP. Rotational motion of the knee. *Am J Sports Med*. 1983;11:152–156.
19. Hamberg J, Bjorklund M, Nordgren B, Sahistedt B. Stretchability of the rectus femoris muscle: investigation of validity and intratester reliability of two methods including x-ray analysis of pelvic tilt. *Arch Phys Med Rehab*. 1993;74:263–270.
20. Smith LK, Weiss EL, Lehmkuhl LD. *Brunnstrom's Clinical Kinesiology*. 5th ed. Philadelphia: FA Davis; 1996.
21. Edelstein JE. Biomechanics of normal ambulation. *J Can Physiother Assoc*. 1965;17:174–185.
22. Inman VT, Ralston HJ, Todd F. *Human Walking*. Baltimore: Williams & Wilkins; 1981.
23. Laubenthal KN, Smidt GL, Kettelkamp DB. A quantitative analysis of knee motion during activities of daily living. *Phys Ther*. 1972;52:34–42.
24. Livingston LA, Stevenson JM, Olney SJ. Stairclimbing kinematics on stairs of differing dimensions. *Arch Phys Med Rehabil*. 1991;72:398–402.
25. Pink M, Perry J, Houglum PA, Devine DJ. Lower extremity range of motion in the recreational sport runner. *Am J Sports Med*. 1994;22:541–549.
26. Mann RA, Hagy JL. The popliteus muscle. *J Bone Joint Surg [Am]*. 1977;59:924–927.
27. Kettelkamp DB, Johnson RJ, Smidt GL, et al. An electrogoniometric study of knee motion in normal gait. *J Bone Joint Surg [Am]*. 1970;52:775–790.

EXERCISES AND QUESTIONS

See the Answer Guide in Appendix F for suggested answers to the following exercises and questions.

1. PALPATION

A. Identify the anatomical reference points a therapist would use to align the universal goniometer axis and stationary and moveable arms when measuring the following ROM or muscle length at the knee:

i. Knee flexion/extension:
Goniometer axis _____
Stationary arm _____
Moveable arm _____

ii. Hamstrings or rectus femoris:
Goniometer axis _____
Stationary arm _____
Moveable arm _____

iii. Whether measuring knee flexion or extension ROM or muscle length at the knee for hamstrings or rectus femoris, the alignment of the goniometer is the same. True or false?

B. i. Palpate the anatomical reference points used to align the goniometer when measuring knee flexion/extension ROM on a skeleton and on a partner.

ii. Palpate the following anatomical structures on a skeleton and on a partner.

Borders of the patella   Tibial tuberosity
Ligamentum patellae   Head of the fibula

2. ASSESSMENT PROCESS

List the 10 main components of the assessment process performed by the therapist to assess the knee joint.

3. ASSESSMENT OF AROM AT THE KNEE ARTICULATIONS

A. Identify and describe the shape of the articular components that make up the femorotibial and patellofemoral articulations.

B. Demonstrate, define, and describe* the femorotibial joint movements.
*(i.e., identify the axis/plane of movement)

C. **Tibial Rotation**

i. The purpose of the first exercise is to demonstrate the presence of **active** internal and external rotation of the tibia.

- Have a partner sit with the knees flexed 90° and the feet flat on the floor.
- Instruct your partner to raise the right or left forefoot off the floor and move the toes inward toward the midline of the body by pivoting on the heel to position the tibia in full internal rotation.
- Using your index finger, palpate your partner's tibial tuberosity.
- Now instruct your partner to move the toes outward by pivoting on the heel to position the tibia in full external rotation.
- Observe and feel the tibial tuberosity move externally under your index finger as this motion is performed.
- From the position of full external rotation, have your partner internally rotate the tibia.
- Observe and feel the tibial tuberosity move as your partner slowly repeats full tibial rotation.
- Have your partner repeat these motions slowly several times to observe and feel the tuberosity move in the described directions.

ii. The purpose of the second exercise is to demonstrate the **automatic** external and internal rotation of the tibia, which occurs at the end of knee extension and at the beginning of knee flexion, respectively. This automatic rotation of the tibia is necessary for normal knee motion.

- Have your partner sit with the knee flexed 90° and the foot flat on the floor.
- Using your index finger, palpate your partner's tibial tuberosity.
- Instruct your partner to slowly extend the knee fully (to 0°). In a normal knee, you should observe and feel the tibial tuberosity move in a lateral direction (i.e., external rotation of the tibia) under your finger as the knee approaches full extension.
- Instruct your partner to move from the position of full extension to 90° flexion.
- Observe and feel the tibial tuberosity move in a medial direction (i.e., internal rotation of the tibia) under your finger at the beginning of the knee flexion motion.
- Have your partner repeat the above movements several times to observe and feel the tuberosity move under your finger in the described directions.

4. ASSESSMENT AND MEASUREMENT OF PROM AT THE KNEE

For each of the movements listed below, demonstrate the assessment and measurement of PROM on a partner and answer the questions that follow. Record your findings on the PROM Recording Form on page 193 (i.e., record excessive, normal, or restricted tibial rotation and patellar mobility). Have a third partner evaluate your performance using the appropriate practical test form in Appendix E.

Knee Flexion

i. What normal end feel(s) would be expected when assessing knee flexion?
ii. What end feel for knee flexion did you identify on your partner?
iii. Identify the normal limiting factor(s) that create the knee flexion end feel on your partner.
iv. If knee flexion ROM were assessed with the patient's hip in 0° extension, what muscle would be stretched at the hip and could then restrict knee flexion ROM?

Knee Extension

i. Identify the two-joint muscle(s) that cross the hip and knee joints that if placed on stretch by placing the hip in _____ could restrict knee extension ROM.
ii. If a patient presents with decreased knee extension PROM, what glide of the tibia would be decreased? Explain the reason for the glide being decreased in the direction indicated.

Tibial Rotation

i. What normal end feels would be expected when assessing tibial internal and external rotation?
ii. What end feel for tibial rotation did you identify on your partner?
iii. Identify the normal limiting factor(s) that create the normal end feels for tibial internal and external rotation.

Patellar Mobility

i. Identify the patellar glides a therapist assesses to determine patellar mobility.
ii. What is the magnitude of the normal vertical displacement of the patella from full flexion to full extension of the knee?
iii. With the knee in extension, what is the normal PROM for medial and lateral movement of the patella?

PROM RECORDING FORM

Patient's Name_____   Therapist_____

	Left Side				Date of Measurement		Right Side		
	*		*		**Date of Measurement**	*		*	
					Knee				
					Flexion (0–135°)				
					Tibial rotation				
					Patellar mobility—Distal glide				
					Patellar mobility—Medial-lateral glide				
					Hypermobility:				
					Comments:				

5. MUSCLE LENGTH ASSESSMENT AND MEASUREMENT

For the hamstrings and the rectus femoris, demonstrate the assessment and measurement of muscle length on a partner. Have a third partner evaluate your performance using the appropriate practical test form in Appendix E.

Rectus Femoris

i.   The therapist stabilizes the femur and the _____ in all tests used to evaluate rectus femoris length.

ii. Identify the means used to stabilize the pelvis when using the following start positions to assess rectus femoris muscle length:
   a. supine
   b. prone (two test positions)

6. FUNCTIONAL ROM AT THE KNEE

A. Have a partner perform or simulate the following functional activities. Use a universal goniometer and measure the maximum knee flexion ROM required to complete each activity:

i.   Lifting a light object from the floor, bending the knees with the back straight.

ii. Sitting in a chair.

iii. Tying a shoe: sitting and bringing the foot up from the floor.

iv. Climbing stairs.

v.   Going down stairs.

B. Walking requires a ROM from about ____° of knee extension as the leg advances forward to make _____ with the ground to a maximum of about ____° of knee flexion at _____ so that the foot _____ the ground as the extremity is advanced forward.

C. In general terms, tibial rotation occurs in ADL that require _____ .

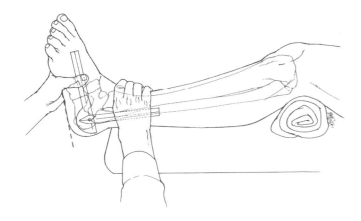

Ankle and Foot

ARTICULATIONS AND MOVEMENTS

Articulations of the ankle and foot are illustrated in Figure 8-1. The articulations at which range of motion (ROM) is commonly measured are the talocrural (ankle) joint, the subtalar joint, and the metatarsophalangeal (MTP) and interphalangeal (IP) joints of the great toe. The movements of these joints are described in Tables 8-1 and 8-2.

The ankle joint is classified as a hinge joint. The proximal concave articulating surface of the joint, commonly referred to as the ankle mortise, is formed by the medial aspect of the lateral malleolus, the distal tibia, and the lateral aspect of the medial malleolus. This concave surface is mated with the convex surface of the body of the talus. The primary movements at the ankle, dorsiflexion and plantarflexion, occur around an oblique frontal axis in an oblique sagittal plane (Fig. 8-2). With the ankle in plantarflexion, the narrower posterior aspect of the body of the talus lies within the mortise and allows additional motion to occur at the joint. This movement is slight and includes side-to-side gliding, rotation, and abduction and adduction (2).

The subtalar joint consists of two separate articulations between the talus and calcaneus that are separated by the tarsal canal. Posterior to the tarsal canal, the concave surface on the inferior aspect of the talus articulates with the convex posterior facet on the superior surface of the calcaneus. Anterior to the canal, the convex head of the talus articulates with the concave middle and anterior facets on the superior surface of the calcaneus. The subtalar joint axis runs posteroanteriorly, obliquely upward from the transverse plane and medial to the sagittal plane (Fig. 8-3). Owing to the obliquity of the joint axis and the opposite shapes of the surfaces of

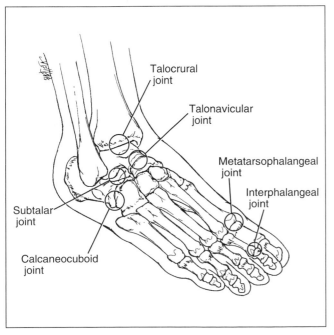

Figure 8-1 Ankle and foot articulations.

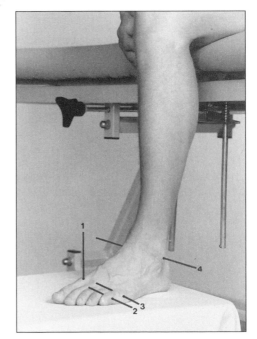

Figure 8-2 Ankle and foot axes: (*1*) metatarsophalangeal (MTP) joint abduction-adduction; (*2*) interphalangeal (IP) joint flexion-extension; (*3*) MTP joint flexion-extension; (*4*) talocrural joint dorsiflexion-plantarflexion.

TABLE 8-1   Joint Structure: Ankle and Foot Movements

	Plantarflexion	Dorsiflexion	Inversion	Eversion
Articulation[1,2]	Talocrural	Talocrural	Subtalar	Subtalar
Plane	Oblique sagittal	Oblique sagittal	Oblique frontal	Oblique frontal
Axis	Oblique frontal	Oblique frontal	Oblique sagittal	Oblique sagittal
Normal limiting factors[1–6]* (See Figs. 8-4 and 8-5)	Tension in the anterior joint capsule, anterior portion of the deltoid, anterior talofibular ligaments, and the ankle dorsiflexors; contact between the talus and the tibia	Tension in the posterior joint capsule, the deltoid, calcane-ofibular and posterior talofibular ligaments, and the soleus; contact between the talus and the tibia	Tension in the lateral collateral ligament, ankle evertors, lateral talocalcaneal ligaments, cervical ligament, and the lateral joint capsule	Contact between the talus and calcaneus; tension in the medial joint capsule, medial collateral ligaments, medial talocalcaneal ligament, tibialis posterior, flexor hallucis longus and flexor digitorum longus
Normal end feel[3,7]	Firm/hard	Firm/hard	Firm	Hard/firm
Normal AROM[8]† (AROM[9])	0–50° (0–40° to 50°)	0–20° (0–15° to 20°)	0–5°: forefoot 0–35° (0–30° to 35°)	0–5°: forefoot 0–15° (0–20°)
Capsular pattern[7,10]	Talocrural joint: plantarflexion, dorsiflexion Subtalar joint: varus (i.e., inversion), valgus (i.e., eversion)			

*Note: There is a paucity of definitive research that identifies the normal limiting factors (NLF) of joint motion. The NLF and end feels listed here are based on knowledge of anatomy, clinical experience, and available references.
†AROM, active range of motion.

the two joints (i.e., talar surfaces: posteriorly concave, anteriorly convex; calcaneal surfaces: posteriorly convex, anteriorly concave) that make up the subtalar joint, movement at the subtalar joint occurs in three planes and is identified as supination and pronation. In non–weight-bearing conditions, when the subtalar joint is supinated, the calcaneus inverts in the frontal plane around a sagittal axis, adducts in the transverse plane around a vertical axis, and plantarflexes in the sagittal plane around a frontal axis (5). Pronation includes calcaneal eversion, abduction, and dorsiflexion. In the clinical setting it is not possible to directly measure triplanar subtalar ROM. "By convention, single-axis calcaneal inversion and eversion is considered representative of triplanar motion of the subtalar joint" (11, p. 430). Therefore, the more easily observed movements of inversion and eversion (5) are assessed and measured in the clinical setting to indicate subtalar joint ROM.

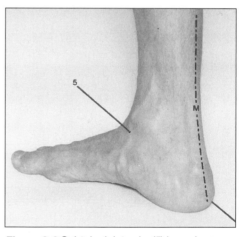

Figure 8-3 Subtalar joint axis: (5) inversion-eversion (*M*, midline of leg and heel).

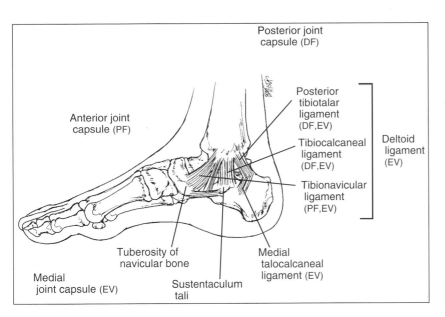

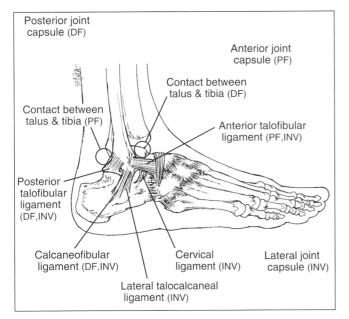

Figure 8-4 Medial view of the ankle and foot showing noncontractile structures that normally limit motion at the ankle and subtalar joints.*

Figure 8-5 Lateral view of the ankle and foot showing noncontractile structures that normally limit motion at the ankle and subtalar joints.*

*Motion limited by structures is identified in brackets, using the following abbreviations: F, flexion; E, extension; Abd, abduction; Add, adduction. Muscles normally limiting motion are not illustrated.

Movement at the transverse tarsal (i.e., talocalcaneonavicular and calcaneocuboid articulations), intertarsal, tarsometatarsal, and intermetatarsal joints (see Fig. 8-1) is essential for normal ankle and foot function. These joints function to accommodate motions between the hindfoot and forefoot to either raise or flatten the arch of the foot, and thus enable the foot to conform to the supporting surface. In the clinical setting, it is not possible to directly measure movements at these joints.

The MTP and IP joints of the toes make up the distal articulations of the foot (see Fig. 8-1). The MTP joints are ellipsoidal joints (2), each formed proximally by the convex head of the metatarsal articulating with the concave base of the adjacent proximal phalanx. The movements at the MTP articulations include flexion, extension, abduction, and adduction. Flexion and extension movements occur in the sagittal plane around a frontal axis, and the movements of abduction/adduction occur in the transverse plane around a vertical axis (see Fig. 8-5). The IP joints are classified as hinge joints, formed by the convex head of the proximal phalanx articulating with the concave base of the adjacent distal phalanx. The IP joints allow flexion and extension movements of the toes.

TABLE 8-2   Joint Structure: Toe Movements

	Flexion	Extension	Abduction	Adduction
Articulation[1,2]	Metatarsophalangeal (MTP), proximal interphalangeal (PIP), distal interphalangeal (DIP) (second to fifth toes)	MTP PIP DIP	MTP	MTP
Plane	Sagittal	Sagittal	Transverse	Transverse
Axis	Frontal	Frontal	Vertical	Vertical
Normal limiting factors[1,3,4,6*] (See Fig. 8-6)	MTP: tension in the dorsal joint capsule, extensor muscles, collateral ligaments PIP: soft tissue apposition between the plantar aspects of the phalanges; tension in the dorsal joint capsule, collateral ligaments DIP: tension in the dorsal joint capsule, collateral ligaments, and oblique retinacular ligaments	MTP: tension in the plantar joint capsule, plantar ligament, flexor muscles PIP: tension in the plantar joint capsule plantar ligament DIP: tension in the plantar joint capsule, plantar ligament	MTP: tension in the medial joint capsule, collateral ligaments, adductor muscles, fascia and skin of the web spaces, and the plantar interosseous muscles	MTP: contact between the toes
Normal end feel[3,7]	MTP firm PIP soft/firm DIP firm	MTP firm PIP firm DIP firm	Firm	

Normal AROM[8]	Great toe
	  MTP 0–45°
	  IP 0–90°
	Toes 2–5
	  MTP 0–40°
	  PIP 0–35°
	  DIP 0–60°
		Great toe
		  MTP 0–70°
		  IP 0°
		Toes 2–5
		  MTP 0–40°
		  IP 0°		

Capsular pattern[7,10]	First MTP joint: extension, flexion Second to fifth MTP joints: variable, tend to fix in extension with the IP joints in flexion			

*Note: There is a paucity of definitive research that identifies the normal limiting factors (NLF) of joint motion. The NLF and end feels listed here are based on knowledge of anatomy, clinical experience, and available references.

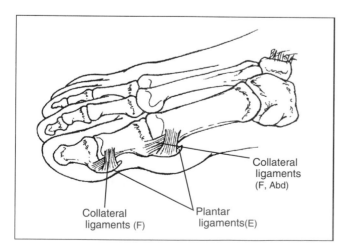

Collateral ligaments (F, Abd)

Collateral ligaments (F)

Plantar ligaments(E)

Figure 8-6 Anteromedial view of the foot showing noncontractile structures that normally limit motion at the MTP and IP joints (medial collateral ligaments not shown). Motion limited by structures is identified in brackets, using the following abbreviations: F, flexion; E, extension; Abd, abduction; Add, adduction. Muscles normally limiting motion are not illustrated.

SURFACE ANATOMY

(Figs. 8-7 through 8-9)

Structure	Location
1. Head of the fibula	Round bony prominence on the lateral aspect of the leg level with the tibial tuberosity.
2. Anterior border of the tibia	Subcutaneous bony ridge along the anterior aspect of the leg.
3. Achilles tendon	Prominent ridge on the posterior aspect of the ankle; tendon edges are palpable proximal to the posterior aspect of the calcaneus.
4. Medial malleolus	Prominent distal end of the tibia on the medial aspect of the ankle.
5. Lateral malleolus	Prominent distal end of the fibula on the lateral aspect of the ankle.
6. Tuberosity of the navicular bone	About 2.5 cm inferior and anterior to the medial malleolus.
7. Base of the fifth metatarsal bone	Small bony prominence at the midpoint of the lateral border of the foot.
8. Head of the first metatarsal	Round bony prominence at the medial aspect of the ball of the foot, at the base of the great toe.
9. Calcaneus	Posterior aspect of the heel.

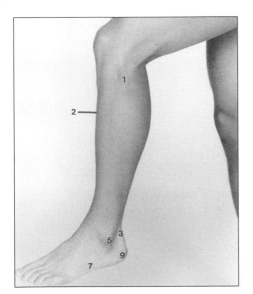

Figure 8-7 Anterolateral aspect of the leg and foot.

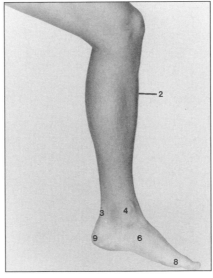

Figure 8-8 Medial aspect of the leg and foot.

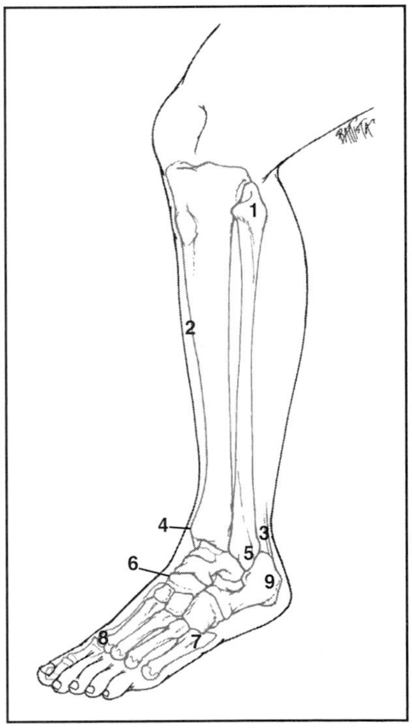

Figure 8-9 Bony anatomy, anterolateral aspect of the leg and foot.

RANGE OF MOTION ASSESSMENT AND MEASUREMENT

Ankle Dorsiflexion and Plantarflexion

AROM Assessment

Substitute Movement. Dorsiflexion—Knee extension, toe extension. Plantarflexion—Knee flexion, toe flexion.

PROM Assessment

Ankle Dorsiflexion

Start Position. The patient is supine. A roll is placed under the knee to position the knee in about 20° to 30° flexion and place the gastrocnemius on slack (Fig. 8-10A). The an-

kle is in the anatomical or neutral position with the foot perpendicular to the lower leg (see Fig. 8-10B).

Stabilization. The therapist stabilizes the tibia and fibula.

Therapist's Distal Hand Placement. The therapist grasps the posterior aspect of the calcaneus and places the forearm against the plantar aspect of the forefoot.

End Position. The therapist applies traction to the calcaneus and using the forearm moves the dorsal aspect of the foot toward the anterior aspect of the lower leg to the limit of ankle dorsiflexion (Fig. 8-11).

End Feel. Dorsiflexion—firm/hard.

Joint Glide. Dorsiflexion—convex body of the talus glides posteriorly on the fixed concave ankle mortise.

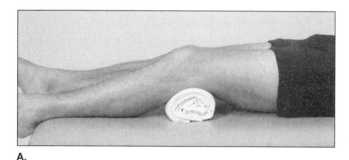

A.

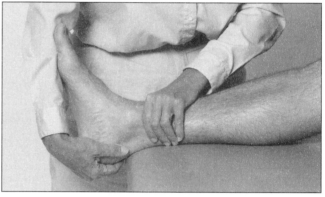

B.

Figure 8-10 A. Position of knee in 20° to 30° flexion for assessment of ankle dorsiflexion. **B.** Start position: ankle dorsiflexion.

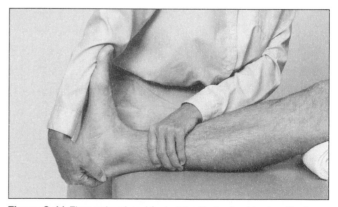

Figure 8-11 Firm or hard end feel at the limit of ankle dorsiflexion.

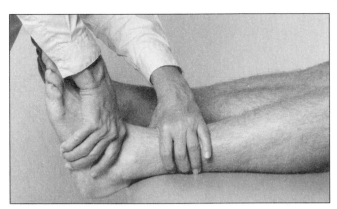

Figure 8-12 Start position for ankle plantarflexion.

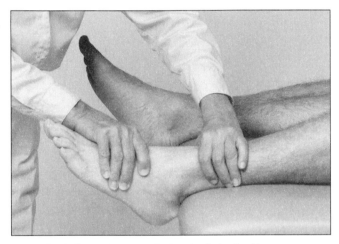

Figure 8-13 Firm or hard end feel at the limit of ankle plantarflexion.

Ankle Plantarflexion

Start Position. The patient is supine. A roll is placed under the knee to maintain about 20° to 30° knee flexion, and the ankle is in the neutral position (Fig. 8-12).

Stabilization. The therapist stabilizes the tibia and fibula.

Therapist's Distal Hand Placement. The therapist grasps the dorsum of the foot with the radial border of the index finger over the anterior aspects of the talus and calcaneus.

End Position. The therapist applies slight traction to and moves the talus and calcaneus in a downward direction to the limit of ankle plantarflexion (Fig. 8-13).

End Feel. Plantarflexion—firm/hard.

Joint Glide. Plantarflexion—convex body of the talus glides anteriorly on the fixed concave ankle mortise.

Measurement: Universal Goniometer

Ankle Dorsiflexion and Plantarflexion

Start Position. The patient is supine with a roll placed under the knee to maintain about 20° to 30° knee flexion and place the gastrocnemius on slack (see Fig. 8-10A). The ankle is in the anatomical position 0° (Fig. 8-14). Alternatively, the patient may be sitting with the knee flexed to 90° and the ankle in anatomical position (Fig. 8-15).

Stabilization. The therapist stabilizes the tibia and fibula.

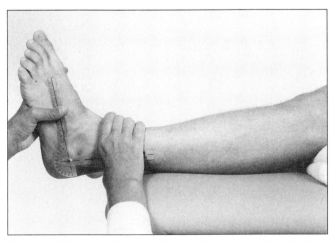

Figure 8-14 Start position for ankle dorsiflexion and plantarflexion.

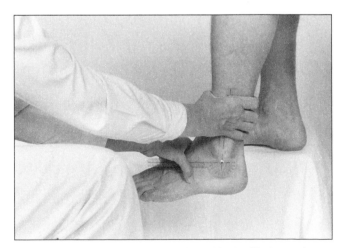

Figure 8-15 Alternate start position for ankle dorsiflexion and plantarflexion.

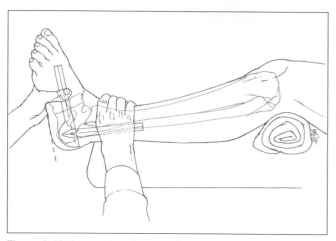

Figure 8-16 Goniometer alignment for ankle dorsiflexion and plantarflexion.

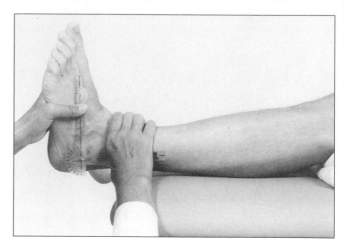

Figure 8-17 Dorsiflexion.

Goniometer Axis. The axis is placed inferior to the lateral malleolus (Fig. 8-16). This measurement may also be obtained by placing the axis inferior to the medial malleolus (not shown).

Stationary Arm. Parallel to the longitudinal axis of the fibula, pointing toward the head of the fibula.

Movable Arm. Parallel to the sole of the heel, to eliminate forefoot movement from the measurement. In the start position described, the goniometer will indicate 90°. This is recorded as 0°. For example, if the goniometer reads 90° at the start position for ankle dorsiflexion and 80° at the end position, ankle dorsiflexion PROM would be 10°.

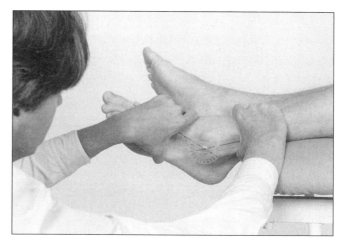

Figure 8-18 Plantarflexion.

End Positions. *Dorsiflexion* (Fig. 8-17): The ankle is flexed with the dorsal aspect of the foot approximating the anterior aspect of the lower leg (20°). *Plantarflexion* (Fig. 8-18): The ankle is extended to the limit of motion (50°).

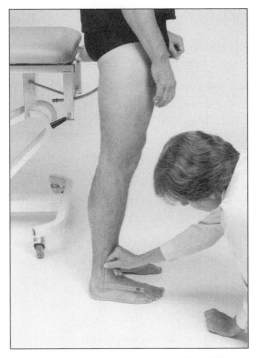

Figure 8-19 Alternate start position for ankle dorsiflexion.

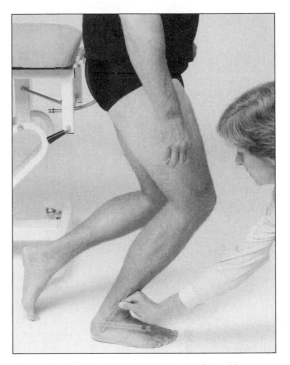

Figure 8-20 Goniometer measurement for ankle dorsiflexion.

Alternate Measurement

This test may be contraindicated for patients with poor standing balance or generalized or specific lower extremity weakness.

Start Position. The patient is standing erect (Fig. 8-19). The nontest foot is off the ground or only lightly touching the ground to assist with balance (Fig. 8-20).

Stabilization. The patient uses the parallel bars or other stable structure for balance. The foot on the test side is stabilized by the patient's body weight.

End Position. The patient is instructed to maintain the foot on the test side flat on the floor, with the toes point-ing forward, and to flex the knee as far as possible (see Fig. 8-20). *Note:* If the soleus muscle is shortened, the patient will feel a muscle stretch over the posterior aspect of the calf and ankle dorsiflexion ROM will be restricted proportional to the decrease in muscle length.

Measurement: Universal Goniometer

The therapist measures and records the available ankle dorsiflexion PROM. The goniometer is placed as described for measuring ankle dorsiflexion ROM (see Fig. 8-16). Ankle dorsiflexion PROM measured in weight-bearing is greater than in non–weight-bearing positions. If dorsiflexion is measured in weight-bearing, this is noted when recording the ROM.

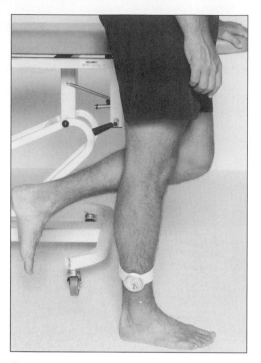

Figure 8-21 Start position for OB goniometer measurement of ankle dorsiflexion.

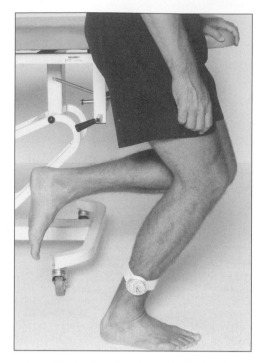

Figure 8-22 End position for ankle dorsiflexion.

Measurement: OB Goniometer

Goniometer Placement. The strap is placed around the lower leg proximal to the ankle. The dial is placed on the lateral aspect of the lower leg (Fig. 8-21). With the patient in the start position, the inclination needle is aligned with the 0° arrow of the fluid-filled container. At the end posi-

tion, the number of degrees the inclination needle moves away from the 0° arrow on the inclinometer dial is recorded as the ankle dorsiflexion PROM (Fig. 8-22). (Alternatively, a standard inclinometer can be placed on the anterior border of the tibia to measure ankle dorsiflexion in standing [not shown].)

Subtalar Inversion and Eversion

AROM Assessment

Substitute Movement. Inversion—hip external rotation. Eversion—hip internal rotation.

Measurement: Universal Goniometer

Start Position. The patient is supine (Fig. 8-23). A roll is placed under the knee to maintain slight flexion. The ankle is in the neutral position. A piece of paper, adhered to a flat surface, is placed under the heel. A flat-surfaced object (Plexiglass or book) is placed against the full sole of the foot. A line is drawn along the Plexiglass or book as shown in Figure 8-23.

Stabilization. The therapist stabilizes the tibia and fibula.

End Positions. The foot is placed in inversion to the limit of motion (Fig. 8-24). The Plexiglass is again positioned against the full sole of the foot in this position and a line is again drawn along the Plexiglass (Fig. 8-25). The process is repeated at the limit of eversion AROM (Figs. 8-26 and 8-27).

Goniometer Axis and Arms. The goniometer is placed on the line graphics to obtain a measure of the arc of movement (Figs. 8-28 and 8-29).

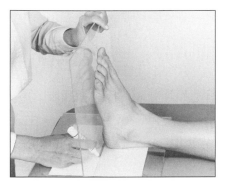

Figure 8-23 Start position for foot inversion and eversion AROM.

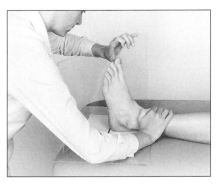

Figure 8-24 Placement of the foot in inversion.

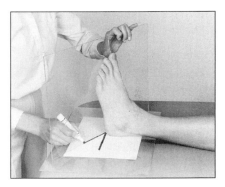

Figure 8-25 Inversion.

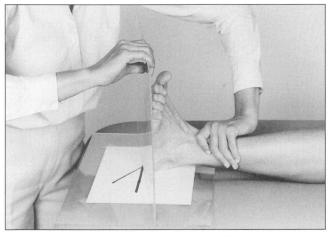

Figure 8-26 Placement of the foot in eversion.

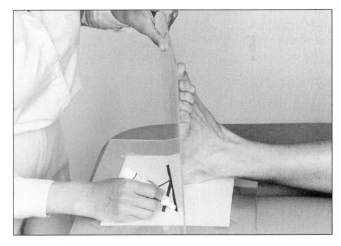

Figure 8-27 Eversion.

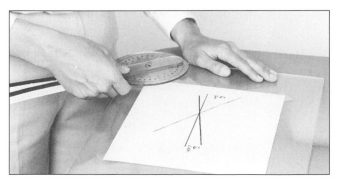

Figure 8-28 Completed measurements of inversion and eversion AROM.

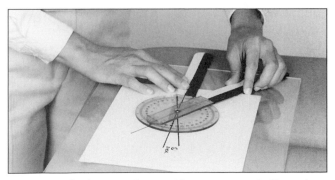

Figure 8-29 Goniometer placement for measurement of inversion AROM.

PROM Assessment

Start Position. The patient is supine. The ankle is in the neutral position (Fig. 8-30).

Stabilization. The therapist stabilizes the talus immediately anterior and inferior to the medial and lateral malleoli. Current research (11) appears to support positioning the ankle in dorsiflexion to assist in stabilizing the talus, as the wider anterior aspect of the body of the talus is wedged within the mortise.

Therapist's Distal Hand Placement. The therapist grasps the posterior aspect and sides of the calcaneus.

End Positions. The therapist applies slight traction to the calcaneus and moves the calcaneus inward to the limit of inversion (Fig. 8-31) and outward to the limit of eversion (Fig. 8-32).

End Feels. Inversion—firm; eversion—hard/firm.

Joint Glides. *Inversion*—(a) posterior subtalar joint surfaces: the convex surface of the calcaneus glides laterally on the fixed concave surface of the talus; (b) anterior subtalar joint surfaces: the concave surfaces of the middle and anterior facets of the calcaneus glide medially on the fixed convex surface of the head of the talus. *Eversion*—(a) posterior subtalar joint surfaces: the convex surface of the calcaneus glides medially on the fixed concave surface of the talus; (b) anterior subtalar joint surfaces: the concave surfaces of the middle and anterior facets of the calcaneus glide laterally on the fixed convex surface of the head of the talus.

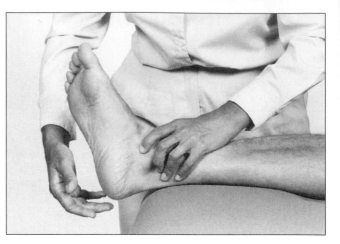

Figure 8-30 Start position for inversion and eversion.

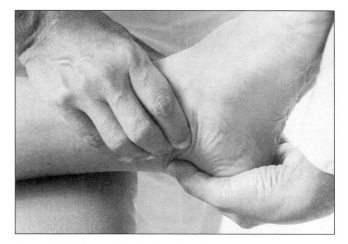

Figure 8-31 Firm end feel at the limit of inversion.

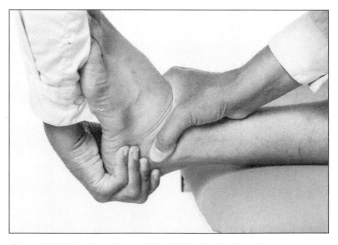

Figure 8-32 Hard or firm end feel at the limit of eversion.

Measurement: Universal Goniometer

Start Position. The patient is prone with the feet off the end of the plinth and the ankle in the neutral position. For alignment of the goniometer, the therapist marks the skin over the midlines of the superior aspect of the calcaneus posteriorly and the inferior aspect of the heel pad posteriorly (Fig. 8-33A).

Stabilization. The therapist stabilizes the tibia and fibula.

Goniometer Axis. The axis is placed over the mark placed at the midline of the superior aspect of the calcaneus (Figs. 8-33B and 8-34).

Stationary Arm. Parallel to the longitudinal axis of the lower leg.

Movable Arm. Lies along the midline of the posterior aspect of the calcaneus. Use the mark on the heel pad posteriorly to assist in maintaining alignment of the movable arm.

End Positions. The calcaneus is passively inverted (Fig. 8-35) and then passively everted (Fig. 8-36) to the limits of motion.

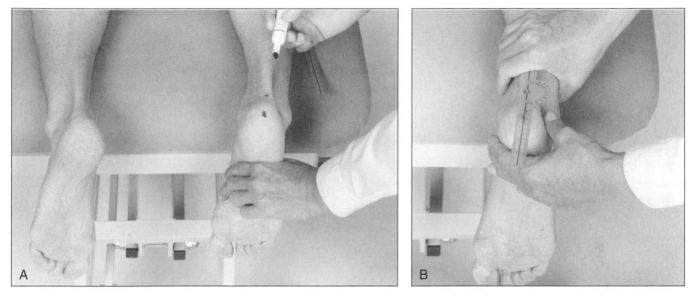

Figure 8-33 A. Subtalar inversion and eversion. Points marked for alignment of goniometer. **B.** Goniometer alignment for subtalar joint inversion and eversion.

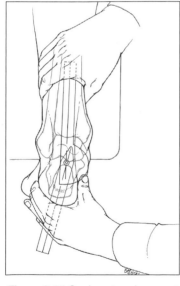

Figure 8-34 Goniometer placement for inversion and eversion, shown with the subtalar joint in eversion.

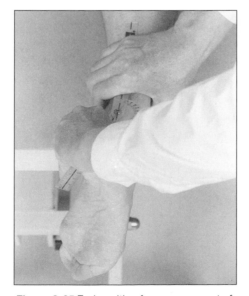

Figure 8-35 End position for measurement of inversion.

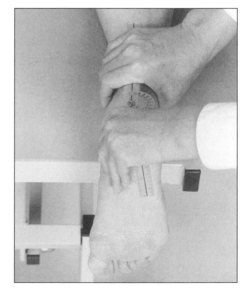

Figure 8-36 End position for measurement of eversion.

MTP Joint Flexion and Extension of the Great Toe

AROM Assessment

PROM Assessment

Start Position. The patient is supine. The ankle and toes are in the neutral position (Fig. 8-37).

Stabilization. The therapist stabilizes the first metatarsal.

Therapist's Distal Hand Placement. The therapist grasps the proximal phalanx.

End Positions. The therapist applies slight traction to and moves the proximal phalanx of the great toe to the limit of MTP joint flexion (Fig. 8-38) and MTP joint extension (Fig. 8-39).

End Feels. MTP joint flexion—firm; MTP joint extension—firm.

Joint Glides. *MTP joint flexion*—the concave base of the proximal phalanx glides in a plantar direction on the fixed convex head of the adjacent metatarsal. *MTP joint extension*—the concave base of the proximal phalanx glides in a dorsal direction on the fixed convex head of the adjacent metatarsal.

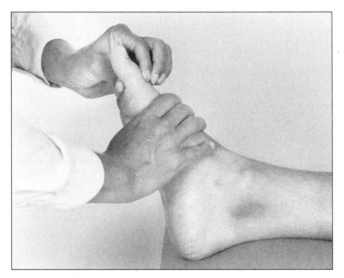

Figure 8-37 Start position for MTP joint flexion and extension.

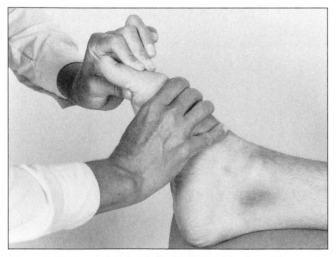

Figure 8-38 Firm end feel at limit of MTP joint flexion of the great toe.

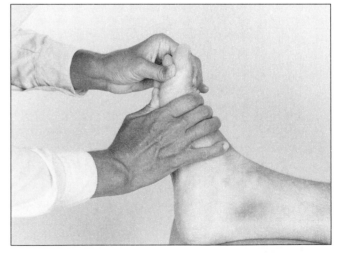

Figure 8-39 Firm end feel at limit of MTP joint extension of the great toe.

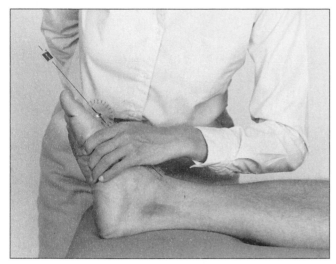

Figure 8-40 Start position for MTP joint flexion.

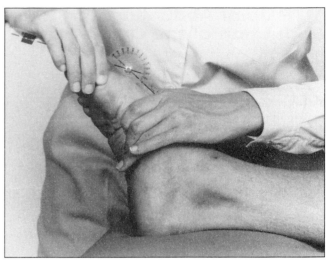

Figure 8-42 MTP joint flexion of the great toe.

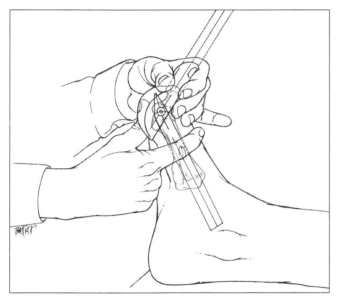

Figure 8-41 Goniometer alignment for MTP joint flexion and extension.

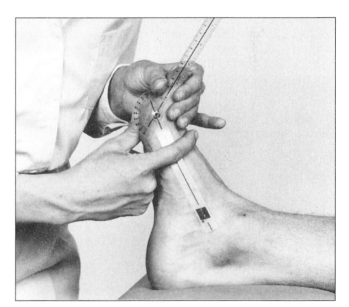

Figure 8-43 MTP joint extension of the great toe.

Measurement: Universal Goniometer

Start Position. The patient is supine or sitting. The ankle and toes are in the neutral position (Fig. 8-40).

Stabilization. The therapist stabilizes the metatarsal of the MTP joint.

Goniometer Axis. For MTP joint flexion, the axis is placed over the dorsum of the MTP joint (see Fig. 8-40). For MTP joint extension, the goniometer axis is placed over the plantar aspect of the MTP joint (not shown). Alternatively, the axis can be placed over the MTP joint axis on the medial aspect of the great toe (Fig. 8-41 and 8-43).

Stationary Arm. Parallel to the longitudinal axis of the first metatarsal.

Movable Arm. Parallel to the longitudinal axis of the proximal phalanx of the great toe.

End Positions. The MTP joint is flexed to the limit of motion (45° for the great toe) (Fig. 8-42). The MTP joint of the toe being measured is extended to the limit of motion (70° for the great toe) (Fig. 8-43).

MTP Joint Flexion/Extension of the Lesser Four Toes

Flexion and extension at the MTP joints of the lesser four toes is normally not measured using a universal goniometer. The MTP joints of the lesser four toes are flexed to the limit of motion (40°) and extended to the limit of motion (40°). The ROM is observed and recorded as either full or decreased.

MTP Joint Abduction and Adduction of the Great Toe

PROM Assessment (MTP Joint Abduction)

Start Position. The patient is supine. The ankle and great toe are in the neutral position.

Stabilization. The therapist stabilizes the first metatarsal.

Therapist's Distal Hand Placement. The therapist grasps the proximal phalanx of the great toe.

End Position. The therapist applies slight traction to and moves the proximal phalanx to the limit of MTP joint abduction (Fig. 8-44).

End Feel. MTP joint abduction—firm.

Joint Glide. *MTP joint abduction*—the concave base of the proximal phalanx glides laterally (relative to the midline of the foot that passes through the second toe) on the fixed convex head of the first metatarsal.

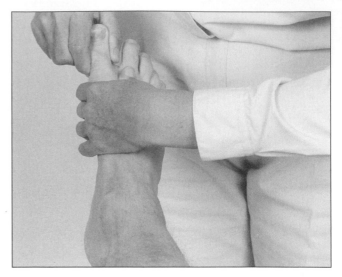

Figure 8-44 Firm end feel at limit of MTP joint abduction.

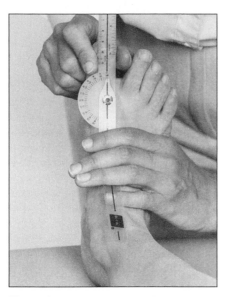

Figure 8-45 Start position for MTP joint abduction and adduction.

Measurement: Universal Goniometer

Start Position. The patient is supine or sitting. The ankle and toes are in the neutral position (Fig. 8-45).

Stabilization. The therapist stabilizes the first metatarsal and the foot proximal to the MTP joint.

Goniometer Axis. The axis is placed on the dorsum of the first MTP joint (Figs. 8-45 and 8-46).

Stationary Arm. Parallel to the longitudinal axis of the first metatarsal.

Movable Arm. Parallel to the longitudinal axis of the proximal phalanx of the great toe.

End Position. The MTP joint is abducted to the limit of motion (Fig. 8-47) and adducted to the limit of motion (Fig. 8-48).

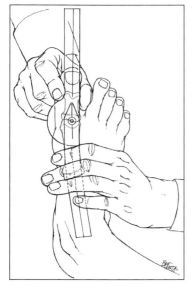

Figure 8-46 Start position and goniometer alignment for MTP joint abduction and adduction.

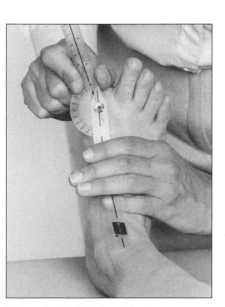

Figure 8-47 MTP joint abduction.

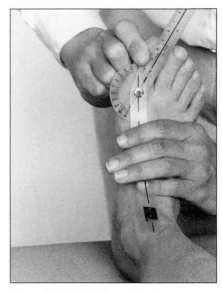

Figure 8-48 MTP joint adduction.

IP Joint Flexion/Extension of the Great Toe

AROM Assessment

PROM Assessment

Start Position. The patient is supine. The ankle and great toe are in the neutral position.

Stabilization. The therapist stabilizes the proximal phalanx of the great toe.

Therapist's Distal Hand Placement. The therapist grasps the distal phalanx of the great toe.

End Positions. The therapist applies slight traction to and moves the distal phalanx to the limit of IP joint flexion (Fig. 8-49) and IP joint extension (Fig. 8-50).

End Feels. IP joint flexion—soft or firm; IP joint extension—firm.

Joint Glides. *IP joint flexion*—the concave base of the distal phalanx of the great toe glides in a plantar direction on the fixed convex head of the proximal phalanx of the great toe. *IP joint extension*—the concave base of the distal phalanx of the great toe glides in a dorsal direction on the fixed convex head of the proximal phalanx of the great toe.

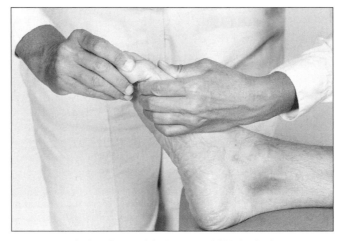

Figure 8-49 Soft or firm end feel at limit of IP joint flexion.

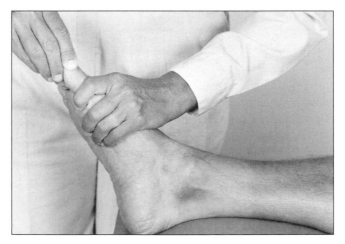

Figure 8-50 Firm end feel at limit of IP joint extension.

Measurement: Universal Goniometer

Start Position. The patient is supine or sitting. The ankle and toes are in the neutral position (Fig. 8-51).

Stabilization. The therapist stabilizes the proximal phalanx.

Goniometer Axis. The axis is placed over the dorsal aspect of the IP joint for flexion and the plantar aspect of the IP joint for extension (not shown).

Stationary Arm. Parallel to the longitudinal axis of the proximal phalanx.

Movable Arm. Parallel to the longitudinal axis of the distal phalanx.

End Positions. The IP joint is flexed to the limit of motion (90° for the great toe) (Fig. 8-52). The IP joint is extended to the limit of motion (0° for the great toe; not shown).

MTP and IP Joint Flexion/Extension of the Lesser Four Toes

Flexion and extension at the MTP and IP joints of the lesser four toes is normally not measured using a universal goniometer. The lesser four toes are flexed and extended as a group, and the ROM is observed and recorded as either full or decreased (not shown).

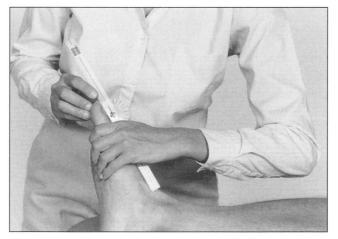

Figure 8-51 Start position for great toe IP joint flexion.

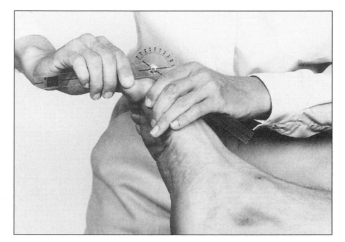

Figure 8-52 IP joint flexion of the great toe.

MUSCLE LENGTH ASSESSMENT AND MEASUREMENT

Gastrocnemius

Origins (2)	Insertion (2)
Gastrocnemius	
a. Medial head: proximal and posterior aspect of the medial condyle of the femur posterior to the adductor tubercle.	Via the Achilles tendon into the calcaneus.
b. Lateral head: lateral and posterior aspect of the lateral condyle of the femur; lower part of the supracondylar line.	

Start Position. The patient is standing erect with the lower extremity in the anatomical position. The patient is positioned facing a stable plinth or wall.

End Position. The patient places the nontest leg ahead of the test leg and leans forward to place the hands on the plinth or wall (Fig. 8-53). The patient is instructed to maintain the foot on the test side flat on the floor, with the toes pointing forward, and to keep the knee in full extension as the leg moves over the foot. The gastrocnemius is placed on full stretch as the patient leans closer toward the supporting surface.

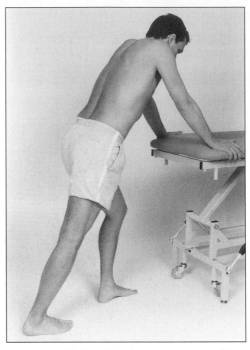

Figure 8-53 End position for measurement of the length of gastrocnemius.

Measurement: Universal Goniometer

If the gastrocnemius is shortened, ankle dorsiflexion ROM will be restricted proportional to the decrease in muscle length. The therapist measures and records the available ankle dorsiflexion PROM. The goniometer is placed as described for measuring ankle dorsiflexion ROM (Fig. 8-54 and 8-55). The patient may flex the knee during the test

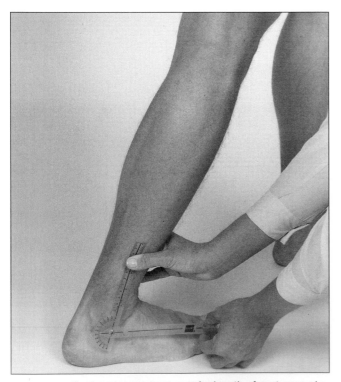

Figure 8-54 Goniometer measurement for length of gastrocnemius.

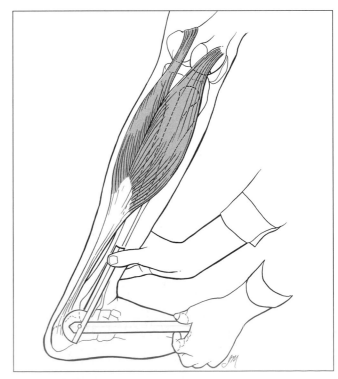

Figure 8-55 Gastrocnemius on stretch.

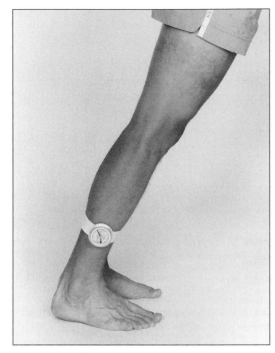

Figure 8-56 OB goniometer measurement for gastrocnemius muscle length.

to place the gastrocnemius on slack. The knee must be maintained in extension.

Measurement: OB Goniometer

Goniometer Placement. The strap is placed around the lower leg proximal to the ankle (Fig. 8-56). The dial is placed on the lateral aspect of the lower leg. With the patient in the start position, the inclination needle is aligned with the 0° arrow of the fluid-filled container. At the end position, the number of degrees the inclination needle moves away from the 0° arrow on the inclinometer dial is recorded to represent the length of the gastrocnemius muscle.

Note: If the contralateral (i.e., nontest) leg is not placed ahead of the test leg, ensure the heel of the nontest leg is raised slightly off the floor. This position ensures a true test for gastrocnemius tightness on the test side because the amount of forward lean the patient achieves will not be limited by contralateral gastrocnemius tightness, if present.

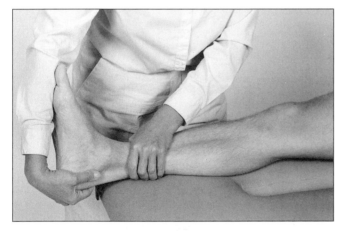

Figure 8-57 Alternate start position for gastrocnemius length.

Alternate Test

Start Position. The patient is supine. The leg is in the anatomical position with the knee in extension (0°) (Fig. 8-57).

Stabilization. The therapist stabilizes the lower leg.

End Position. The foot is moved to the limit of ankle dorsiflexion (Fig. 8-58).

End Feel. Gastrocnemius on stretch—firm.

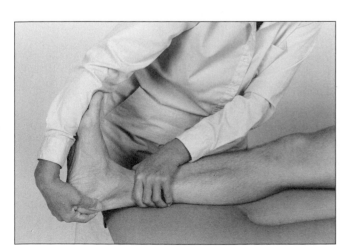

Figure 8-58 Gastrocnemius on stretch.

FUNCTIONAL APPLICATION

Joint Function

The foot functions as a flexible base to accommodate rough terrain (12) and functions as a rigid lever during terminal stance of the walking pattern (5). In transmitting forces between the ground and the leg, the foot absorbs shock (12). With the foot planted, the ankle and foot elevate the body, and when off the ground, the foot is used to manipulate machinery (12). When weight is taken through the foot, the MTP joints allow movement of the rigid foot over the toes (5).

Functional Range of Motion (Table 8-3)

Ankle Dorsiflexion and Plantarflexion

The normal AROM of the ankle joint is 20° dorsiflexion and 50° plantarflexion. However, ankle dorsiflexion ROM measured in weight-bearing (e.g., on stairs, when rising from sitting) is greater than in non–weight-bearing positions.

The full range of ankle dorsiflexion is necessary to descend stairs (Fig. 8-59). Rising from sitting (Fig. 8-60) also requires significant ankle dorsiflexion ROM (i.e., an average of 28° [13]).

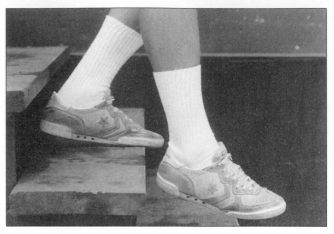

Figure 8-59 Full range of ankle dorsiflexion is required to descend stairs.

Full ankle plantarflexion may be required when climbing, jumping, or reaching high objects (Fig. 8-61). Less than the full range of ankle plantarflexion may be used to perform activities such as depressing the accelerator of a motor vehicle (Fig. 8-62) or the foot pedals of a piano and wearing high-heeled shoes.

Livingston and colleagues (14) found that maximum ankle dorsiflexion ROM requirements to ascend and descend ranged between averages of 14° and 27° to ascend and 21° and 36° to descend stairs. The average maximum ankle plantarflexion ROM requirements ranged from 23° to 30° to ascend and 24° to 31° to descend stairs (14).

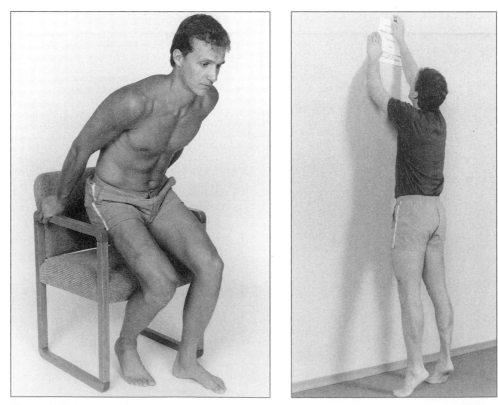

Figure 8-60 Ankle dorsiflexion is required to rise from sitting.

Figure 8-61 Ankle plantarflexion and toe extension.

TABLE 8-3 Ankle and Great Toe ROM Required for Selected ADL

Activity	Ankle Dorsiflexion	Ankle Plantarflexion	Great Toe MTP Extension
Rising from sitting*	28°		
Ascending stairs[†]	14–27°	23–30°	
Descending stairs[†]	21–36°	24–31°	
Walking	10°[‡]	20°[‡]	90°[15]
Running[§]	17°	32°	

*Average of young and elderly average values from original source.[13]

[†]Ankle dorsiflexion and plantarflexion ROM values for 15 subjects during ascent and descent of three stairs of different dimensions. Maximum ankle dorsiflexion and plantarflexion requirements varied depending on the stair dimensions and subject height.[14]

[‡]Data from the Rancho Los Amigos gait analysis forms as cited in the work of Levangie and Norkin.[5]

[§]There were no differences in average ankle ROM at fast-paced (faster than a 7.5-minute mile) and slow-paced (slower than an 8-minute mile) running.[16]

Movements of the Foot

The AROM of the subtalar joint is 5° each for inversion and eversion without forefoot movement. The ranges of inversion and eversion may be augmented by forefoot movement of 35° and 15°, respectively. The subtalar, transverse tarsal joints, and joints of the forefoot must be fully mobile to allow the foot to accommodate to varying degrees of rough terrain (Fig. 8-63). With the foot across the opposite thigh, inversion is required to inspect the foot.

In standing, the MTP joints are in at least 25° extension due to the downward slope of the metatarsals (2). Ranges approximating the full 90° of extension of the MTP joint of the great toe are required for many activities of daily living (ADL) (15). Extension of the great toe and lesser four toes is essential for activities such as rising onto the

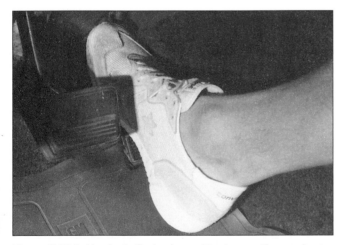

Figure 8-62 Ankle plantarflexion is used to depress the accelerator of a motor vehicle.

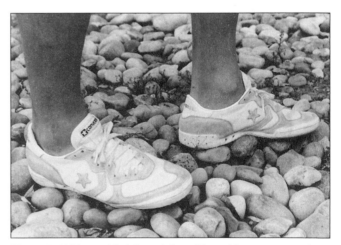

Figure 8-63 The mobile joints of the ankle and foot accommodate rough terrain.

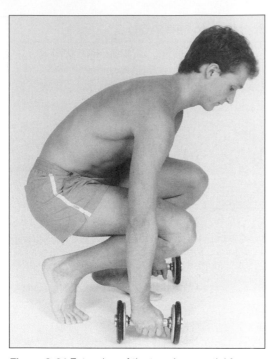

Figure 8-64 Extension of the toes is essential for squatting.

Running requires a range of ankle joint motion from an average of 17° dorsiflexion at midstance to an average 32° maximum ankle plantarflexion at early swing (16). Ankle ROM was the same when fast-paced running was compared to slow-paced running (16).

References

1. Kapandji IA. *The Physiology of the Joints*. Vol. 1. 5th ed. New York: Churchill Livingstone; 1982.
2. Soames RW. Skeletal system. Salmon S, ed. Muscle. In: *Gray's Anatomy*. 38th ed. New York: Churchill Livingstone; 1995.
3. Norkin CC, White DJ. *Measurement of Joint Motion: A Guide to Goniometry*. 3rd ed. Philadelphia: FA Davis; 2003.
4. Daniels L, Worthingham C. *Muscle Testing: Techniques of Manual Examination*. 5th ed. Philadelphia: WB Saunders; 1986.
5. Levangie PK, Norkin CC. *Joint Structure & Function: A Comprehensive Analysis*. 3rd ed. Philadelphia: FA Davis; 2001.
6. Woodburne RT. *Essentials of Human Anatomy*. 5th ed. London: Oxford University Press; 1973.
7. Magee DJ. *Orthopedic Physical Assessment*. 4th ed. Philadelphia: WB Saunders; 2002.
8. American Academy of Orthopaedic Surgeons. *Joint Motion: Method of Measuring and Recording*. Chicago: AAOS; 1965.
9. Berryman Reese N, Bandy WD. *Joint Range of Motion and Muscle Length Testing*. Philadelphia: WB Saunders; 2002.
10. Cyriax J. *Textbook of Orthopaedic Medicine. Vol. 1. Diagnosis of Soft Tissue Lesions*. 8th ed. London: Bailliere Tindall; 1982.
11. Taylor Major KF, Bojescul Captain JA, Howard RS, et al. Measurement of isolated subtalar range of motion: a cadaver study. *Foot Ankle Int*. 2001;22:426–432.
12. Smith LK, Weiss EL, Lehmkuhl LD. *Brunnstrom's Clinical Kinesiology*. 5th ed. Philadelphia: FA Davis; 1996.
13. Ikeda ER, Schenkman ML, Riley PO, Hodge WA. Influence of age on dynamics of rising from a chair. *Phys Ther*. 1991;71:473–481.
14. Livingston LA, Stevenson JM, Olney SJ. Stairclimbing kinematics on stairs of differing dimensions. *Arch Phys Med Rehabil*. 1991;72:398–402.
15. Sammarco GJ, Hockenbury RT. Biomechanics of the foot and ankle. In: Nordin M, Frankel VH. *Basic Biomechanics of the Musculoskeletal System*. 3rd ed. Philadelphia: Lippincott Williams & Wilkins; 2001.
16. Pink M, Perry J, Houglum PA, Devine DJ. Lower extremity range of motion in the recreational sport runner. *Am J Sports Med*. 1994;22:541–549.
17. Thordarson DB, Schmotzer H, Chon J, Peters J. Dynamic support of the human longitudinal arch. *Clin Orthop Relat Res*. 1995;316:165–172.

toes to reach high objects (see Fig. 8-61) and squatting (Fig. 8-64). For most ADL, only a few degrees of flexion are required at the great toe (15). There appears to be no significant function that can be attributed to abduction and adduction at the MTP joints (5).

Gait

Normal walking (see Appendix D) requires a maximum of 10° of ankle dorsiflexion at midstance to terminal stance as the tibia advances over the fixed foot and a maximum of 20° of plantarflexion at the end of preswing (from the Rancho Los Amigos gait analysis forms as cited in the work of Levangie and Norkin [5]). At the MTP joint of the great toe, almost 90° of extension is required at preswing (15). Extension is also required of the lesser four toes (15). Extension of the toes stretches the plantar aponeurosis, resulting in significant longitudinal arch support (17).

EXERCISES AND QUESTIONS

See the Answer Guide in Appendix F for suggested answers to the following exercises and questions.

1. PALPATION

A. For each anatomical structure listed below, identify the ROM at the ankle or foot that would be measured using the structure to align the universal goniometer. Also identify the part of the goniometer (i.e., axis, stationary arm, or moveable arm) that would be aligned with the anatomical structure for the purpose of the measurement.

   i. Proximal phalanx of the great toe. _____

   ii. Mark placed at the midline of the posterior superior aspect of the calcaneus._____

   iii. Head of the fibula. _____

B. On a skeleton and on a partner, palpate the following anatomical structures.

First MTP joint line   Tip of the lateral malleolus

Posterior surface of the calcaneus   Head of the first metatarsal

Head of the fibula

2. ASSESSMENT PROCESS

Identify whether the following statements are true or false:

   i. AROM is assessed prior to assessing PROM at a joint.

   ii. End feels are determined when assessing PROM at a joint.

   iii. The presence or absence of pain is noted when assessing AROM and PROM at a joint.

   iv. The therapist always measures all PROM through goniometry when assessing a joint.

3. ASSESSMENT OF AROM AT THE ANKLE AND FOOT

For the ankle joint, subtalar joint, and IP joints:

   i. List the AROM a therapist would assess.

   ii. For each AROM listed, identify the axis and plane of movement.

   iii. Assume the start position for the assessment and measurement of the AROM and demonstrate the full available AROM at the joint.

4. ASSESSMENT AND MEASUREMENT OF PROM AT THE ANKLE AND FOOT

For each of the movements listed below, demonstrate the assessment and measurement of PROM on a partner and answer the questions that follow. Have a third partner evaluate your performance using the appropriate practical test form in Appendix E. Record your findings on the PROM Recording Form on pages 220 and 221.

Ankle Dorsiflexion

   i. What normal end feel(s) would be expected when assessing ankle dorsiflexion? Identify the end feel for ankle dorsiflexion on your partner.

   ii. What position is the knee placed in when assessing ankle dorsiflexion ROM? Explain why the knee is placed in this position.

   iii. Identify and describe the shape of the articular components that make up the ankle joint.

Ankle Plantarflexion

   i. Have your partner assume the start position for assessment of ankle dorsiflexion/plantarflexion. Have your partner perform full ankle dorsiflexion and plantarflexion and observe the contour of the lateral border of the foot. What part of the lateral border of the foot is mobile and what part is immobile? Using the universal goniometer to measure ankle joint dorsiflexion/plantarflexion, to what part of the lateral border of the foot would the therapist align the moveable arm of the goniometer to avoid an erroneous measurement due to substitute motion?

ii. Identify the direction of glide of the talus during ankle plantarflexion.

iii. Identify the normal limiting factors that create the normal end feel(s) for ankle plantarflexion. What normal end feel(s) is/are produced by these normal limiting factors?

Subtalar Inversion

If a patient presented with decreased subtalar joint inversion PROM:

i. Identify the glide of the posterior facet of the calcaneus that would be limited.

ii. Identify the glide of the anterior and middle facets of the calcaneus that would be limited.

iii. Explain the reason for the glides being decreased in the direction(s) indicated in i. and ii.

Great Toe MTP Joint Extension

i. When assessing great toe MTP joint extension PROM, you note decreased PROM and a firm end feel. Would the firm end feel be considered a normal finding? Explain.

ii. If a patient has decreased passive great toe MTP joint extension ROM, what glide of the base of the proximal phalanx of the great toe would be decreased? Explain the reason for the glide being decreased in the direction indicated.

iii. Identify the pattern of movement restriction at the MTP joint in the presence of a capsular pattern.

PROM RECORDING FORM

Patient's Name _____   Therapist _____

Left Side				Date of Measurement	Right Side			
*		*		**Date of Measurement**	*		*	
				Ankle				
				Dorsiflexion (0–20°)				
				Plantarflexion (0–50°)				
				Inversion (0–35°)				
				Eversion (0–15°)				
				Hypermobility:				
				Comments:				
				Toes				
				MTP great toe flexion (0–45°)				
				extension (0–70°)				
				abduction				
				MTP digit 2 flexion (0–40°)				
				extension (0–40°)				
				MTP digit 3 flexion (0–40°)				
				extension (0–40°)				

				MTP digit 4 flexion	(0–40°)				
				extension	(0–40°)				
				MTP digit 5 flexion	(0–40°)				
				extension	(0–40°)				
				IP great toe flexion	(0–90°)				
				PIP digit 2 flexion	(0–35°)				
				PIP digit 3 flexion	(0–35°)				
				PIP digit 4 flexion	(0–35°)				
				PIP digit 5 flexion	(0–35°)				
				Hypermobility: Comments:					

Summary of Limitation:

Additional Comments:

5. MUSCLE LENGTH ASSESSMENT AND MEASUREMENT

Gastrocnemius

i.   Identify the origin and insertion of the gastrocnemius muscle.

ii. What movements of the lower extremity would move the origin and insertion of the gastrocnemius muscle farther apart and thus place the muscle on stretch?

iii. Demonstrate the assessment and measurement of gastrocnemius muscle length on a partner. Have a third partner evaluate your performance using the appropriate practical test form in Appendix E.

iv. If the gastrocnemius muscle is shortened, what end feel would the therapist note at the limit of ankle PROM when assessing gastrocnemius muscle length?

6. FUNCTIONAL ROM AT THE KNEE

A. Normal walking requires a maximum of _____° of ankle dorsiflexion at midstance to terminal stance as the tibia advances over the fixed foot and a maximum of ___° of plantarflexion at the end of preswing.

B. For each movement listed below, identify three daily activities that require the specified movement, and demonstrate each activity:

i.   ankle dorsiflexion

ii. ankle plantarflexion

iii. toe extension

C. Have a partner perform the following activities and, using a universal goniometer, determine the maximum ankle dorsiflexion ROM required to perform each activity in a normal manner.

i.   Rise from sitting on a standard-height chair

ii. Descend a standard-height step

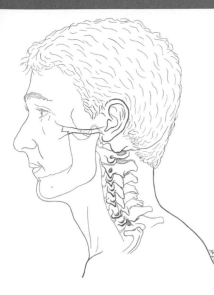

Head, Neck, and Trunk

ARTICULATIONS AND MOVEMENTS

The articulations and joint axes of the temporomandibular joint (TMJ) and cervical spine are illustrated in Figures 9-1, 9-2, and 9-3. The joint structure and movements of the TMJ and cervical spine are described below and summarized in Tables 9-1 and 9-2.

The Temporomandibular Joints

The TMJs, located on each side of the head just anterior to the ears, are individually described as condylar joints and together form a bicondylar articulation (2), being linked via the mandible (lower jaw). The TMJs are evaluated together as a functional unit. The articular surfaces of the TMJ are incongruent mates, but an articular disc positioned between

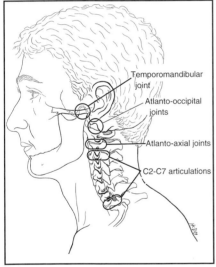

Figure 9-1 TMJ and cervical spine articulations.

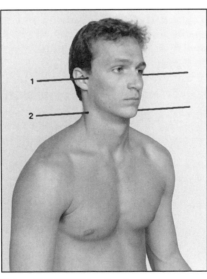

Figure 9-2 (1) TMJ axis: elevation-depression. (2) Cervical spine axis: flexion-extension.

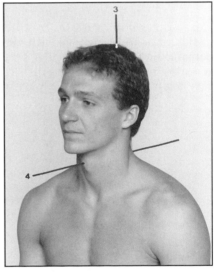

Figure 9-3 Cervical spine axes: (3) rotation; (4) lateral flexion.

TABLE 9-1   Joint Structure: Jaw Movements

	Opening of the Mouth (Depression of the Mandible)	Closing of the Mouth (Occlusion)	Protrusion	Retrusion	Lateral Deviation
Articulation[1,2]	Temporomandibular (TM)	TM	TM	TM	TM
Plane	Sagittal	Sagittal	Horizontal	Horizontal	Horizontal
Axis	Frontal	Frontal			
Normal limiting factors* (See Figs. 9-4 9-5, and 9-6)	Tension in the lateral/ temporomandibular ligament and the retrodiscal tissue[2]	Occlusion or contact of the teeth[3]	Tension in the sphenomandibular and stylomandibular ligaments		
Normal AROM† (tape measure)	35–50 cm[4]	Contact of teeth	3–7 mm[5]		5–12 mm[6]
Capsular pattern[4,7]	Limitation of mouth opening				

*Note: There is a paucity of definitive research that identifies the normal limiting factors (NLF) of joint motion. The NLF and end feels listed here are based on knowledge of anatomy, clinical experience, and available references.
†AROM, active range of motion.

these surfaces promotes congruency and divides the TMJ into upper and lower compartments (Fig. 9-6).

The upper compartment of each TMJ is formed superiorly by the concave mandibular fossa and the convex temporal articular eminence that lies anterior to the fossa. These bony surfaces together form the superior TMJ surface and articulate with the reciprocally shaped superior surface of the articular disc, which is anteroposteriorly concavoconvex. The inferior surface of the articular disc is concave and is mated with the condyle of the mandible, which is convex, to form the lower compartment of the TMJ.

Simultaneous movement of the TMJs produce depression (to open the mouth), elevation (to close the mouth), protrusion, retraction, or lateral deviation of the mandible. Elevation and depression of the mandible occur in the sagittal plane with movement around a frontal axis (see Fig. 9-2). On mouth opening, a two-part sequence of motion occurs within the lower joint compartment of each TMJ. First, the mandibular condyle rotates

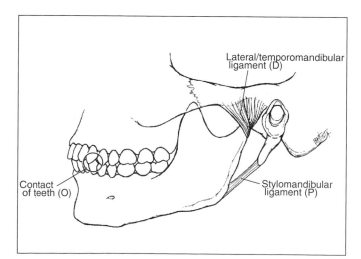

Figure 9-4 Lateral view of the TMJ.*

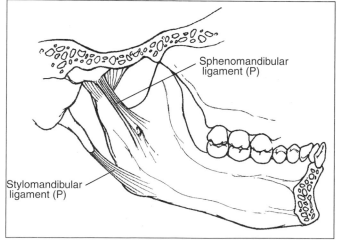

Figure 9-5 Medial view (sagittal section) of the TMJ showing noncontractile structures that normally limit motion.

*Motion limited by structures is identified in brackets, using the following abbreviations: D, depression of mandible; O, occlusion; P, protrusion.

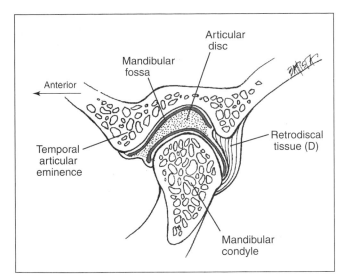

Figure 9-6 Sagittal section of the TMJ showing noncontractile structures that normally limit motion. Motion limited by structures is identified in brackets, using the following abbreviations: D, depression of mandible; O, occlusion; P, protrusion.

and glides forward and downward on the articular disc. Second, because of the posterior attachment of the disc to the mandibular condyle, both structures move together anteriorly (2). This motion results in the anterior gliding of the articular disc over the temporal joint surfaces within the upper compartment (2). These motions are reversed with mouth closing.

When the lower jaw is protracted and retracted, the articular disc of each TMJ moves with the mandibular condyle (2) as the mandible moves in the transverse plane anteriorly and posteriorly, respectively. Movement within the upper compartment of each TMJ occurs between the articular disc and the temporal bone (15).

Lateral deviation of the mandible includes rotation of the mandibular condyle in the mandibular fossa on the side toward which the deviation occurs and a gliding forward of the contralateral mandibular condyle over the mandibular fossa and temporal articular eminence (2).

The Neck: Cervical Spine

There are seven vertebrae that make up the cervical spine (see Fig. 9-1). The third through seventh vertebrae (C3–C7) have a similar structure, but C1 and C2 have a different structure.

The first cervical vertebra (C1) articulates with the occiput of the skull via the atlanto-occipital joints (Figs. 9-1 and 9-7). These joints are formed superiorly by the convex condyles of the occiput articulating with the concave superior articular facets of C1, which lie in the transverse plane and face superiorly and medially. The orientation of the facets determines the motion at the atlanto-occipital articulations. The main movement at the atlanto-occipital joints is flexion and extension and slight lateral flexion (15), with no rotation (16).

There are three atlanto-axial articulations between the atlas (C1) and the axis (C2) (Figs. 9-1 and 9-8). A pivot is formed (2) between the odontoid process (dens) of C2 as it articulates anteriorly with the concave posterior surface of the anterior arch of C1, and posteriorly with the cartilaginous posterior surface of the transverse ligament. The transverse ligament retains the odontoid process in place. There are two facet joints, one on each side between C1 and C2, that lie posterior to the transverse ligament in the transverse plane. Each of the inferior facets of C1 articulates with a superior facet of C2. The orientation of the facets results in rotation being the primary motion at the atlanto-axial joints. Most of the rotation of the cervical spine occurs at the atlanto-axial joints (16).

From C2 to C7, a vertebral segment consists of two vertebrae and the three articulations between these vertebrae (see Fig. 9-1). Anteriorly the intervertebral disc is positioned between the adjacent vertebral bodies (see Fig. 9-8). Two facet joints are located posteriorly on each side of the vertebral segment. Each facet joint is formed by the inferior facet of the superior vertebra (oriented inferiorly and anteriorly) and the superior facet of the inferior vertebra (oriented superiorly and posteriorly). The surfaces of the facet joints lie at an angle of about 45° to the transverse plane. The orientation of the facets permits cervical spine flexion, extension, lateral flexion, and rotation from C2 through C7.

When assessing cervical spine ROM, the combined motions of the segments between the occiput and C7 are assessed and measured, since segmental motion cannot be measured clinically. Cervical spine movements include neck flexion and extension, which occur in the sagittal plane about a frontal axis (see Fig. 9-2); lateral flexion, which occurs in the frontal plane around a sagittal axis (see Fig. 9-3); and rotation, which occurs in the transverse plane around a vertical axis (see Fig. 9-3). About 40% of cervical flexion and 60% of cervical rotation occur at the occiput/C1/C2 complex of the cervical spine (17).

TABLE 9-2   Joint Structure: Cervical Spine Movements

	Flexion	Extension	Lateral Flexion	Rotation
Articulation[1,2]	Atlanto-occipital Atlantoaxial Intervertebral	Atlanto-occipital Atlantoaxial Intervertebral	Atlanto-occipital Intervertebral (with rotation)	Atlanto-occipital Atlantoaxial Intervertebral (with lateral flexion)
Plane	Sagittal	Sagittal	Frontal	Transverse
Axis	Frontal	Frontal	Sagittal	Vertical
Normal limiting factors[8,9]* (See Figs. 9-7 and 9-8)	Tension in the tectorial membrane, posterior atlantoaxial ligament, posterior longitudinal ligament, ligamentum nuchae, ligamentum flavum, posterior neck muscles, and posterior fibers of annulus; contact between anterior rim of foramen magnum of skull and dens (atlanto-occipital joint)	Tension in the anterior longitudinal ligament and anterior atlantoaxial ligament; anterior neck muscles; anterior fibers of annulus; bony contact between the spinous processes	Tension in the alar ligament limits lateral flexion to the contralateral side; lateral fibers of annulus; uncinate processes	Tension in the alar ligament limits rotation to the ipsilateral side; tension in the annulus fibrosis
Normal AROM CROM[10]† Tape Measure[11,12]‡ Inclinometer[13]	0–45° 3 cm 0–50°	0–65° 20 cm 0–60°	0–35° 13 cm 0–45°	0–60° 11 cm 0–80°
Universal Goniometer[14]	0–45°	0–45°	0–45°	

*Note: There is a paucity of definitive research that identifies the normal limiting factors (NLF) of joint motion. The NLF and end feels listed here are based on knowledge of anatomy, clinical experience, and available references.
†AROM for 337 healthy subjects between 11 and 97 years of age. Values represent the means of the mean values (rounded to the nearest 5°) from each age group as derived from the original source.[10]
‡Values represent the mean (rounded to the nearest cm) of the mean values derived from both studies.[11,12]

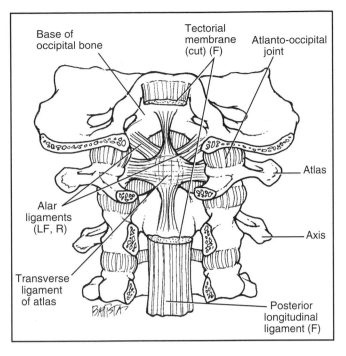

Figure 9-7 label references:
- Base of occipital bone
- Tectorial membrane (cut) (F)
- Atlanto-occipital joint
- Atlas
- Axis
- Posterior longitudinal ligament (F)
- Alar ligaments (LF, R)
- Transverse ligament of atlas

Figure 9-7 Posterior view (frontal section) of the occiput and upper cervical spine showing noncontractile structures that normally limit movement.*

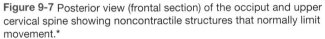

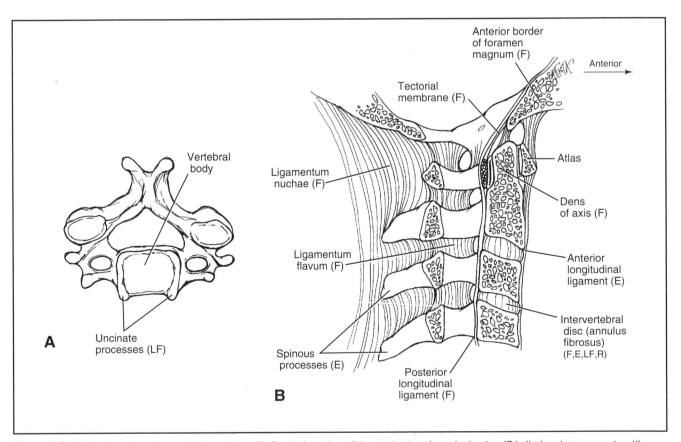

A. label references:
- Vertebral body
- Uncinate processes (LF)

B. label references:
- Anterior border of foramen magnum (F)
- Anterior
- Tectorial membrane (F)
- Ligamentum nuchae (F)
- Atlas
- Dens of axis (F)
- Ligamentum flavum (F)
- Anterior longitudinal ligament (E)
- Intervertebral disc (annulus fibrosus) (F,E,LF,R)
- Spinous processes (E)
- Posterior longitudinal ligament (F)

Figure 9-8 A. Superior view of a cervical vertebra. **B.** Sagittal section of the occiput and cervical spine (C1-4) showing noncontractile structures that normally limit motion.*

*Motion limited by structures is identified in brackets, using the following abbreviations: F, flexion; E, extension; LF, lateral flexion; R, rotation. Muscles normally limiting motion are not illustrated.

SURFACE ANATOMY

(Figs. 9-9 through 9-12)

Structure	Location
1. Suprasternal (jugular) notch	The rounded depression at the superior border of the sternum and between the medial ends of each clavicle.
2. Thyroid cartilage	The most prominent laryngeal cartilage located at the level of the 4th and 5th cervical vertebrae; subcutaneous projection (Adam's apple).
3. Hyoid bone	A submandibular U-shaped bone located above the thyroid cartilage at the level of the 3rd cervical vertebra; the body is felt in the midline below the chin at the angle formed between the floor of the mouth and the front of the neck.
4. Angle of the mandible	The angle of the lower jaw located medially and distally to the earlobe.
5. Angle of the mouth	The lateral angle formed by the upper and lower lips.
6. Nasolabial fold	The fold of skin extending from the nose to the angle of the mouth.
7. Temporomandibular joint	The joint may be palpated anterior to the tragus of the external ear during opening and closing of the mouth.
8. Mastoid process	Bony prominence of the skull located behind the ear.
9. Acromion process	Lateral aspect of the spine of the scapula at the tip or point of the shoulder.
10. Spine of the scapula	The bony ridge running obliquely across the upper four fifths of the scapula.
11. C7 spinous process	Often the most prominent spinous process at the base of the neck.
12. T1 spinous process	The next spinous process inferior to the C7 spinous process.
13. Lobule of the ear	The soft lowermost portion of the auricle of the ear.

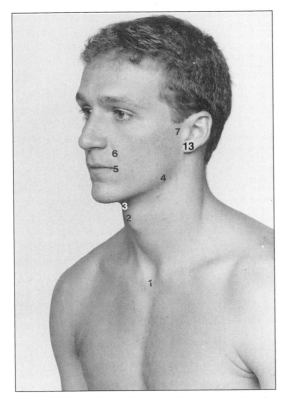

Figure 9-9 Anterolateral aspect of the head and neck.

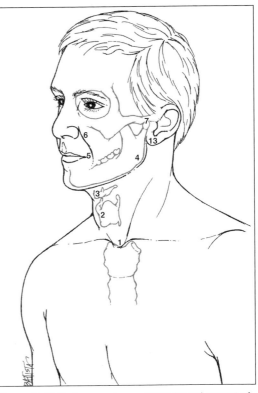

Figure 9-10 Surface anatomy, anterolateral aspect of the head and neck.

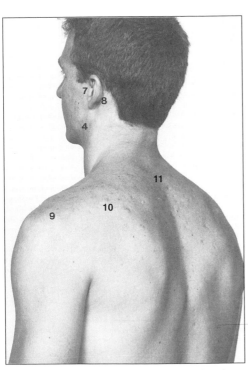

Figure 9-11 Posterolateral aspect of the head and neck.

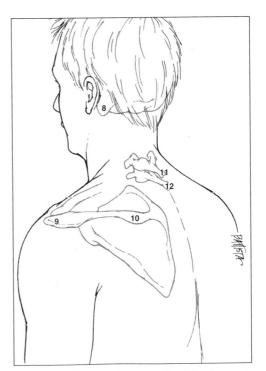

Figure 9-12 Bony anatomy, posterolateral aspect of the head and neck.

ACTIVE RANGE OF MOTION ASSESSMENT AND MEASUREMENT: HEAD AND NECK

AROM measurements of the TMJs are made using a ruler or calipers. The tape measure (see Fig. 1-28), standard inclinometer (see Fig. 1-29), Cervical Range-of-Motion Instrument (CROM) (18) (Performance Attainment Associates, Roseville, MN) (see Fig. 1-30), and the universal goniometer (as described in Chapter 1) are the instruments used to measure neck AROM as presented in this text. These instruments and the measurement procedure for each instrument are described and illustrated. Summaries of the validity and reliability research for the instruments used to measure TMJ and neck AROM are presented in this chapter. Many studies evaluate more than one instrument for the measurement of joint ROM, so some repetition occurs between the summaries. In some cases there is a wide difference between the subjects and methods used to evaluate validity and reliability in these studies and a paucity of research. This should be taken into consideration when reviewing the research summaries. For this reason, the research summaries presented in this chapter appear in more detail in Appendix B.

Instrumentation and Measurement Procedures

Tape Measure/Ruler

ROM is measured by observing a change in distance from one anatomical landmark to a second anatomical landmark, or to a stationary external surface such as the floor or the plinth. The tape measure or ruler is commonly used to measure AROM of the TMJs and spine.

Measurement Procedure: Tape Measure/Ruler

A linear measurement of ROM is obtained using a tape measure and one of the following three methods:

Method 1: The patient moves to the end position for the motion being tested. Using a tape measure, the therapist measures the distance between two specified anatomical landmarks (e.g., see Fig. 9-22) or a specified anatomical landmark and the plinth or floor (e.g., see Figs. 9-66 and 9-76) to determine the ROM in centimeters.

Method 2: The distance is measured between two specified vertebral levels at the start position (e.g., see Fig. 9-57) and at the end position (e.g., see Fig. 9-59) for the ROM being measured. The difference between the two measures is the ROM in centimeters.

Method 3: In the start position for the ROM being assessed, the position of an anatomical landmark is marked on a part of the body that remains stationary during the measurement process (e.g., see Fig. 9-77). The patient moves to the end position for the ROM being assessed and the new position of the anatomical landmark is marked on the stationary body part (e.g., see Fig. 9-78). The distance between the marks on the stationary body part at the start and at the end positions for the ROM being assessed is the ROM in centimeters (e.g., see Fig. 9-79).

Inclinometry

The inclinometer is a device used to measure ROM through measurement of either (a) the inclination of a body part in relation to the vertical, using a pendular inclination needle influenced by the force of gravity or a bubble within a fluid-filled chamber, to measure movement occurring in the frontal or sagittal planes, or (b) the rotational change in position of a body part as movement occurs in a horizontal plane, using a compass inclination needle within a fluid-filled chamber, that reacts to Earth's magnetic field.

The inclinometer can be held in place over an anatomical landmark by the therapist (i.e., standard inclinometer; see Figs. 1-29 and 9-23) or positioned on the body by means of straps and/or extension plates (i.e., OB goniometer as described in Chapter 1; see Figs. 1-27 and 7-16) or a frame (i.e., CROM; see Figs. 1-30 and 9-29). An inclinometer contains a 360° protractor and a gravity inclination needle and/or compass inclination needle. The protractor scale on some inclinometers can be rotated so that the gravity or compass inclination needle can be zeroed (i.e., aligned to zero degrees at the start position for the measured motion). In this case, the final position of the gravity or compass inclination needle or bubble relative to the protractor scale provides the ROM or joint position in degrees. If the needle cannot be zeroed at the start position, the ROM will be recorded as the difference in degrees between the readings on the inclinometer at the start and end positions for the assessed motion.

Standard Inclinometer

The standard inclinometer consists of a gravity-dependent needle and a 360° protractor. The surface of the inclinometer that is placed in contact with the patient can consist of a fixed flat surface, fixed feet, or adjustable feet. Adjustable feet or mounts (see Fig. 1-29) facilitate placement of the inclinometer over curved body surfaces. The American Medical Association (AMA) (13) advocates using the inclinometer to evaluate spinal ROM when evaluating permanent impairment of the spine. One or two standard inclinometers may be used to assess ROM.

Measurement Procedure: Standard Inclinometer

Single Inclinometry. One inclinometer is used to assess the AROM when either the proximal or distal joint segment is stabilized. With the patient in the start position, the inclinometer is positioned in relation to a specified anatomical landmark, normally located on the distal end of the moving segment being measured (e.g., see Fig. 9-43). The protractor of the inclinometer is adjusted to 0° in the start position. The patient is instructed to move through the AROM. At the end of the movement, the therapist reads the number of degrees shown on the inclinometer (e.g., see Fig. 9-44). This measurement is the AROM for the spinal movement being assessed.

Double Inclinometry. When two inclinometers are used to assess AROM, the patient is in the start position with one inclinometer placed at a specified anatomical landmark at the inferior (i.e., stationary or stabilized) end of the spinal segments being measured (e.g., see Fig. 9-61). A second inclinometer is placed at a specified anatomical landmark at the superior (i.e., moving) end of the spinal segments being measured. The protractor of each inclinometer is adjusted to 0° in the start position. The patient is instructed to move through the AROM. At the end of the movement, the therapist reads the number of degrees shown on each inclinometer (e.g., see Fig. 9-63). The difference between the two readings at the end position is the AROM for the spinal movement being assessed.

When measuring ROM, the therapist should ensure that sources of error (described in Chapter 1) do not occur or are minimized, so that ROM measurements will be reliable and the patient's progress can be meaningfully monitored. Mayer and colleagues (19) studied the sources of error with inclinometric measurement of spinal ROM and found that "training and practice was the most significant factor (eliminating the largest source of error) improving overall test performance" (19, p. 1981).

Cervical Range-of-Motion Instrument

The CROM (18) (see Fig. 1-30) is designed to measure cervical spine motion. It consists of a headpiece (i.e., frame that holds three inclinometers) and a magnetic yoke. The inclinometers located on the front and side of the CROM each contain an inclination needle that is influenced by the force of gravity. The third inclinometer, situated in the transverse plane, contains a compass needle that reacts to Earth's magnetic field for measurement of cervical spine rotation.

Measurement Procedure: CROM

The CROM is positioned on the patient's head with the bridge of the frame placed comfortably on the nose and the occipital strap snug (see Fig. 9-29). The magnetic yoke is used when measuring cervical spine rotation ROM and serves to eliminate substitute trunk motion from the cervical spine rotation measurement. The magnetic yoke is positioned over the shoulders with the arrow on the yoke pointing north (see Fig. 9-45) (indicated by observing the position of the red needle on the compass inclinometer with the yoke greater than 4 feet away).

With the patient in the start position for movements in either the sagittal plane (i.e., flexion/extension) (see Fig. 9-29) or the frontal plane (i.e., lateral flexion) (see Fig. 9-38), the gravity inclinometer situated in the same plane as that of the motion to be measured should read 0°. With the patient in the start position for movement in the transverse plane (i.e., rotation), both gravity inclinometers should read 0° by adjusting the patient's head position. The compass inclinometer is then rotated to read 0° (see Fig. 9-45).

The patient moves through the AROM to be measured. At the end of the test movement, the therapist reads the appropriate gravity or compass inclinometer and records the angular AROM measurement for the cervical spine movement being assessed.

TMJ Movements

The measurement of TMJ AROM is described and illustrated, followed by a summary of the validity and reliability research of the ruler as used to measure the AROM.

Start Position. The patient assumes a resting position of the TMJs. In this position, there is minimal muscle action potential in the mandibular muscles, and there is no occluded contact between the maxillary and mandibular teeth (3). The patient is sitting. The head, neck and trunk are in the anatomical position and remain in this position throughout the test movements. It is important to maintain a standard position of the head and neck because it has been shown (20,21) that the magnitude of mandibular opening is affected by head and neck position. From the rest position, the patient is asked to occlude the teeth and depress, protrude, and laterally deviate the lower jaw to each side.

Occlusion of the Teeth

The patient elevates the lower jaw to a position where the teeth are in contact (Fig. 9-13) and the relative position of the mandibular teeth in relation to the maxillary teeth is observed.

Depression of the Mandible

The patient is asked to open the mouth (Fig. 9-14). On slow active opening of the mouth, the therapist observes for deviation of the mandible from the midline. In normal mouth opening, the mandible moves in a straight line. Deviation of the mandible to the left in the form of a C-type curve indicates hypomobility of the TMJ situated on

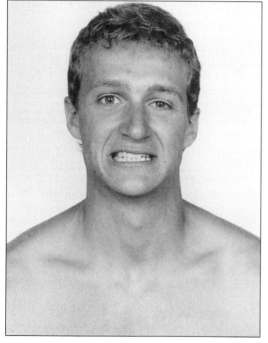

Figure 9-13 Occlusion of the teeth.

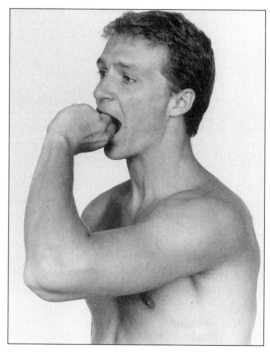

Figure 9-14 Opening of the mouth (depression of the mandible).

the convex side of the C curve, or hypermobility of the joint on the concave side of the curve (4). Deviation in the shape of an S-type curve may indicate a muscular imbalance or displacement of the condyle (4). Functional ROM is determined by placing two or three flexed proximal interphalangeal joints between the upper and lower central incisor teeth (4) (see Fig. 9-14). The fingers represent a distance of about 35 to 50 mm (4). Using a ruler and the edges of the upper and lower central incisor teeth (Fig. 9-15) for reference, a measure of opening can be obtained (22) for recording change (Fig. 9-16). Vernier calipers may also be used to measure the distance between the edges of the upper and lower central incisor teeth to establish the range of mandibular depression (Fig. 9-17).

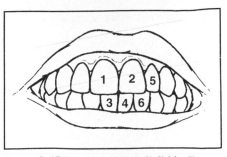

Figure 9-15 Teeth occluded. (1,2) Maxillary central incisors. (3,4) Mandibular central incisors. (5,6) Lateral incisors.

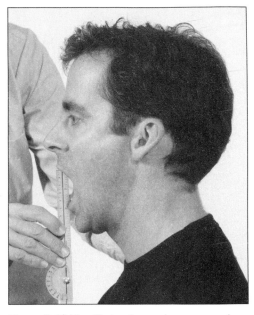

Figure 9-16 Mandibular depression measured with a ruler.

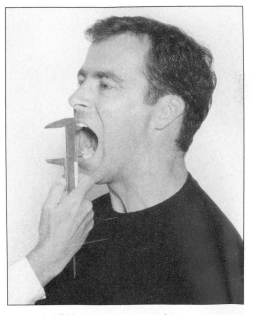

Figure 9-17 Vernier calipers used to measure mandibular depression.

Protrusion of the Mandible

The patient protrudes the lower jaw (Fig. 9-18). The lower jaw should protrude far enough for the patient to place the lower teeth beyond the upper teeth (6). A ruler measurement may be obtained by measuring the distance between the upper and lower central incisors (22) (see Fig. 9-18). Normal protrusion from resting position is 3 to 7 mm (5).

Lateral Deviation of the Mandible

The patient deviates the lower jaw to one side and then the other (Fig. 9-19). A measure can be obtained for recording purposes by measuring the distance between two selected points that are level, one on the upper teeth and one on the lower teeth (4), such as the space between the central incisors. The normal range of motion is 5 to 12 mm (6). Lateral deviation of the mandible should be symmetrical.

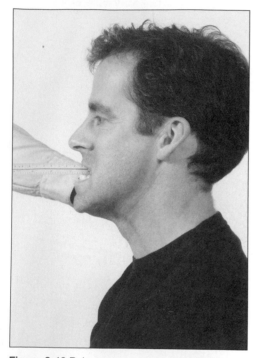

Figure 9-18 Ruler measurement of distance between the upper and lower central incisors, a measure of protrusion of the mandible.

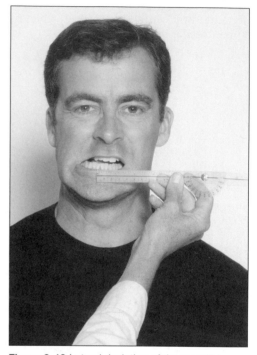

Figure 9-19 Lateral deviation of the mandible.

Neck Movements

Tests of head and neck movement are contraindicated in some instances. Contraindications include pathology that may result in spinal instability and pathology of the vertebral artery. In the absence of contraindications, cervical spine AROM may be assessed using a tape measure, inclinometers, the CROM, or the universal goniometer.

The AMA (13) advocates using the inclinometer to evaluate spinal ROM when evaluating permanent impairment of the spine. The present author (Clarkson) advocates using the tape measure, inclinometry, or the CROM to evaluate spinal AROM.

The measurement of cervical spine AROM is described and illustrated, followed by description of the validity and reliability research of the instruments used to measure the AROM.

When measuring cervical spine AROM, the start position (i.e., sitting) and stabilization are the same for all movements regardless of the instrument used to measure the AROM, with one exception: active cervical spine rotation (i.e., start position is supine) when measured using an inclinometer.

Start Position. The patient is sitting in a chair with a back support. The feet are flat on the floor and the arms are relaxed at the sides. The head and neck are in the anatomical (neutral zero) position (Fig. 9-20).

Stabilization. The back of the chair provides support for the thoracic and lumbar spines. The patient is instructed to avoid substitute movement and the therapist can stabilize the trunk.

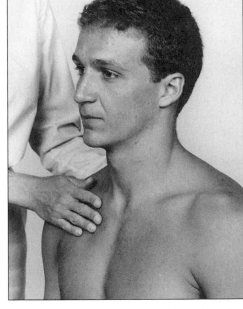

Figure 9-20 Start position for all movements of the neck with the exception of rotation when measured using the inclinometer.

Neck Flexion-Extension

End Positions. *Flexion*: The patient flexes the neck to the limit of the motion. *Extension*: The patient extends the neck to the limit of motion.

Substitute Movement. Mouth opening (for tape measurements), trunk flexion-extension.

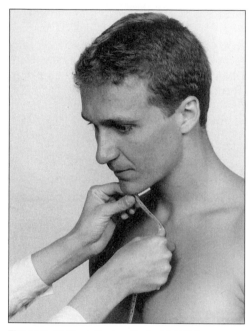

Figure 9-21 Neck flexion: limited AROM.

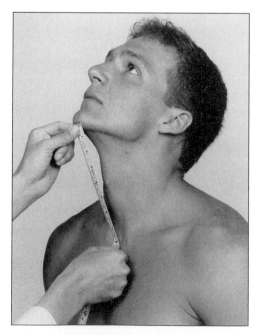

Figure 9-22 Neck extension: full AROM.

Tape Measure Measurement

Flexion. The distance is measured between the tip of the chin and the suprasternal notch. A measure is taken in the flexed position (Fig. 9-21). The linear measure reflects the neck flexion ROM.

Extension. The same reference points are used. A measure is taken in the extended position (Fig. 9-22). The linear measure reflects the range of neck extension.

Inclinometer Measurement

Inclinometer Placement. *Superior*: On the vertex (i.e., top [26]) of the head. *Inferior*: On the spine of T1. In the start position (Fig. 9-23), the inclinometers are zeroed.

Flexion. At the limit of neck flexion (Fig. 9-24) the therapist records the angle measurements from both inclinometers. The neck flexion ROM is the difference between the two inclinometer readings.

Extension. At the limit of neck extension (Fig. 9-25) the therapist records the angle measurements from both inclinometers. The neck extension ROM is the difference between the two inclinometer readings.

Alternate Inclinometer Measurement

The inferior inclinometer may be positioned over the spine of the scapula (27) if the position of the inclinometer over T1 hinders neck extension ROM or a large neck extension ROM displaces the inclinometer.

Inclinometer Placement. *Superior*: On the vertex (i.e., top) of the head. *Inferior*: Over the spine of the scapula. In the start position (Fig. 9-26), the inclinometers are zeroed.

Flexion. At the limit of neck flexion (Fig. 9-27) the therapist records the angle measurements from both inclinometers. The neck flexion ROM is the difference between the two inclinometer readings.

Extension. At the limit of neck extension (Fig. 9-28) the therapist records the angle measurements from both inclinometers. The neck extension ROM is the difference between the two inclinometer readings.

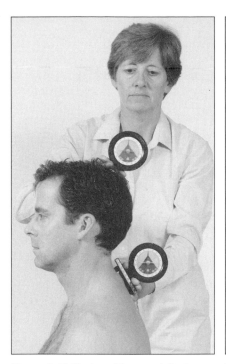

Figure 9-23 Start position: neck flexion and extension with inclinometers positioned on the vertex of the head and over the spine of T1.

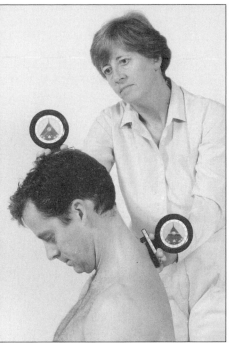

Figure 9-24 End position: neck flexion.

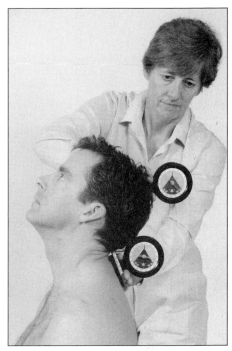

Figure 9-25 End position: neck extension.

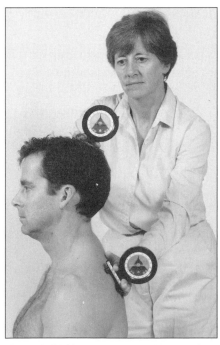

Figure 9-26 Alternate start position: neck flexion and extension with inclinometers positioned on the vertex of the head and over the spine of the scapula.

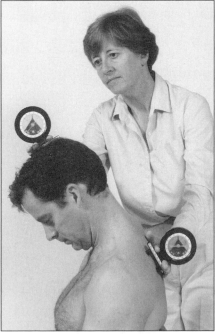

Figure 9-27 End position: neck flexion.

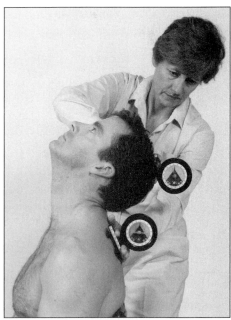

Figure 9-28 End position: neck extension.

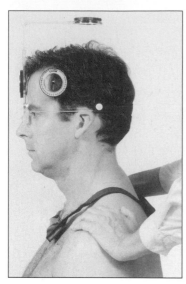

Figure 9-29 Start position: neck flexion and extension.

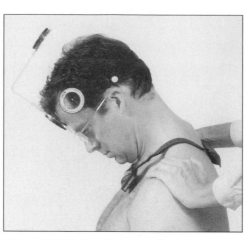

Figure 9-30 End position: neck flexion.

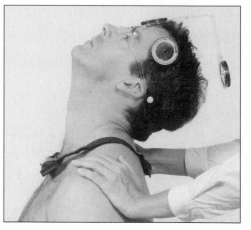

Figure 9-31 End position: neck extension.

CROM Measurement

By positioning the patient's head, the inclinometer on the lateral aspect of the CROM is zeroed in the start position (Fig. 9-29).

Flexion. The neck is flexed to the limit of motion and the reading on the lateral inclinometer is the neck flexion ROM (Fig. 9-30).

Extension. The neck is extended to the limit of motion and the reading on the lateral inclinometer is the neck extension ROM (Fig. 9-31).

Universal Goniometer Measurement

Goniometer Axis. Over the lobule of the ear (Fig. 9-32).

Stationary Arm. Perpendicular to the floor.

Movable Arm. Lies parallel to the base of the nares. In the start position (Fig. 9-32) the goniometer will indicate 90°. This is recorded as 0°.

Flexion. The goniometer is realigned at the limit of neck flexion (Fig. 9-33). The number of degrees the movable arm lies away from the 90° position is recorded as the neck flexion ROM.

Extension. The goniometer is realigned at the limit of neck extension (Fig. 9-34). The number of degrees the movable arm lies away from the 90° position is recorded as the neck extension ROM.

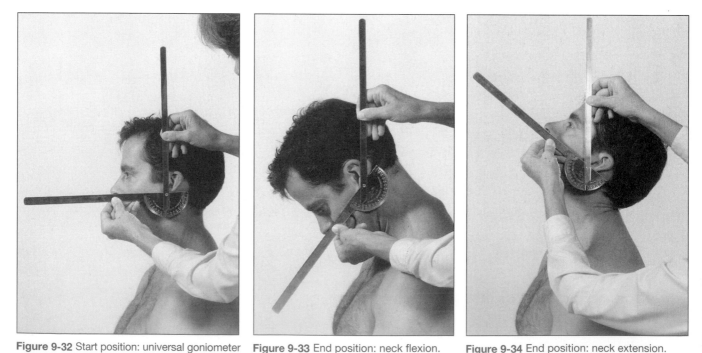

Figure 9-32 Start position: universal goniometer placement for neck flexion and extension.

Figure 9-33 End position: neck flexion.

Figure 9-34 End position: neck extension.

Neck Lateral Flexion

End Positions. The patient flexes the neck to the left side (without rotatlon) to the limit of motion (Fig. 9-35). The patient flexes the neck to the right side (without rotation) to the limit of motion.

Substitute Movement. Elevation of the shoulder girdle to approximate the ear; ipsilateral trunk lateral flexion.

Tape Measure Measurement

Lateral Flexion. The distance is measured between the mastoid process of the skull and the lateral aspect of the acromion process (see Fig. 9-35). The linear measure reflects the range of neck lateral flexion to the side measured.

Inclinometer Measurement

Inclinometer Placement. *Superior*: On the vertex (i.e., top) of the head. *Inferior*: On the spine of T1. In the start position (Fig. 9-36), the inclinometers are zeroed.

Lateral Flexion. At the limit of neck lateral flexion (Fig. 9-37), the therapist records the angle measurements from both inclinometers. The neck lateral flexion ROM is the difference between the two inclinometer readings.

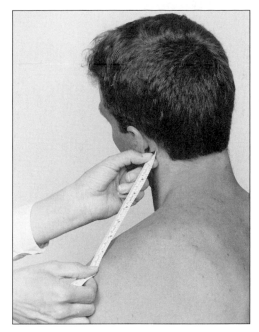

Figure 9-35 Neck lateral flexion.

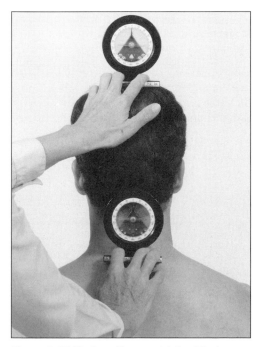

Figure 9-36 Start position: neck lateral flexion.

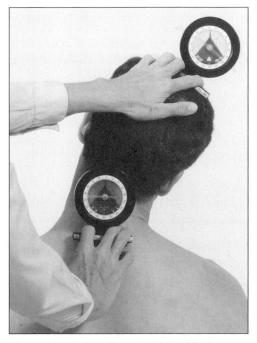

Figure 9-37 End position: neck lateral flexion.

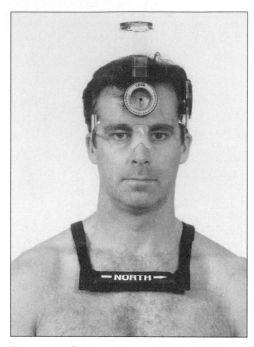

Figure 9-38 Start position: neck lateral flexion.

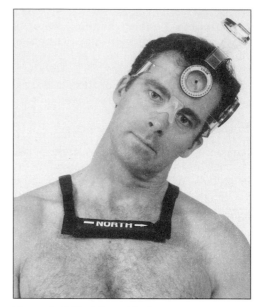

Figure 9-39 Neck lateral flexion.

CROM Measurement

By positioning the patient's head, the inclinometer on the anterior aspect of the CROM is zeroed in the start position (Fig. 9-38).

Lateral Flexion. The neck is laterally flexed to the limit of motion, and the reading on the anterior inclinometer is the neck lateral flexion ROM to the side measured (Fig. 9-39).

Universal Goniometer Measurement

Goniometer Axis. Over the C7 spinous process (Fig. 9-40).

Stationary Arm. Along the spine and perpendicular to the floor.

Movable Arm. Points toward the midpoint of the head. In the start position (Fig. 9-40), the goniometer will indicate 0°.

Lateral Flexion. The goniometer is realigned at the limit of neck lateral flexion (Fig. 9-41). The number of degrees the movable arm lies away from the 0° position is recorded as the neck lateral flexion ROM to the side measured.

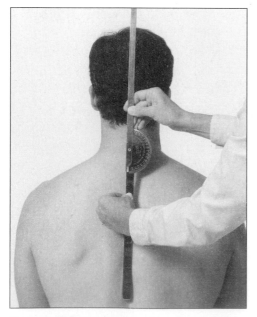

Figure 9-40 Start position: universal goniometer alignment neck lateral flexion.

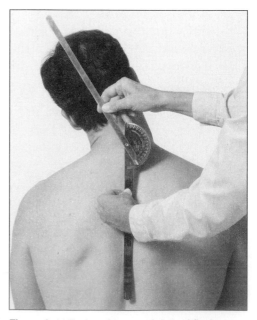

Figure 9-41 End position: neck lateral flexion.

Neck Rotation

End Position. The patient rotates the head to the left to the limit of motion (Fig. 9-42). The patient rotates the head to the right side to the limit of motion.

Substitute Movement. Elevation and/or protrusion of the shoulder girdle to approximate the chin (tape measure); trunk rotation.

Tape Measure Measurement

Rotation. The distance is measured between the tip of the chin and the lateral aspect of the acromion process (see Fig. 9-42). The linear measure reflects the range of neck rotation to the side measured.

Inclinometer Measurement

Start Position. The patient is supine with the head and neck in anatomical position (Fig. 9-43).

Inclinometer Placement. In the midline at the base of the forehead. In the start position, the inclinometer is zeroed.

Rotation. At the limit of neck rotation (Fig. 9-44), the therapist records the inclinometer reading as the neck rotation AROM to the side measured.

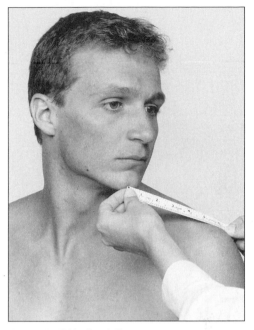

Figure 9-42 Neck rotation.

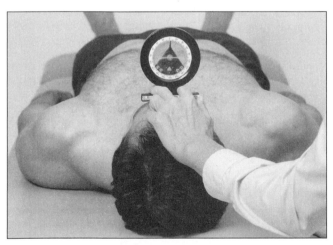

Figure 9-43 Start position for neck rotation with the inclinometer placed in the midline at the base of the forehead.

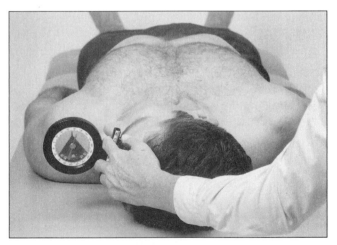

Figure 9-44 End position: neck rotation.

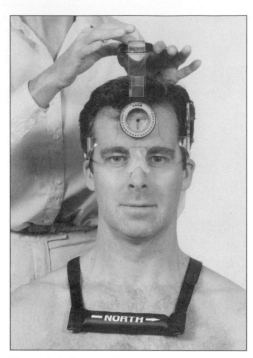

Figure 9-45 Start position: neck rotation.

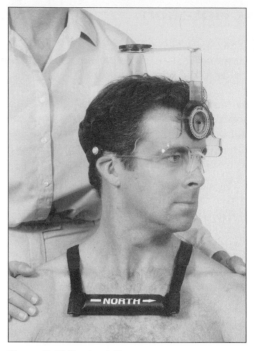

Figure 9-46 Neck rotation.

CROM Measurement

The magnetic yoke is positioned over the shoulders with the arrow on the yoke pointing north. With the patient in the start position, both gravity inclinometers should read 0° (accomplished by adjusting the patient's head position). The compass inclinometer is then rotated to read 0° (Fig. 9-45).

Rotation. The neck is rotated to the limit of motion, and the reading on the compass inclinometer is the neck rotation ROM to the side measured (Fig. 9-46).

Universal Goniometer Measurement

Goniometer Axis. Over the midpoint of the top of the head (Fig. 9-47).

Stationary Arm. Parallel to a line joining the two acromion processes.

Movable Arm. Aligned with the nose. In the start position (Fig. 9-47), the goniometer will indicate 90°. This is recorded as 0°.

Rotation. The goniometer is realigned at the limit of neck rotation (Fig. 9-48). The number of degrees the movable arm lies away from the 90° position is recorded as the neck rotation ROM.

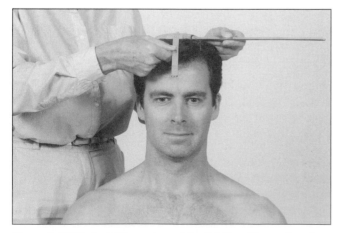

Figure 9-47 Start position: universal goniometer alignment neck rotation.

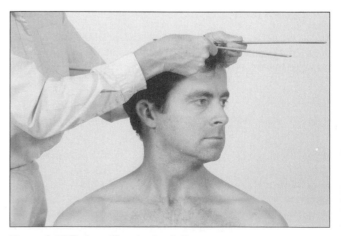

Figure 9-48 End position: neck rotation.

VALIDITY AND RELIABILITY: MEASUREMENT OF THE TMJ AND CERVICAL SPINE AROM

TMJ

Ruler

Walker and colleagues (23) evaluated the construct validity of using a ruler to measure AROM of the TMJs for mandibular depression, lateral deviation, and protrusion. The measurement of mouth opening was the only measure that demonstrated construct validity for identifying TMJ pathology. Therefore, the authors concluded that mouth opening measured by ruler might be a possible method for documenting and monitoring the status of patients with TMJ disorders.

Evaluating the intra- and intertester reliability of the ruler for measuring mouth opening AROM, researchers (21,23–25) found the ruler to be reliable. In addition, Dijkstra and coworkers (24) pointed out that mandibular length may influence how much the mouth can be opened. Therefore, when comparing different subjects with the same linear mouth opening, one cannot conclude similar TMJ mobility. However, using a ruler to measure the distance between the central incisors in maximal mouth opening is a reliable and accurate measure of TMJ mobility when evaluating progress in the same subject over time.

For measurements of lateral deviation and protrusion of the TMJs using the ruler, Walker and associates (23) found acceptable intratester reliability and good to excellent intertester reliability, but Dworkin and colleagues (25) found less-than-desirable intertester reliability. Dworkin and colleagues (25) also found that examiners trained in the standardized procedure for the measurement of TMJ AROM demonstrated better intertester reliability than untrained examiners, supporting the importance of using standardized procedures for reliable clinical measurement of TMJ AROM.

Cervical Spine

Tape Measure

In reviewing the literature, no studies were found that examined the validity of measuring cervical spine ROM using a tape measure. Several studies (11,12,28,29) assessed the reliability of using the tape measure to assess cervical spine ROM. The reliability of the tape measure was evaluated measuring healthy subjects (11,12) and patients with ankylosing spondylitis (28,29) and, in general, the reliability was reported to be good.

Jordan (30) assessed the literature on the reliability of tools used to measure cervical spine ROM in clinical settings; Jordan could give "no strong recommendation for any tool" (30, p. 194) but suggested the tape measure as possibly being the preferred clinical option. The tape measure is inexpensive, portable, and clinically acceptable, but Jordan (30) found that the tape measure needs more support in the literature.

Chibnall and colleagues (31) demonstrated that linear measurements of neck ROM depend on body size. Therefore, when comparing different patients with the same linear neck AROM, one cannot conclude similar neck mobility.

Inclinometry

Bush and associates (32) assessed the validity of measuring cervical spine AROM using single and double inclinometry techniques and a single inclinometry stabilization technique. The inclinometry measurements were compared to radiologic measurements and computerized tomography scan measurements of cervical spine motions. Based on the criteria used by the researchers, the only valid methods of measurement were single inclinometry for flexion and extension, double inclinometry for flexion, and the single inclinometry stabilization measurement of extension.

Herrmann (33) compared radiographic measurements and inclinometric measurements of the total neck flexion and extension PROM. The inclinometer was strapped to the lateral aspect of the head just above the ears. The investigator concluded the inclinometer could be used as a valid tool for measuring passive head and neck motion in the sagittal plane.

Hole and colleagues (34) evaluated the concurrent validity of the CROM and the single inclinometer and showed good agreement for flexion, extension, and lateral flexion measurements but not for rotation.

Studies (11,32,34–40) conducted to determine the intra- and intertester reliability of the inclinometer for measuring cervical spine ROM included only healthy subjects. These studies, using different types of inclinometers, in nearly all instances showed the inclinometer to be a reliable tool for measuring cervical spine AROM.

CROM

When CROM measurements were compared with radiographic measurements (41–43), the CROM was found to be a valid tool for measuring flexion, extension, and lateral flexion. Hole and colleagues (34) showed the CROM and single inclinometer to be concurrently valid for all neck motions except rotation.

Several studies examined the reliability of the CROM for measuring the cervical spine flexion, extension, lateral flexion, and rotation AROM of subjects with cervical spine pathology (44,45) and healthy subjects (10,34,46,47). The results of these studies support Tousignant and colleagues' statement that "reliability of the cervical range of motion device has been well established." (43, p. 812)

Jordan (30) reviewed the literature to assess the reliability of tools to measure cervical spine ROM in clinical settings and identified the CROM to be the most reliable tool, adding that the CROM may not be the most practical tool in the clinical setting owing to cost, portability, and specificity for use in measuring only cervical spine ROM. Jordan (30) concluded that reliability appears to be good for a population of mixed pathologic conditions, but more research is needed using normal subjects and those with specific neck pathology.

Universal Goniometer

Several investigators (28,37,39,44) compared the reliability of the universal goniometer to other ROM measurement tools for measuring cervical spine AROM. Pile and associates (28) compared the tape measure and a universal goniometer. Despite results showing what appeared to be good intertester reliability for both the tape measure

and universal goniometer, they recommended the use of the universal goniometer because it was easier to use. Studies (37,39,44) comparing the intertester reliability of the universal goniometer with that of the inclinometer or CROM showed greater reliability for the inclinometer or CROM than the universal goniometer. Zachman and coworkers (37) found the inclinometer showed greater intertester reliability than the universal goniometer and noted the inclinometer does not require the therapist to locate as many landmarks and appears to be quicker and easier to use compared to the universal goniometer. Tucci and associates (39) found better intertester reliability for measures of cervical spine ROM using the inclinometer with an inexperienced and experienced examiner than when cervical ROM was measured using the universal goniometer and two experienced examiners. Youdas and colleagues (44) compared the CROM and the universal goniometer and found both had good to high intratester reliability, but the CROM proved to be the more reliable method of assessing the cervical spine ROM when different therapists measured the same patient.

ARTICULATIONS AND MOVEMENTS

The Trunk: Thoracic and Lumbar Spines

The articulations and joint axes of the trunk are illustrated in Figures 9-49, 9-50, and 9-51. The joint structure and movements of the trunk are described below and summarized in Table 9-3.

There are 12 vertebrae in the thoracic spine and 5 in the lumbar spine (see Fig. 9-49). Vertebral segments are referred to when describing the articulations of the spine. A vertebral segment consists of two vertebrae and the three articulations between them (Fig. 9-52). Anteriorly, intervertebral discs are positioned between the adjacent vertebral bodies. However, it is the orientation of the facet joints, located posteriorly on each side of the

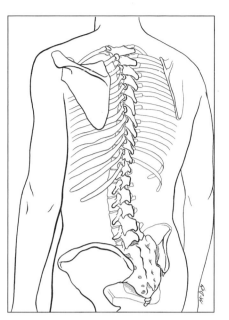

Figure 9-49 Trunk articulations.

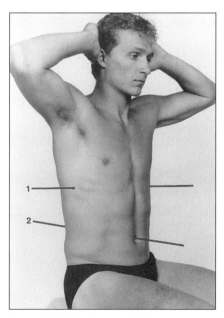

Figure 9-50 Trunk axes: (1) flexion-extension; (2) lateral flexion.

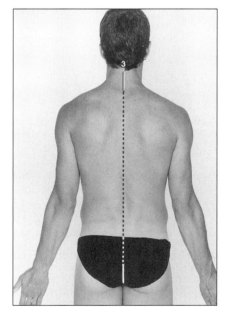

Figure 9-51 Trunk axis: (3) rotation.

TABLE 9-3   Joint Structure: Trunk Movements

	Flexion	Extension	Lateral Flexion	Rotation
Articulation[48]	Lumbar spine, thoracic spine (mainly T6–12)	Lumbar spine, thoracic spine (mainly T6–12)	Lumbar spine, thoracic spine	Thoracic spine, lumbosacral articulation
Plane	Sagittal	Sagittal	Frontal	Horizontal
Axis	Frontal	Frontal	Sagittal	Vertical
Normal limiting factors[6,8,9]* (See Fig. 9-52)	Tension in the posterior longitudinal, supraspinous, and interspinous ligaments, the ligamentum flavum, facet joint capsules and spinal extensor muscles; compression of the intervertebral discs anteriorly and tension in the posterior fibers of the annulus; apposition of articular facets and spine; rib cage	Tension in the anterior longitudinal ligament, abdominal muscles, facet joint capsules and the anterior fibers of the annulus; contact between adjacent spinous processes; apposition of articular facets and thoracic spine	Contact between the iliac crest and thorax; tension in the contralateral trunk side flexors, intertransverse and iliolumbar ligaments and facet joint capsules; tension in the contralateral fibers of the annulus; apposition of articular facets and lumbar spine	Tension in the costovertebral, supraspinous, interspinous, and iliolumbar ligaments and facet joint capsules lumbar spine and annulus fibrosus of the intervertebral discs; tension in the ipsilateral external and contralateral internal abdominal oblique muscles; apposition of the articular facets lumbar spine
Normal AROM Tape measure	10 cm[5]† 6 cm[49]§		22 cm[50]‡	
Inclinometer[13]	0–60+° L spine	0–25° L spine	0–25° L spine	0–30° T spine
Universal goniometer[51]		0–35°		
Capsular pattern	It is difficult to perform passive movements of the trunk due to its size and weight. It is difficult to determine the capsular pattern for the trunk.[7]			

*Note: There is a paucity of definitive research that identifies the normal limiting factors (NLF) of joint motion. The NLF and end feels listed here are based on knowledge of anatomy, clinical experience, and available references.
†Measured between C7 and S1.
‡Measured between level of middle finger on thigh in anatomical position and at end of lateral flexion ROM. Value represents the mean of mean values from the original source[50] for right and left lateral flexion ROM of 39 healthy subjects.
§Measured between level of PSIS and 15 cm proximal. Value represents the rounded mean of mean values from the original source[49] for L spine flexion ROM of 104 children 13 to 18 years of age.

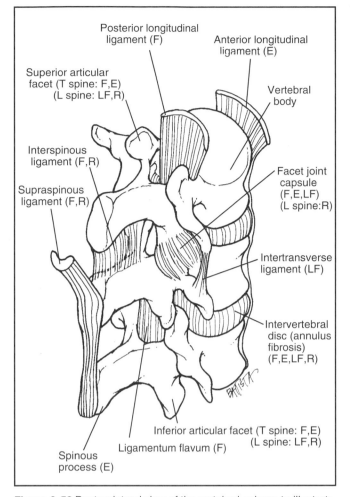

Posterior longitudinal
ligament (F)

Anterior longitudinal
ligament (E)

Superior articular
facet (T spine: F,E)
(L spine: LF,R)

Vertebral
body

Interspinous
ligament (F,R)

Facet joint
capsule
(F,E,LF)
(L spine:R)

Supraspinous
ligament (F,R)

Intertransverse
ligament (LF)

Intervertebral
disc (annulus
fibrosis)
(F,E,LF,R)

Inferior articular facet (T spine: F,E)
(L spine: LF,R)

Ligamentum flavum (F)

Spinous
process (E)

Figure 9-52 Posterolateral view of the vertebral column to illustrate noncontractile structures that normally limit motion in the thoracic and lumbar spines. Motion limited by structures is identified in brackets, using the following abbreviations: F, flexion; E, extension; LF, lateral flexion; R, rotation. Muscles normally limiting motion are not illustrated.

vertebral segment, that determines the predominant motions that occur between the vertebral segments. Each facet joint is formed by the inferior facet of the superior vertebra articulating with the superior facet of the inferior vertebra.

Although all segments of the thoracic and lumbar spines contribute to flexion, extension, lateral flexion, and rotation of the trunk, the regional contribution to these motions varies. The surfaces of the facets in the thoracic spine lie in the frontal plane, favoring the motions of lateral flexion and rotation. The facet joint surfaces of

the lumbar spine are oriented in the sagittal plane, favoring flexion and extension.

When assessing thoracic and lumbar spine ROM, the combined motions of the segments are assessed and measured since segmental motion cannot be measured clinically. Thoracic and lumbar spine movements include flexion and extension, which occur in the sagittal plane around a frontal axis (see Fig. 9-50); lateral flexion, which occurs in the frontal plane around a sagittal axis (Fig. 9-50); and rotation, which occurs in the transverse plane around a vertical axis (see Fig. 9-51).

SURFACE ANATOMY

(Figs. 9-53 through 9-56)

Structure	Location
1. Suprasternal (jugular) notch	The rounded depression at the superior border of the sternum, between the medial ends of each clavicle.
2. Xiphoid process	The lower end of the body of the sternum.
3. Anterior superior iliac spine (ASIS)	Round bony prominence at the anterior end of the iliac crest.
4. Iliac crest	Upper border of the ilium; a convex bony ridge, the top of which is level with the space between the spines of L4 and L5.
5. Posterior superior iliac spine (PSIS)	Round bony prominence at the posterior end of the iliac crest, felt subcutaneously at the dimples on the proximal aspect of the buttocks.
6. S2 spinous process	At the midpoint of a line drawn between each PSIS.
7. Inferior angle of the scapula	At the inferior aspect of the vertebral border of the scapula.
8. Spine of the scapula	The bony ridge running obliquely across the upper four fifths of the scapula.
9. T7 spinous process	Midline of the body at the level of the inferior angle of the scapula with the body in the anatomical position.
10. T3 spinous process	With the body in the anatomical position, it is at the midpoint of a line drawn between the roots of the spines of each scapula.
11. C7 spinous process	Often the most prominent spinous process at the base of the neck.
12. T1 spinous process	The next spinous process inferior to the C7 spinous process.
13. Acromion process	Lateral aspect of the spine of the scapula at the tip or point of the shoulder.
14. Greater trochanter	With the tip of the thumb on the lateral aspect of the iliac crest, the tip of the third digit placed distally on the lateral aspect of the thigh locates the upper border of the greater trochanter.

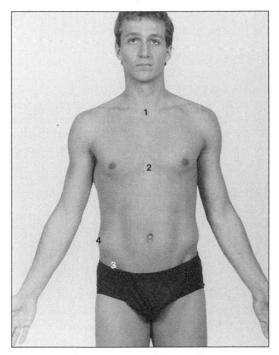

Figure 9-53 Anterior aspect of the trunk.

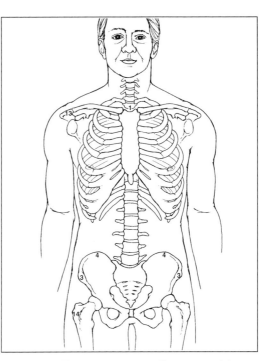

Figure 9-54 Bony anatomy, anterior aspect of the trunk.

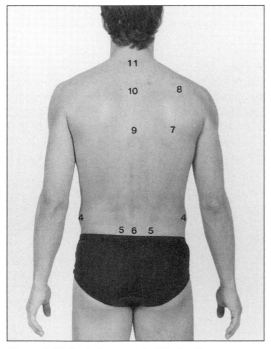

Figure 9-55 Posterior aspect of the trunk.

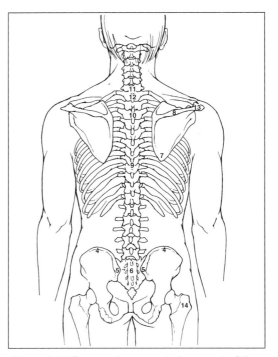

Figure 9-56 Bony anatomy, posterior aspect of the trunk.

ACTIVE RANGE OF MOTION ASSESSMENT AND MEASUREMENT: TRUNK

The tape measure, universal goniometer, and standard inclinometers are the tools used to objectively measure spinal AROM as presented in this text. However, in the clinic, the therapist often prefers to observe the patient to assess spinal movements, any deviations from normal, and the presence or absence of a rib hump. The measurement of spinal AROM is described and illustrated, followed by description of the validity and reliability research of the instruments used to measure spinal AROM. Summaries of the validity and reliability research for instruments used to measure spinal AROM are presented in this chapter. In some cases, there is a wide difference between the subjects and methods used to evaluate validity and reliability in these studies and a paucity of research. This should be taken into consideration when reviewing the research summaries. For this reason, the research summaries presented in this chapter appear in more detail in Appendix B.

Trunk Flexion and Extension: Thoracolumbar Spine

Tape Measure Measurement

Start Positions. *Flexion.* The patient is standing with feet shoulder width apart (Fig. 9-57). A tape measure is used to measure the distance between the spinous processes of C7 and S2. *Extension.* For thoracolumbar extension, the patient's hands are placed on the iliac crests and into the small of the back (Fig. 9-58). A tape measure is used to measure the distance between the spinous processes of C7 and S2. The patient is instructed to keep the knees straight when performing the test movements.

Substitute Movement. None.

End Positions. *Flexion.* The patient flexes the trunk forward to the limit of motion for thoracolumbar flexion (Fig. 9-59). The distance between the spinous processes of C7 and S2 is measured again. The difference between the start and end position measures is the thoracolumbar flexion ROM. *Extension.* The patient extends the trunk backward to the limit of motion for thoracolumbar extension (Fig. 9-60). The distance between the spinous processes of C7 and S2 is measured again. The difference between the start and end position measures is the thoracolumbar extension ROM.

Inclinometer Measurement

Start Positions. The patient is standing with feet shoulder width apart (Fig. 9-61). For thoracolumbar extension, the patient's hands are placed on the iliac crests and into the small of the back (Fig. 9-62). The inclinometers are positioned and zeroed in each start position. The patient is instructed to keep the knees straight when performing the test movements.

Substitute Movement. None.

Inclinometer Placement. *Superior*: On the spine of C7. *Inferior*: On the spine of S2.

End Positions. The patient flexes the trunk forward to the limit of motion for thoracolumbar flexion (Fig. 9-63). The patient extends the trunk backward to the limit of motion for thoracolumbar extension (Fig. 9-64). At the end position for each movement, the therapist records the angle measurements from both inclinometers. The AROM for the movement measured is the difference between the inclinometer readings.

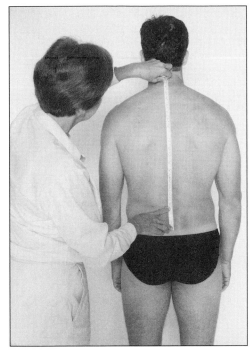

Figure 9-57 Start position: thoracolumbar spinal flexion. The distance is measured between the spinous processes of C7 and S2.

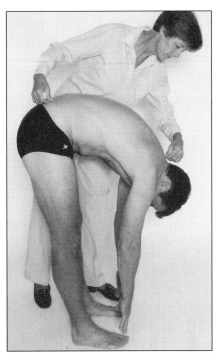

Figure 9-59 End position: thoracolumbar spinal flexion.

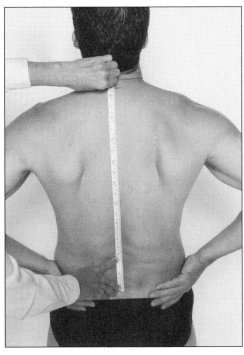

Figure 9-58 Start position for thoracolumbar extension.

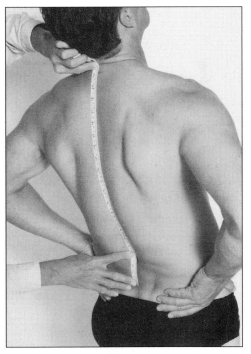

Figure 9-60 End position: thoracolumbar extension.

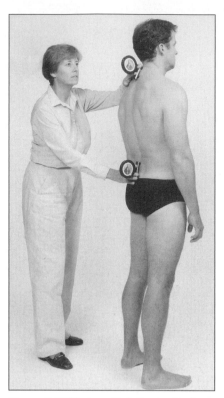

Figure 9-61 Start position: thoracolumbar flexion with inclinometer placement over the spines of C7 and S2.

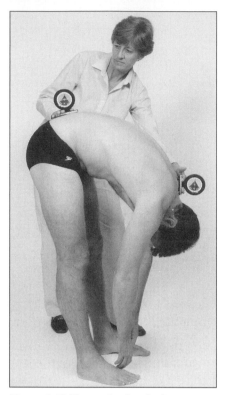

Figure 9-63 Thoracolumbar flexion.

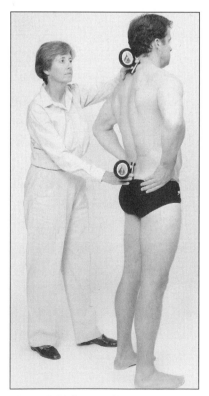

Figure 9-62 Start position: thoracolumbar extension.

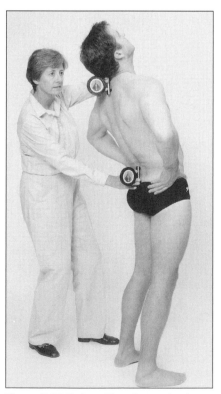

Figure 9-64 End position: thoracolumbar spine extension.

Trunk Extension: Thoracolumbar Spine

Tape Measure Measurement (Prone Press-Up)

Start Position. The patient is prone (Fig. 9-65). The hands are positioned on the plinth at shoulder level.

Stabilization. A strap is placed over the pelvis.

Substitute Movement. Lifting the pelvis from the plinth.

End Position. The patient extends the elbows to raise the trunk and extends the thoracolumbar spine (Fig. 9-66). A tape measure is used to measure the perpendicular distance between the suprasternal notch and the plinth at the limit of motion. This method is unsuitable for patients who have upper extremity muscle weakness or find the prone position uncomfortable. In these cases spinal extension is assessed in standing using a tape measure.

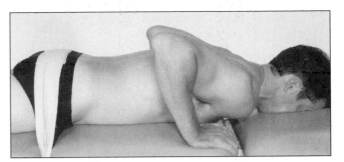

Figure 9-65 Start position: thoracolumbar spinal extension.

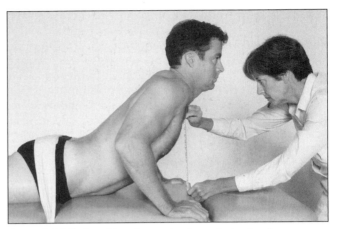

Figure 9-66 End position: thoracolumbar spinal extension.

Hip Adduction

AROM Assessment

Substitute Movement. Hip internal rotation, hiking of the contralateral pelvis.

PROM Assessment

Start Position. The patient is supine; the pelvis is level and the lower extremity is in the anatomical position. The hip on the nontest side is abducted to allow full ROM in adduction on the test side (Fig. 6-29).

Stabilization. The therapist stabilizes the ipsilateral pelvis.

Therapist's Distal Hand Placement. The therapist grasps the distal femur.

End Position. The therapist applies slight traction and moves the femur to the limit of hip adduction ROM (30°) (Fig. 6-30).

End Feel. Hip adduction—soft or firm.

Joint Glide. *Hip adduction*—the convex femoral head glides superiorly on the fixed concave acetabulum.

Measurement: Universal Goniometer

Start Position. The patient is supine with the lower extremity in the anatomical position. The hip on the nontest side is abducted to allow full range of hip adduction on the test side (see Fig. 6-29). The pelvis is level.

Stabilization. The therapist stabilizes the ipsilateral pelvis.

Goniometer Axis. The axis is placed over the ASIS on the side being measured. The goniometer is aligned the same as for hip abduction ROM measurement (see Figs. 6-26 and 6-27).

Stationary Arm. Along a line that joins the two ASISs.

Movable Arm. Parallel to the longitudinal axis of the femur, pointing toward the midline of the patella. In the start position described, the goniometer will indicate 90°. This is recorded as 0°. For example, if the goniometer reads 90° at the start position for hip adduction and 105° at the end position, hip adduction PROM would be 15°.

End Position. The hip is adducted to the limit of motion (30°) (Fig. 6-31).

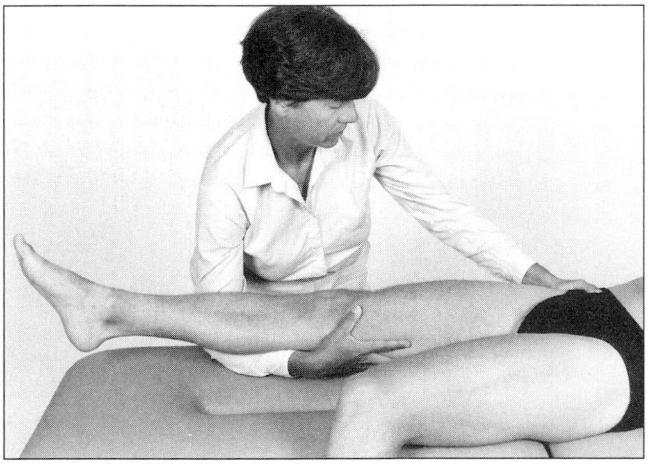

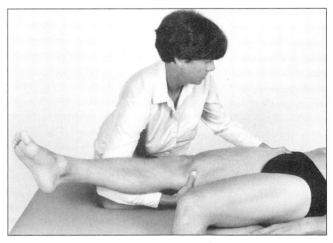

Figure 6-29 Start position: hip adduction.

Figure 6-30 Soft or firm end feel at limit of hip adduction.

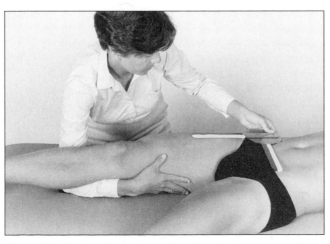

Figure 6-31 End position: universal goniometer measurement for hip adduction.

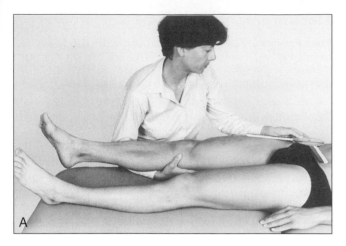

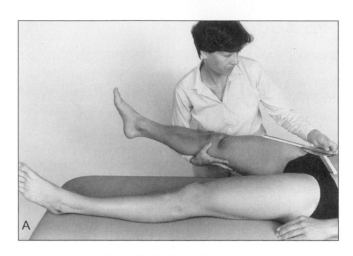

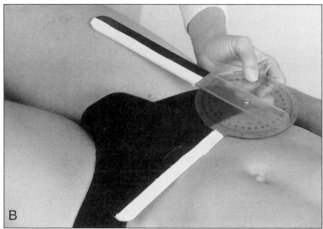

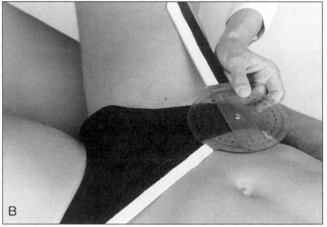

Figure 6-26 A. Start position: hip abduction. **B.** Goniometer alignment.

Figure 6-28 A. End position: hip abduction. **B.** Goniometer alignment.

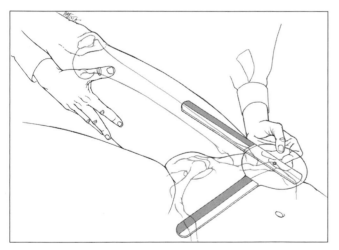

Figure 6-27 Goniometer alignment: hip abduction and adduction.

Hip Abduction

AROM Assessment

Substitute Movement. External rotation and flexion of the hip, hiking of the ipsilateral pelvis.

PROM Assessment

Start Position. The patient is supine; the pelvis is level and the lower extremities are in the anatomical position (Fig. 6-24).

Stabilization. The therapist stabilizes the ipsilateral pelvis. If additional stabilization of the trunk and pelvis is required, the contralateral lower extremity may be positioned in hip abduction with the knee flexed over the edge of the plinth and the foot supported on a stool (see Fig. 6-29).

Therapist's Distal Hand Placement. The therapist grasps the medial aspect of the distal femur.

End Position. The therapist applies slight traction to and moves the femur to the limit of hip abduction motion (Fig. 6-25).

End Feel. Hip abduction—firm.

Joint Glide. *Hip abduction*—the convex femoral head glides inferiorly on the fixed concave acetabulum.

Measurement: Universal Goniometer

Start Position. The patient is supine with the lower extremities in the anatomical position (Fig. 6-26A). Ensure the pelvis is level.

Stabilization. The therapist stabilizes the ipsilateral pelvis. If additional stabilization of the trunk and pelvis is required, the contralateral lower extremity may be positioned in hip abduction with the knee flexed over the edge of the plinth and the foot supported on a stool (see Fig. 6-29).

Goniometer Axis. The axis is placed over the ASIS on the side being measured (Figs. 6-26B and 6-27).

Stationary Arm. Along a line that joins the two ASISs.

Movable Arm. Parallel to the longitudinal axis of the femur, pointing toward the midline of the patella. In the start position described, the goniometer will indicate 90°. This is recorded as 0°. For example, if the goniometer reads 90° at the start position for hip abduction and 60° at the end position, hip abduction PROM would be 30°.

End Position. The hip is abducted to the limit of motion (45°) (Fig. 6-28).

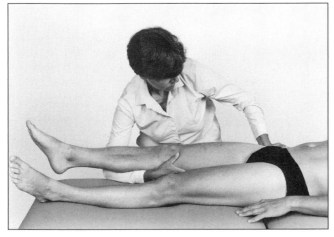

Figure 6-24 Start position for hip abduction.

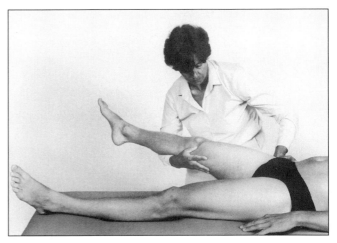

Figure 6-25 Firm end feel at the limit of hip abduction.

Hip Extension

AROM Assessment

Substitute Movement. Anterior pelvic tilt and extension of the lumbar spine.

PROM Assessment

Start Position. The patient is prone. Both hips and knees are in the neutral position. The feet are over the end of the plinth (Fig. 6-20).

Stabilization. The therapist stabilizes the pelvis.

Therapist's Distal Hand Placement. The therapist grasps the anterior aspect of the distal femur.

End Position. The therapist applies slight traction to and moves the femur posteriorly to the limit of hip extension (Fig. 6-21).

End Feel. Hip extension—firm.

Joint Spin (15). *Hip extension*—the convex femoral head spins in the fixed concave acetabulum.

Measurement: Universal Goniometer

Start Position. The patient is prone. The hips and knees are in the neutral position. The feet are over the end of the plinth (Fig. 6-22).

Stabilization. The pelvis is stabilized through strapping. Alternatively, a second therapist may assist to manually stabilize the pelvis.

Goniometer Axis. The axis is placed over the greater trochanter of the femur (see Fig. 6-18).

Stationary Arm. Parallel to the midaxillary line of the trunk.

Movable Arm. Parallel to the longitudinal axis of the femur, pointing toward the lateral epicondyle.

End Position. The patient's knee is maintained in extension to place the rectus femoris on slack. The hip is extended to the limit of motion (30°) (Fig. 6-23).

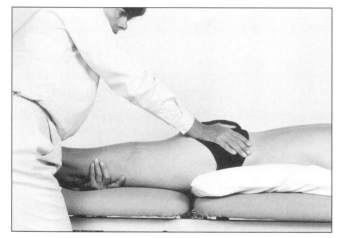

Figure 6-20 Start position: hip extension.

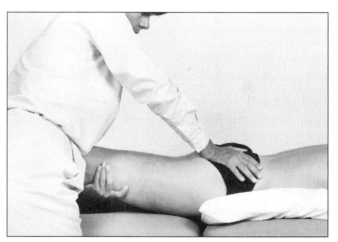

Figure 6-21 Firm end feel at limit of hip extension.

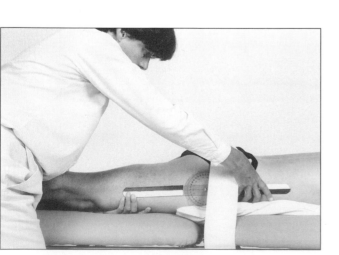

Figure 6-22 Start position: hip extension.

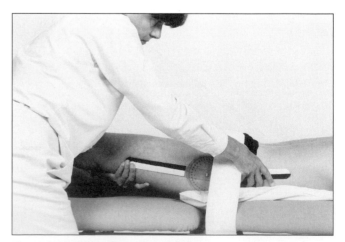

Figure 6-23 End position: hip extension.

Trunk Flexion and Extension: Lumbar Spine

Tape Measure Measurement

Start Positions. *Flexion* (49): The patient is standing with feet shoulder width apart. A tape measure is used to measure a distance and mark a point 15 cm above the midpoint of the line connecting the PSISs (i.e., the spinous process of S2) with the patient in the start position (Fig. 9-67). *Extension:* For lumbar extension, the patient's hands are placed on the iliac crests and into the small of the back (Fig. 9-68). The patient is instructed to keep the knees straight when performing the test movements.

End Positions. *Flexion:* The patient flexes the trunk forward to the limit of lumbar flexion motion (Fig. 9-69). A second measure is taken to measure the distance between the PSIS and the 15-cm skin mark at the limit of lumbar flexion ROM. The difference between the start and end measures is the lumbar spinal flexion ROM. This method of measurement is referred to as the modified-modified Schöber method. *Extension:* The patient extends the trunk backward to the limit of motion for lumbar extension (Fig. 9-70). A second measure is taken to measure the distance between the PSIS and the 15-cm skin mark at the limit of lumbar extension ROM. The difference between the start and end measures is the lumbar spinal extension ROM.

Inclinometer Measurement

Start Positions. *Flexion:* For lumbar flexion, the patient is standing with feet shoulder width apart (Fig. 9-71). *Extension:* For lumbar extension, the patient's hands are placed on the iliac crests and into the small of the back (Fig. 9-72). The inclinometers are positioned and zeroed in each start position. The patient is instructed to keep the knees straight when performing the test movements.

Inclinometer Placement. *Superior*: On a mark 15 cm above the spinous process of S2. *Inferior:* On the spine of S2.

End Positions. *Flexion:* The patient flexes the trunk forward to the limit of motion for lumbar flexion (Fig. 9-73). *Extension:* The patient extends the trunk backward to the limit of motion for lumbar extension (Fig. 9-74). At the end position for each movement, the therapist records the angle measurements from both inclinometers. The AROM for lumbar spine flexion or extension is the difference between the inclinometer readings in the end position for the movement being measured.

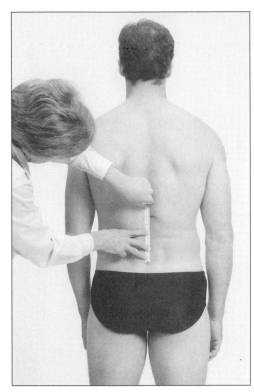

Figure 9-67 Start position: lumbar flexion, modified-modified Schöber method. The distance measured is between the spine of S2 and a point 15 cm above S2.

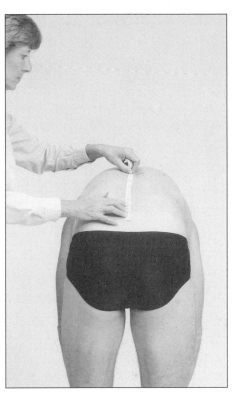

Figure 9-69 End position: lumbar flexion, modified-modified Schöber method.

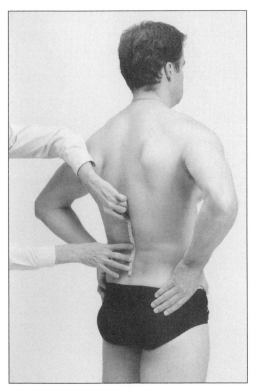

Figure 9-68 Start position: lumbar extension.

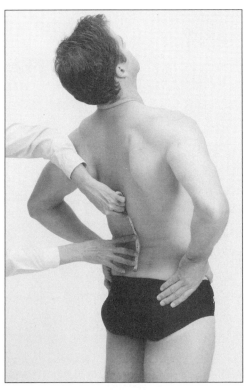

Figure 9-70 End position: lumbar extension.

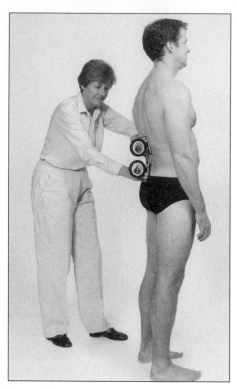

Figure 9-71 Start position: lumbar flexion with inclinometer placement over the spine of S2 and over a mark 15 cm above the spine of S2.

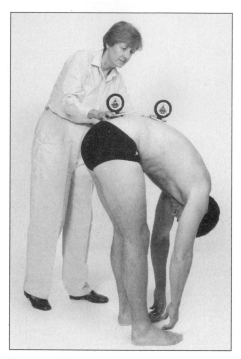

Figure 9-73 Lumbar spine flexion.

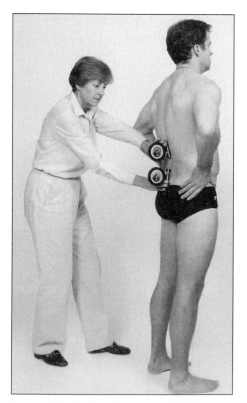

Figure 9-72 Start position: lumbar spine extension.

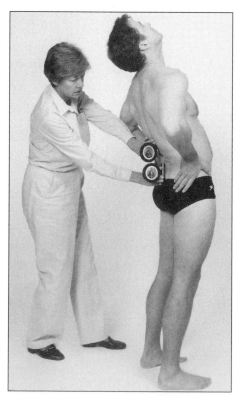

Figure 9-74 Lumbar spine extension.

Trunk Lateral Flexion

Tape Measure Measurement

Start Position. The patient is standing with the feet shoulder width apart (Fig. 9-75). The patient is instructed to keep both feet flat on the floor when performing the test movements.

Stabilization. None.

Substitute Movement. Trunk flexion, trunk extension, ipsilateral hip and knee flexion, raising the contralateral or ipsilateral foot from the floor.

End Position. The patient laterally flexes the trunk to the limit of motion (Fig. 9-76). A tape measure is used to measure the distance between the tip of the third digit and the floor.

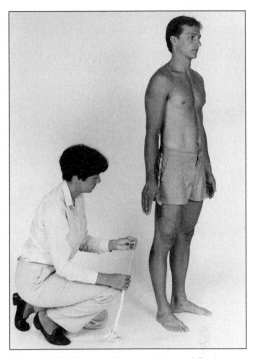

Figure 9-75 Start position: trunk lateral flexion.

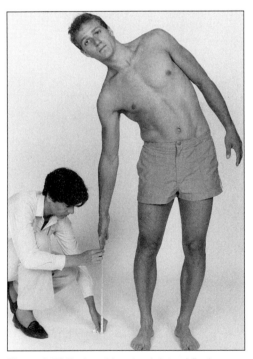

Figure 9-76 End position: trunk lateral flexion.

Alternate Tape Measure Measurement (50)

Start Position. The patient is standing with the feet shoulder width apart. A mark is placed on the thigh at the level of the tip of the middle finger (Fig. 9-77). The patient is instructed to keep both feet flat on the floor when performing the test movements.

Stabilization. None.

End Position. The patient laterally flexes the trunk to the limit of motion. A second mark is placed on the thigh at the level of the tip of the middle finger (Fig. 9-78).

Measurement. A tape measure is used to measure the distance between the marks placed on the thigh at the level of the tip of the middle finger at the start position and at the end position (Fig. 9-79). The distance measured represents the lateral flexion ROM.

Inclinometer Measurement

Start Position. The patient stands with feet shoulder width apart. The inclinometers are positioned and zeroed (Fig. 9-80). The patient is instructed to keep both feet flat on the floor when performing the test movements.

Inclinometer placement. *Superior:* On the spine of T1. *Inferior:* On the spine of S2.

End Position. The patient laterally flexes the trunk to the limit of motion (Fig. 9-81). At the end position, the therapist records the angle measurements from both inclinometers. The AROM for lateral flexion is the difference between the inclinometer readings.

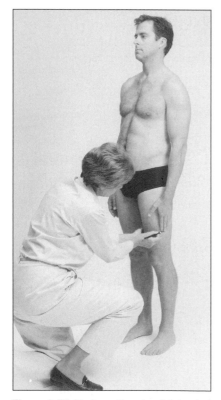

Figure 9-77 Start position: trunk lateral flexion.

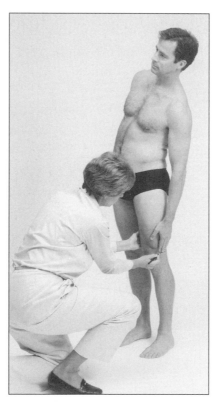

Figure 9-78 End position: trunk lateral flexion.

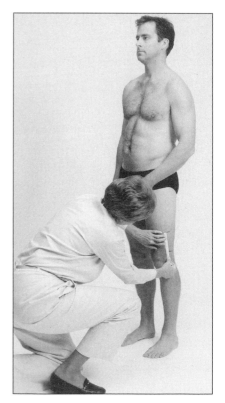

Figure 9-79 Measurement: trunk lateral flexion.

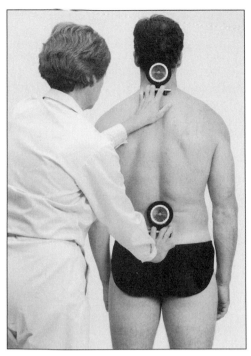

Figure 9-80 Inclinometer placement (spines of T1 and S2) for trunk lateral flexion.

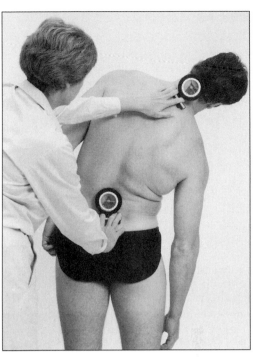

Figure 9-81 End position: trunk lateral flexion.

Universal Goniometer Measurement

Start Position. Standing (Fig. 9-82).

Goniometer Axis. In the midline at the level of the PSIS (i.e., over the S2 spinous process).

Stationary Arm. Perpendicular to the floor.

Movable Arm. Points toward the spine of C7.

Lateral Flexion. The goniometer is realigned at the limit of trunk lateral flexion (Fig. 9-83). The number of degrees the movable arm lies away from the 0° position is recorded as the thoracolumbar lateral flexion ROM to the side measured.

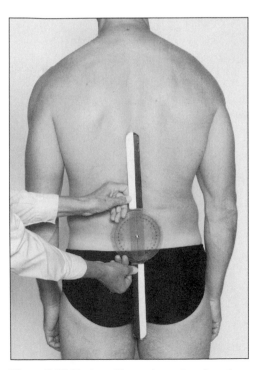

Figure 9-82 Start position: universal goniometer placement trunk lateral flexion.

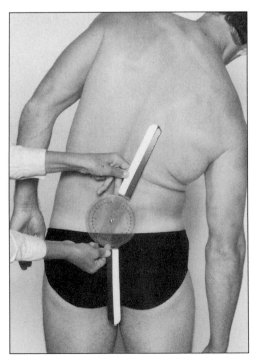

Figure 9-83 End position: trunk lateral flexion.

Trunk Rotation: Thoracolumbar Spine

Tape Measure Measurement

Start Position. The patient is sitting with the feet supported on a stool and the arms crossed in front of the chest. The patient holds the end of the tape measure on the lateral aspect of the acromion process. The therapist holds the other end of the tape measure on either the uppermost point of the iliac crest at the midaxillary line (not shown) or on the upper border of the greater trochanter (Fig. 9-84). The distance between the lateral aspect of the acromion process and the uppermost point of the iliac crest at the midaxillary line or the upper border of the greater trochanter is measured.

Stabilization. The body weight on the pelvis; the therapist can also stabilize the pelvis.

Substitute Movement. Trunk flexion, trunk extension, and shoulder girdle protraction (on the side the tape measure is held).

End Position. The patient rotates the trunk to the limit of motion (Fig. 9-85). The distance between the lateral aspect of the acromion process and either the uppermost point of the iliac crest at the midaxillary line or the upper border of the greater trochanter is measured at the limit of rotation. The difference between the start position and end position measures is the thoracolumbar rotation ROM. The surface landmarks used in the assessment should be documented.

Frost and colleagues (52) described the use of the tape measure to measure trunk rotation (using the posterior clavicular prominence and the greater trochanter as landmarks) and noted that the accurate definition and palpation of the landmarks used in the assessment are critical for reliable assessment.

The present author (Clarkson) recommends using the lateral aspect of the acromion process and the uppermost point of the iliac crest as the preferred surface landmarks, as these are easily palpable.

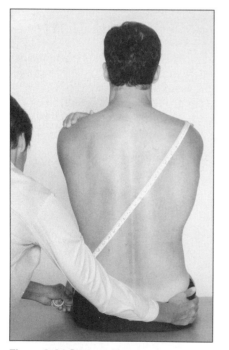

Figure 9-84 Start position: trunk rotation.

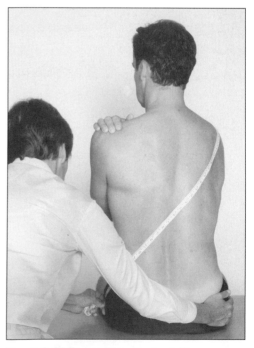

Figure 9-85 End position: trunk rotation.

Trunk Rotation: Thoracic Spine

Inclinometer Measurement

Start Position. The patient is standing with the arms crossed in front of the chest. The patient leans forward with the head and trunk parallel to the floor or as close to this position as possible. The inclinometers are positioned and zeroed (Fig. 9-86).

Inclinometer Placement. *Superior:* On the spine of T1. *Inferior:* On the spine of T12.

End Positions. The patient rotates the trunk to the limit of motion (Fig. 9-87). At the end position, the therapist records the angle measurements from both inclinometers. The AROM for thoracic spine rotation is the difference between the inclinometer readings.

Substitute Movement. Trunk flexion and trunk extension. The range of trunk rotation when measured in the forward lean or stooped posture is less than when measured in sitting (53). This may be caused by the contraction of the back muscles required to sustain the stooped posture that splint the spine and restrict trunk rotation (53).

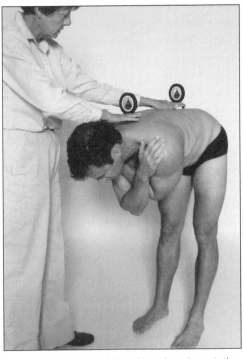

Figure 9-86 Start position: thoracic spine rotation with inclinometers placed over the spines of T1 and T12.

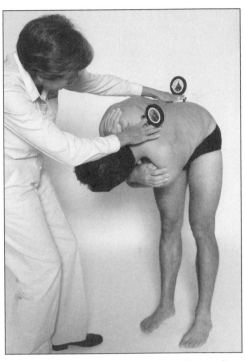

Figure 9-87 End position: thoracic spine rotation.

Chest Expansion

Tape Measure Measurement

Start Position. The patient is sitting. The patient makes a full expiration (Fig. 9-88).

End Position. The patient makes a full inspiration (Fig. 9-89).

Measurement. A tape measure is used to measure the circumference of the chest at the level of the xiphisternal joint. Measures are taken at full expiration and at full inspiration. The difference between the two measures is the chest expansion. The chest expansion may also be mea-

sured at the levels of the nipple line and anterior axillary fold. The chest expansion measured at the latter points is slightly less than that at the xiphisternal joint. It is recommended (54) that two measurement sites, specifically the xiphoid and axilla, and a consistent patient position be used to provide a thorough evaluation of pulmonary status. A wide range of normal values exists for normal chest expansion and, beginning in the late 30s, chest expansion gradually decreases with increasing age (55). Decreased chest expansion may indicate costovertebral joint involvement in certain pathological conditions (56) or may occur with chronic obstructive pulmonary disease (e.g., emphysema).

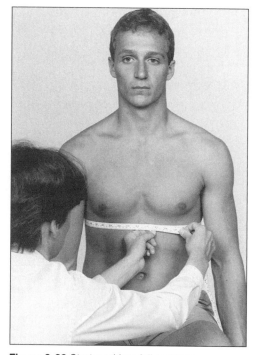

Figure 9-88 Start position: full expiration measured at the level of the xiphisternal joint.

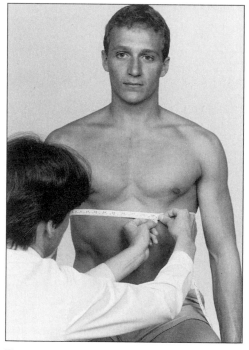

Figure 9-89 End position: full inspiration measured at the level of the xiphisternal joint.

MUSCLE LENGTH ASSESSMENT AND MEASUREMENT

Trunk Extensors and Hamstrings (Toe-Touch Test)

The trunk extensors are the erector spinae (iliocostalis thoracis and lumborum, longissimus thoracis, spinalis thoracis, semispinalis thoracis, multifidus); the hip extensor and knee flexor muscles are the hamstrings (semitendinosus, semimembranosus, biceps femoris). The toe-touch test provides a composite measure of hip, spine, and shoulder girdle ROM.

Start Position. The patient is standing (Fig. 9-90).

Substitute Movement. Knee flexion.

Stabilization. None.

End Position. The patient flexes the trunk and hips and reaches toward the toes to the limit of motion (Fig. 9-91).

Measurement. A tape measure is used to measure the distance between the floor and the most distant point reached by both hands. Normal ROM is present if the patient can touch the toes. If the patient can reach beyond floor level, the test can be carried out with the patient standing on a step or platform to measure reach distance beyond the supporting surface.

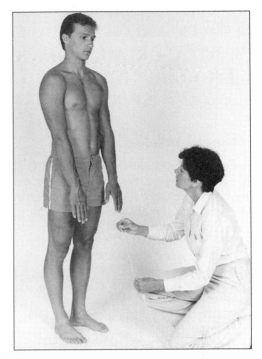

Figure 9-90 Start position: toe-touch test.

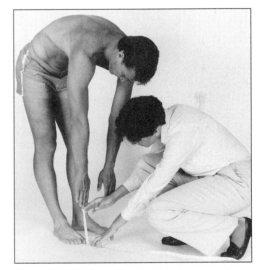

Figure 9-91 End position: trunk extensor and hamstring muscle length.

VALIDITY AND RELIABILITY: MEASUREMENT OF THORACIC SPINE AND LUMBAR SPINE AROM

Tape Measure/Ruler

Two research teams (57,58) investigated the validity of using the tape measure to evaluate lumbar spine flexion AROM by comparing tape measurements with measures obtained by radiography. Macrae and Wright (58) used the Schöber and modified Schöber methods to measure subjects' lumbar flexion ROM; Portek and colleagues (57) used the modified Schöber method.

To measure lumbar flexion AROM using a tape measure and the Schöber or modified Schöber methods, the subject is in standing position. For the Schöber method, the skin is marked over the spine at the level of the lumbosacral junction and a point 10 cm superior to the lumbosacral junction. For the modified Schöber method, the skin is marked in the midline at points 5 cm inferior and 10 cm superior to the lumbosacral junction. At the end of the forward flexion ROM, distances are remeasured between the superior and inferior marks for each method. The increase in distance between the marks at the end of the ROM (i.e., the increase from 10 cm for the Schöber method and from 15 cm for the modified Schöber method) represents the lumbar flexion AROM.

Portek and colleagues (57) concluded that the modified Schöber method gives only a linear index of movement and does not reflect true spinal movement. Assessing subjects with and without spinal disease, Macrae and Wright (58) found a linear relationship between the lumbar flexion measurements obtained using the Schöber and modified Schöber methods and radiographic measurements. However, using the modified Schöber method, the accuracy of the measurement of lumbar flexion was superior.

Research conducted to establish the reliability of using the tape measure for thoracic and/or lumbar spine AROM measurement is presented by spinal region and motion assessed and is summarized below.

Thoracolumbar Extension

PSIS to C7 Method (see Figs. 9-58 and 9-60). Frost and colleagues (52) examined the intra- and intertester reliability of measuring thoracolumbar spine extension AROM using a tape measure to assess the change in distance between the points at the midline at the level of the PSIS and the C7 spinous process. The results showed poor intra- and intertester measurement reliability. The research group suggested that more accurate palpation of bony landmarks would lessen the amount of error.

Prone Press-Up (see Figs. 9-65 and 9-66). Bandy and Reese (59) assessed the intra- and intertester reliability of using the tape measure to quantify the range of lumbar spine extension using the prone press-up position. The researchers found the tape measure to be reliable for mea-

suring lumbar extension using the prone press-up, with and without the use of the pelvic stabilization strap, for both experienced and inexperienced examiners. However, the ROM values were found to be greater when the subject's pelvis was stabilized with the strap. Therefore, these two methods of assessing lumbar spine extension ROM should not be used interchangeably. In addition, with the pelvis unstrapped, the researchers noted the subjects were concerned with keeping the pelvis against the plinth and therefore were unable "to attain full range of lumbar extension."

Lumbar Flexion/Extension

Schöber Method. The intertester reliability of measuring lumbar flexion AROM using the Schöber method was investigated by Fitzgerald and associates (60). The Schöber method showed high intertester reliability.

Modified Schöber Method. The modified Schöber method is used to measure the lumbar spine flexion as previously described. This method can also be used to measure lumbar extension ROM by recording the decrease in the 15-cm distance between the landmarks at the end of the lumbar extension ROM. This method of measuring lumbar spine extension is the modified Schöber attraction method.

Several researchers examined the intratester reliability of measuring lumbar flexion (57,61,62) and lumbar extension (61,63) AROM using the tape measure and the modified Schöber method, and all found the measurements were reliable. However, the majority of research, carried out on healthy subjects to determine the intertester reliability for measuring lumbar flexion (57,62) using the modified Schöber method—or a slightly modified version of the method (64)—found the measurement method to have low intertester reliability. The one study by Oksanen and Salminen (65) that reported high intertester reliability for measuring lumbar flexion using the modified Schöber method studied younger subjects (15-year-old school children), 50% of whom had recurrent or continuous low back pain.

Beattie and associates (63) examined the intertester reliability of using the modified Schöber method to measure lumbar extension and found high intertester reliability for the method.

Modified-Modified Schöber Method (see Figs. 9-67 through 9-70). To measure lumbar flexion or extension AROM using the modified-modified Schöber method, the subject is in standing position. The skin is marked over the spine at the level of the PSIS and at a point 15 cm superior to the level of the PSIS. A tape measure is used at the end of the lumbar flexion or extension ROM to measure the increase or decrease, respectively, in the distance between the marks at the level of the PSIS and 15 cm superior. The change in distance represents the lumbar flexion or extension AROM.

Van Adrichem and van der Korst (49) tested the reproducibility of measuring the lumbar flexion AROM using a mark placed in the midline between the PSIS and marks placed 5, 10, 15, and 20 cm superior to the level of the PSIS. The researchers concluded that a mark 15 cm superior seemed to best represent the true length of the lumbar spine; they reported that their findings showed "a simple reliable clinical assessment of lumbar flexibility can be made by measuring the increasing distance between two skin marks 15 cm apart" (49, p. 90) during lumbar flexion.

Williams and coworkers (66) assessed the intra- and intertester reliability of measuring active lumbar flexion and extension using the modified-modified Schöber method in subjects with chronic low back pain. The researchers concluded the modified-modified Schöber method is a reliable and time-efficient method to use for measuring lumbar flexion and extension ROM.

Thoracolumbar Lateral Flexion

Lateral Flexion: Fingertip-to-Floor Measurement Method (see Figs. 9-75 and 9-76). Frost and colleagues (52) evaluated the intra- and intertester reliability of trunk lateral flexion AROM by measuring the distance between the middle fingertip and the floor at the end of the lateral flexion ROM. This method of measuring lateral trunk flexion showed good intra- and intertester measurement reliability.

Lateral Flexion: Thigh Measurement Method (see Figs. 9-77 through 9-79). Several studies (38,50,62,65,67) assessed healthy subjects to evaluate the reliability of measuring lateral trunk flexion using a tape measure to measure the distance between marks placed on the lateral thigh at the level of the tip of the middle finger at the start and end of trunk lateral flexion AROM. In summary, most of these studies (38,50,62,65) reported good to strong intra- and/or intertester reliability for the thigh measurement method for healthy subjects. Hyytiäinen and colleagues (62) also noted that the method proved to be quick and easy to perform; Rose (67), in studying intratester reliability of this measurement technique, found the intratester reliability was poor, but noted that error may have been introduced into the study by several subjects having taken part in an exercise class between measures.

Thoracolumbar Rotation (see Figs. 9-84 and 9-85)

Frost and colleagues (52) evaluated the intra- and intertester reliability of measuring trunk rotation AROM using the tape measure. The researchers reported poor reliability for the measurements and suggested the bony landmarks selected and inaccurate palpation of bony landmarks may have affected the measurement accuracy and reliability.

Toe-Touch Test (see Figs. 9-90 and 9-91)

The toe-touch test or fingertip-to-floor method of assessing ROM provides a composite measure of hip, spine, and shoulder girdle ROM. The majority of studies (52,62,65,68) that examined the intra- and/or intertester reliability of the toe-touch test reported good to strong reliability for this method. However, Gill and coworkers (61) found the fingertip-to-floor method to have poor intratester reliability and suggested this may result from the measurement being less specific to the lumbar vertebral movement and including movement of other parts of the spine and joints of the upper extremity.

Inclinometry

The work by Lee and colleagues (69) was the only study found in the literature that examined the validity of measuring thoracic spine ROM using inclinometry. These researchers compared single inclinometer measures with radiographic measures of thoracic spine lateral flexion. The researchers reported poor to moderate validity for the measurement of thoracic spine lateral flexion by single inclinometry and concluded that due to the low validity, the usefulness of the technique in the clinic should be "minimized" until further research establishes validity.

Studies (57,64,70–73) conducted to determine the validity of measuring lumbar spine AROM using the inclinometer examined lumbar flexion and extension. These studies compared the inclinometer measurements to radiographic measurements. The study findings were mixed, with three research groups (57,64,70) reporting low validity and an equal number (71–73) finding the inclinometer to be a valid means of assessing the lumbar spine AROM.

Many researchers have employed various types of inclinometers to determine the reliability of using the inclinometer to measure thoracolumbar and lumbar spine ROM.

Thoracic Flexion/Extension/Lateral Flexion

Lee and colleagues (69) examined the intra- and intertester reliability of measuring the thoracic spine flexion, extension, and lateral flexion ROM of 31 healthy subjects using single inclinometry. The testers positioned the inclinometer over the spine of T1 and then T12 to take the measurements. The authors interpreted the intra- and intertester reliability to be generally good, but noted that the usefulness of the single inclinometer in the clinical setting is minimal due to the low validity reported in this study.

Thoracolumbar Flexion/Extension/Lateral Flexion

In the late 1960s, Loebl (74) provided a descriptive report of "a new simple method for accurate clinical measurement of spinal posture and movements" using the inclinometer. The inclinometer was placed on the vertebral spines of S1, T12, T1, and a point midway between T1 and T12 to measure the spinal AROM of nine normal subjects. Loebl (74) concluded that the inclinometer method was quick to use and accurate to within 10% of the total ROM for the majority of subjects.

Other studies that examined the reliability of inclinometry for measuring thoracolumbar flexion, extension, and lateral flexion used the pendulum goniometer (75), electronic dual inclinometer (76), and the OB "Myrin" inclinometer (77,78). Reynolds (75), using the pendulum goniometer, found the intra- and intertester reliability to be acceptable for thoracolumbar flexion, extension, total sagittal motion, and lateral flexion. Measurements of thoracolumbar extension and lumbar lateral flexion were found not reproducible. Using the electronic inclinometer, Nitschke and coworkers (76) concluded that the double inclinometer method of measuring low back ROM for patients with chronic low back pain had poor intra- and intertester reliability. Mellin (77) and Mellin and colleagues (78) measured healthy subjects using the OB "Myrin" inclinometer and found the intratester reliability to be acceptable. Mellin (77) also evaluated the intertester reliability and found it to be acceptable. Mellin (77) noted the "accuracy of the methods described makes them useful for measurements of thoracolumbar mobility in the sagittal and frontal planes. However, training is needed in the methods, manipulation of the instruments, and instructions to give the subjects before the measurements can be considered reliable" (77, p. 761).

Lumbar Flexion/Extension/Lateral Flexion

The majority of researchers evaluating the measurement of lumbar flexion (79–81), flexion and extension (57,61,82–84), and lateral flexion (82) ROM using the inclinometer have found good intratester reliability. However, Williams and coworkers (66) and Chen and colleagues (85) concluded that intratester reliability using the inclinometer is questionable and requires improvement or is "mostly clinically undesirable," respectively.

The intertester reliability using the inclinometer when measuring lumbar flexion or extension ROM has been shown to be high by some researchers (38,57,83,84) but poor by others (66,79,80,85). The results of two additional studies, by Saur and colleagues (71) and Burdett and associates (64), showed that using the inclinometer to measure lumbar flexion ROM showed high intertester reliability, but that lumbar extension ROM showed low intertester reliability. Patel (81) reported only moderate intertester reliability for lumbar flexion measured by double inclinometry.

Thoracic and Lumbar Spine Rotation

Alaranta and colleagues (38) assessed the intertester reliability of measuring total right and left trunk rotation ROM with the subjects in sitting, using the OB "Myrin" goniometer positioned at the inferior level of the scapulae. The study showed good intertester reliability for the measurement of total trunk rotation using the OB goniometer.

Boline and associates (86) examined the intertester reliability of the inclinometer, positioned at the T12–L1 level, to measure lumbar rotation with subjects forward flexed to face the floor in the standing position. In this study, two chiropractors measured the lumbar rotation ROM of 25 subjects with chronic low back pain and 25 healthy subjects. Boline and associates (86) found intertester reliability to be moderate to good for measuring lumbar rotation using the inclinometer.

Universal Goniometer

Thoracolumbar Flexion/Extension/Lateral Flexion

The intertester reliability of measuring thoracolumbar extension and right and left lateral flexion ROM using the universal goniometer was investigated by Fitzgerald and associates (60). All spinal movements, as measured by two testers on each of 17 healthy subjects, showed substantial intertester reliability. Nitschke and coworkers (76) researched the intra- and intertester reliability of using a universal goniometer and an electronic dual inclinometer to measure flexion, extension, and lateral flexion ROM of the thoracolumbar and lumbar spinal regions, according to the guidelines set out by the AMA Guides to the Evaluation of Permanent Impairment (14). The researchers concluded that the universal goniometer and double inclinometer methods of measuring low back ROM for patients with chronic low back pain have poor intra- and intertester reliability.

Back Range-of-Motion Instrument

The Back Range-of-Motion Instrument (BROMII) (87) (Performance Attainment Associates, Roseville, MN) is a relatively new tool designed to measure AROM of the lumbar spine. It consists of two units for the measurement of back ROM. First, a frame that contains a protractor scale is positioned over S1 and held in place using Velcro straps. An L-shaped extension arm slides into the frame, and this device is used to measure lumbar flexion and extension ROM. Second, a frame that holds two inclinometers is positioned horizontally over the T12 spinous process and held in place by the therapist during the measurement of lateral flexion and rotation. One inclinometer lies in the frontal plane with a gravity-dependent needle for measurement of lateral flexion; a second, oriented in the transverse plane, contains a compass needle that reacts to Earth's magnetic field for measurement of rotation. A magnetic yoke is positioned around the pelvis to eliminate substitute pelvic motion from the rotation measurement.

Studies (79,88,89) assessing the reliability of the BROMII were all carried out using healthy young subjects. Breum and colleagues (88) examined the intra- and intertester reliability of the BROMII and found it to be reliable for measuring active flexion and lateral flexion, but the reliability for extension and rotation was considered unacceptable.

Rondinelli and associates (79) used two testers to examine eight subjects and obtain reliability estimates of lumbar flexion AROM using the BROMII, single inclinometry, and double inclinometry. For the BROMII, the intratester reliability was reported to be acceptable and intertester reliability unacceptable for lumbar flexion. The BROMII had a median range of measurement error of 16°, compared to 8.5° for single inclinometry and 10.5° for double inclinometry.

Intratester reliability of the BROMII was also studied by Madson and coworkers (89), who found the instrument to be reliable for measuring active lateral flexion and rotation. However, intratester reliability of lumbar spine flexion and extension AROM was reported to be poor and fair, respectively. Madson and coworkers (89) suggested that because of the high reliability of tape measure measurements, the tape measure should be preferred over the BROMII for flexion and extension ROM measurement.

The BROMII is relatively expensive, and from the research to date, it does not appear to be superior to other means of measuring AROM of the lumbar spine. For this reason, the BROMII is not used to demonstrate ROM assessment in this text.

FUNCTIONAL APPLICATION

Joint Function: Neck and Trunk

The trunk complex consists of the vertebral column, thorax, sternum, ribs, sacrum, and coccyx. The vertebral column and its system of linkages have particular significance in functional application of ROM. The stability function of the spine includes resisting compressive forces; supporting the major portion of the body weight; supporting the head, arms, and trunk against the force of gravity; shock absorption; protecting the spinal cord; and providing a stable structure for movement of the extremities (8,90).

The articulations at the intervertebral and facet joints of the vertebral column permit movement in flexion, extension, lateral flexion, and rotation to allow neck and back mobility. The functional range of the spine is increased by the tilt of the pelvis. The total motion of the spine is the result of the collective movements of the articulations of the various segments of the vertebral column (8,15,91), and functional ranges vary between individuals (91). Restriction of motion at any level may result in increased motion at another level (91). Mobility in all planes is the greatest at the cervical spine segment. The thoracic spine has limited mobility in all planes due to the limitations imposed by the thorax (1,8,15). Through movements of the thoracic wall, intrathoracic volume is increased or decreased for inspiration and expiration. The lumbar spine is most mobile in the sagittal plane. Functional ROM is described for the cervical and the thoracic and lumbar spines.

Functional Range of Motion

Cervical Spine

The movement components of the cervical spine allow movement for functioning of the sense organs within the head (92) and expression of nonverbal communication, including affirmative (nodding) or negative responses. Maintenance of ROM in flexion, extension, lateral flexion, and rotation is of particular importance to the individual for interacting with the environment through the sense of vision. The significance of the interdependence between vision and neck movements is demonstrated in many self-care, leisure, and occupational tasks. Full ROM in all planes is not required for most self-care activities (Figs. 9-92 and 9-93). Ranges approximating full values may be required for such activities as shoulder checking in

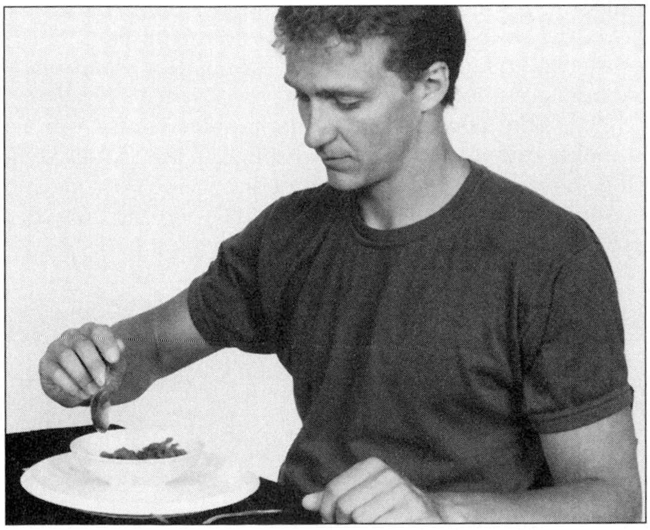

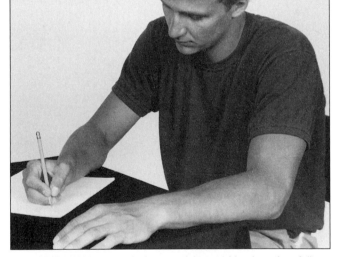

Figure 9-92 Eating: an activity requiring less than full neck flexion ROM.

Figure 9-93 Writing at a desk: an activity requiring less than full neck flexion ROM.

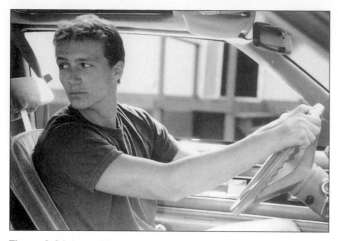

Figure 9-94 An activity requiring full neck rotation ROM.

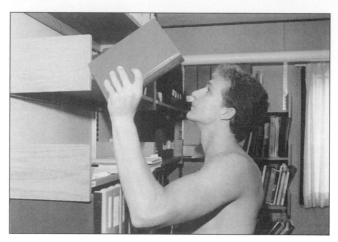

Figure 9-95 An activity requiring full extension ROM.

driving (lateral flexion and rotation [Fig. 9-94]), painting a ceiling, placing an object on a high shelf (Fig. 9-95), gazing at the stars (extension), and many specific leisure and occupational tasks linking vision and neck movements. When eye mobility is restricted, greater cervical spine ROM may be required (93) or head posture may be affected (94) to accommodate for the restricted field of gaze.

Neck extension is required when drinking (Fig. 9-96). The shape of the body of the glass and the diameter of the rim are factors that determine the amount of neck extension required to drink from a glass (95). "Pot-bellied" and narrow-rimmed glasses require more neck extension (95). For example, nearly full neck extension (i.e., a mean of

40°) is required to drink from a narrow champagne flute compared to 0° for a saucer-shaped champagne glass (95).

Thoracic and Lumbar Spines

Rotation of the trunk is achieved through the movement components of the thoracic and lumbar spine and is coupled with slight lateral flexion (90,91,96). Rotation is a movement that is most free in the upper spinal segments and progressively diminishes in the lower segments (96). Rotation of the trunk extends the reach of the hands beyond the contralateral side of the body and permits the individual to face different directions without foot movement (Fig. 9-97).

The major contribution of the mobility in the lumbar spine to daily functioning is through flexion and extension movements. When combined with the thoracic and cervical segments, the individual can reach the more dis-

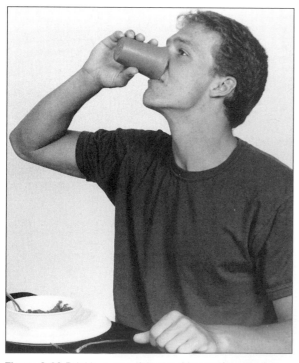

Figure 9-96 Drinking: an activity requiring neck extension.

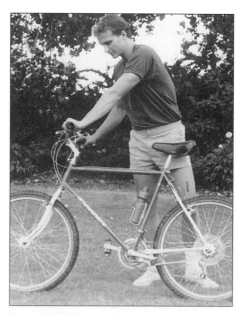

Figure 9-97 Trunk rotation.

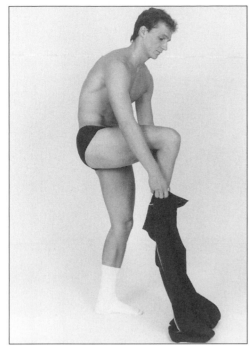

Figure 9-98 Donning a pair of trousers requires flexion of the thoracic and lumbar spines.

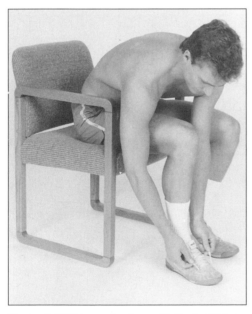

Figure 9-99 Tying a shoelace with the foot flat on the floor requires thoracic and lumbar flexion and neck extension.

tal parts of the lower extremities and objects in the environment (Figs. 9-95, 9-98, 9-99 and 9-100). The final degrees of functional range are achieved through the interaction of the pelvis and hip (8,15).

Coordination of movement in the lumbar and pelvic regions provides smooth movement and a large excursion of movement for the lower extremity and trunk. This special instance of coordinated pattern of movement between the lumbar spine and pelvis is called "lumbar-pelvic rhythm" (97) and occurs when forward flexing to touch the toes (see Figs. 9-90 and 9-91). The first part of the motion consists of lumbar flexion. This is followed by anterior tilting of the pelvis to complete the motion. On return to the upright position, the pelvis tilts posteriorly, followed by extension of the lumbar spine.

Normal ROM for lumbar spine flexion is about 60° (98). Sitting to put on a sock (see Fig. 9-100) and squatting

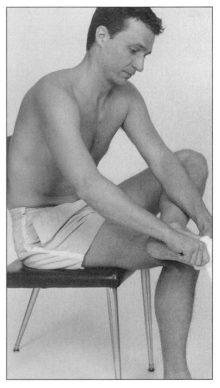

Figure 9-100 Lumbar flexion.

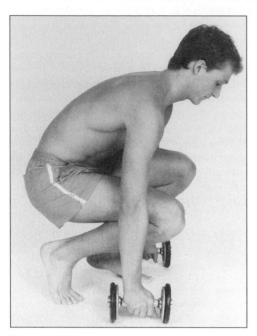

Figure 9-101 Squatting to pick up an object from the floor requires almost full lumbar flexion (i.e., about 95% of full flexion) (98).

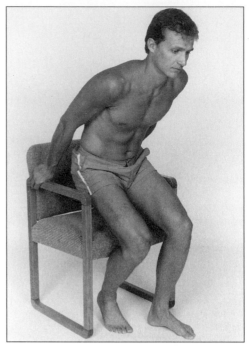

Figure 9-102 Moving from standing to sitting and returning to standing requires about 56% to 66% of full lumbar flexion ROM (98).

to pick up an object from the floor (Fig. 9-101) are examples of activities that require almost full lumbar spine flexion (i.e., about 90% and 95% of full flexion, respectively) (98). Moving from standing to sitting and returning to standing position requires about 56% to 66% of full lumbar flexion ROM (98) (Fig. 9-102).

Activities that require lateral flexion of the spine include reaching down to pick up an object from a low surface at one's side, moving from a side-lying position to sitting on the edge of a bed, and reaching objects overhead (Fig. 9-103). To mount a bicycle, one leg is lifted over the seat of the bicycle and the trunk is laterally flexed to the same side.

Gait (8)

As the pelvis rotates forward on the side of the advancing leg, the upper trunk rotates forward on the opposite side to decrease the motion of the body during the gait cycle.

References

1. Kapandji IA. *The Physiology of the Joints.* Vol 3. 2nd ed. London: Churchill Livingstone; 1974.
2. Soames RW, ed. Skeletal system. In: *Gray's Anatomy. 38th* ed. New York: Churchill Livingstone; 1995.
3. Hertling D. The temporomandibular joint. In: Hertling D, Kessler RM. *Management of Common Musculoskeletal Disorders: Physical Therapy Principles and Methods.* 3rd ed. Philadelphia: Harper & Row; 1996.
4. Magee DJ. *Orthopedic Physical Assessment.* 4th ed. Philadelphia: Saunders; 2002.
5. American Academy of Orthopaedic Surgeons. *Joint Motion: Method of Measuring and Recording.* Chicago: AAOS; 1965.
6. Norkin CC, White DJ. *Measurement of Joint Motion: A Guide to Goniometry.* 3rd ed. Philadelphia: FA Davis; 2003.

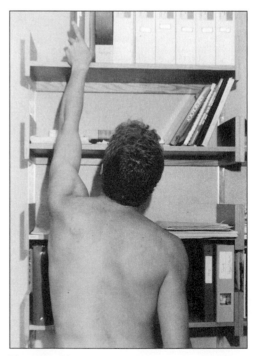

Figure 9-103 Reaching objects overhead requires trunk lateral flexion.

7. Cyriax J. *Textbook of Orthopaedic Medicine, Vol 1. Diagnosis of Soft Tissue Lesions.* 8th ed. London: Bailliere Tindall; 1982.
8. Levangie PK, Norkin CC. *Joint Structure & Function: A Comprehensive Analysis.* 3rd ed. Philadelphia: FA Davis; 2001.
9. Daniels L, Worthingham C. *Muscle Testing: Techniques of Manual Examination.* 5th ed. Philadelphia: WB Saunders; 1986.

10. Youdas JW, Garrett TR, Suman VJ, et al. Normal range of motion of the cervical spine: an initial goniometric study. *Phys Ther.* 1992;72:770–780.

11. Balogun JA, Abereoje OK, Olaogun MO, Obajuluwa VA. Inter- and intratester reliability of measuring neck motions with tape measure and Myrin gravity-reference goniometer. *JOSPT.* 1989;10:248–253.

12. Hsieh C-Y, Yeung BW. Active neck motion measurements with a tape measure. *JOSPT.* 1986;8:88–92.

13. American Medical Association. *Guides to the Evaluation of Permanent Impairment.* 5th ed. Chicago: AMA Press; 2001.

14. American Medical Association. *Guides to the Evaluation of Permanent Impairment.* 2nd ed. Chicago: AMA Press; 1984.

15. Soderberg GL. *Kinesiology: Application to Pathological Motion.* 2nd ed. Baltimore: Williams & Wilkins; 1997.

16. Iglarsh ZA, Snyder-Mackler L. Temporomandibular joint and the cervical spine. In: Richardson JK, Iglarsh ZA. *Clinical Orthopaedic Physical Therapy.* Philadelphia: WB Saunders; 1994.

17. Moskovich R. Biomechanics of the cervical spine. In: Nordin M, Frankel VH. *Basic Biomechanics of the Musculoskeletal System.* 3rd ed. Philadelphia: Lippincott Williams & Wilkins; 2001.

18. Performance Attainment Associates. CROM Procedure Manual: Procedure for Measuring Neck Motion with the CROM. St. Paul, MN, 1988 (copyright University of Minnesota).

19. Mayer TG, Kindraske G, Beals SB, Gatchel RJ. Spinal range of motion: accuracy and sources of error with inclinometric measurement. *Spine.* 1997;22:1976–1984.

20. Calder I, Picard J, Chapman M, et al. Mouth opening: a new angle. *Anesthesiology.* 2003;99:799–801.

21. Higbie EJ, Seidel-Cobb D, Taylor LF, Cummings GS. Effect of head position on vertical mandibular opening. *JOSPT.* 1999;29:127–130.

22. Thurnwald PA. The effect of age and gender on normal temporomandibular joint movement. *Physiotherapy Theory and Practice.* 1991;7:209–221.

23. Walker N, Bohannon RW, Cameron D. Discriminant validity of temporomandibular joint range of motion measurements obtained with a ruler. *JOSPT.* 2000;30:484–492.

24. Dijkstra PU, De Bont LGM, Stegenga B, Boering G. Temporomandibular joint mobility assessment: a comparison between four methods. *J Oral Rehab.* 1995;22:439–444.

25. Dworkin SF, LeResche L, DeRouen T, VonKorff M. Assessing clinical signs of temporomandibular disorders: reliability of clinical examiners. *J Prosthetic Dentistry.* 1990;63:574–579.

26. Venes D (Ed.). *Taber's Cyclopedic Medical Dictionary.* 19th ed. Philadelphia: FA Davis; 2001.

27. American Medical Association. *Guides to the Evaluation of Permanent Impairment.* 3rd ed (Revised). Chicago: AMA Press; 1990.

28. Pile KD, Laurent MR, Salmond CE, et al. Clinical assessment of ankylosing spondylitis: a study of observer variation in spinal measurements. *Br J Rheumatol.* 1991;30:29–34.

29. Viitanen JV, Kokko M-L, Heikkilä S, Kautiainen H. Neck mobility assessment in ankylosing spondylitis: a clinical study of nine measurements including new tape methods for cervical rotation and lateral flexion. *Br J Rheumatol.* 1998;37: 377–381.

30. Jordan K. Assessment of published reliability studies for cervical range-of-motion measurement tools. *J Manip Physiol Therapeutics.* 2000;23:180–195.

31. Chibnall JT, Duckro PN, Baumer K. The influence of body size on linear measurements used to reflect cervical range of motion. *Phys Ther.* 1994;74:51–54.

32. Bush KW, Collins N, Portman L, Tillett N. Validity and intertester reliability of cervical range of motion using inclinometer measurements. *J Manip Ther.* 2000;8:52–61.

33. Herrmann DB. Validity study of head and neck flexion-extension motion comparing measurements of a pendulum goniometer and roentgenograms. *JOSPT.* 1990; 11:414–418.

34. Hole DE, Cook JM, Bolton JE. Reliability and concurrent validity of two instruments for measuring cervical range of motion: effects of age and gender. *Man Ther.* 1995;1:36–42.

35. Ålund M, Larsson S-E. Three-dimensional analysis of neck motion a clinical method. *Spine.* 1990;15:87–91.

36. Hagen KB, Harms-Ringdahl K, Enger NO et al. Relationship between subjective neck disorders and cervical spine mobility and motion-related pain in male machine operators. *Spine.* 1997;22:1501–1507.

37. Zachman ZJ, Traina AD, Keating JC Jr., et al. Interexaminer reliability and concurrent validity of two instruments for the measurement of cervical ranges of motion. *J Manip Physiol Therapeutics.* 1989;12:205–210.

38. Alaranta H, Hurri H, Heliövaara M, et al. Flexibility of the spine: normative values of goniometric and tape measurements. *Scand J Rehab Med.* 1994;26:147–154.

39. Tucci SM, Hicks JE, Gross EG, et al. Cervical motion assessment: a new, simple and accurate method. *Arch Phys Med Rehabil.* 1986;67:225–230.

40. Defibaugh JJ. Part II: An experimental study of head motion in adult males. *Phys Ther.* 1964;44:163–168.

41. Ordway N, Seymour R, Donelson RG, et al. Cervical sagittal range-of-motion analysis using three methods. *Spine.* 1997;22:501–508.

42. Tousignant M, de Bellefeuille L, O'Donoughue S, Grahovac S. Criterion validity of the cervical range of motion (CROM) goniometer for cervical flexion and extension. *Spine.* 2000;25:324–330.

43. Tousignant M, Duclos E, Lafleche S, et al. Validity study for the cervical range of motion device used for lateral flexion in patients with neck pain. *Spine.* 2002;27:812–817.

44. Youdas JW, Carey JR, Garrett TR. Reliability of measurements of cervical spine range of motion: comparison of three methods. *Phys Ther.* 1991;71:23–29.

45. Rheault W, Albright B, Byers C, et al. Intertester reliability of the cervical range of motion device. *JOSPT.* 1992;15: 147–150.

46. Peolsson A, Hedlund R, Ertzgaard S, Oberg B. Intra- and inter-tester reliability and range of motion of the neck. *Physiother Can.* 2000; Summer:233–242.

47. Capuano-Pucci D, Rheault W, Aukai J, et al. Intratester and intertester reliability of the cervical range of motion device. *Arch Phys Med Rehabil.* 1991;72:338–340.

48. White AA, Panjabi MM. *Clinical Biomechanics of the Spine.* Philadelphia: JB Lippincott; 1978.

49. van Adrichem JAM, van der Korst JK. Assessment of the flexibility of the lumbar spine. *Scand J Rheumatol.* 1973;2:87–91.

50. Mellin GP. Accuracy of measuring lateral flexion of the spine with a tape. *Clin Biomechanics.* 1986;1:85–89.

51. Berryman Reese N, Bandy WD. *Joint Range of Motion and Muscle Length Testing.* Philadelphia: WB Saunders; 2002.

52. Frost M, Stuckey S, Smalley LA, Dorman G. Reliability of measuring trunk motions in centimeters. *Phys Ther.* 1982; 62:1431–1437.

53. Pearcy MJ. Twisting mobility of the human back in flexed postures. *Spine.* 1993;18:114–119.

54. Harris J, Johansen J, Pedersen S, LaPier TK. Site of measurement and subject position affect chest expansion measurements. *Cardiopulmonary Phys Ther.* 1997;8:12–17.

55. Moll JMH, Wright V. An objective clinical study of chest expansion. *Ann Rheum Dis.* 1972;31:1–8.

56. Neustadt DH. Ankylosing spondylitis. *Postgrad Med.* 1977;61:124–135.

57. Portek I, Pearcy MJ, Reader GP, Mowat AG. Correlation between radiographic and clinical measurement of lumbar spine movement. *Br J Rheumatol.* 1983;22:197–205.

58. Macrae IF, Wright V. Measurement of back movement. *Ann Rheum Dis.* 1969;28:584–589.

59. Bandy WD, Reese NB. Strapped versus unstrapped techniques of the prone press-up for measurement of lumbar extension using a tape measure: differences in magnitude and reliability of measurements. *Arch Phys Med Rehab.* 2004; 85:99–103.

60. Fitzgerald GK, Wynveen KJ, Rheault W, Rothschild B. Objective assessment with establishment of normal values for lumbar spinal range of motion. *Phys Ther.* 1983;63:1776–1781.

61. Gill K, Krag MH, Hohnson GB, et al. Repeatability of four clinical methods for assessment of lumbar spinal motion. *Spine.* 1968;13:50–53.

62. Hyytiäinen K, Salminen JJ, Suvitie T, et al. Reproducibility of nine tests to measure spinal mobility and trunk muscle strength. *Scand J Rehab Med.* 1991;23:3–10.

63. Beattie P, Rothstein JM, Lamb RL. Reliability of the attraction method for measuring lumbar spine backward bending. *Phys Ther.* 1987;67:364–369.

64. Burdett RG, Brown KE, Fall MP. Reliability and validity of four instruments for measuring lumbar spine and pelvic motions. *Phys Ther.* 1986;66:677–684.

65. Oksanen A, Salminen JJ. Tests of spinal mobility and muscle strength in the young: reliability and normative values. *Physiotherapy Theory and Practice.* 1996;12:151–160.

66. Williams R, Binkley J, Bloch R, et al. Reliability of the modified-modified Schöber and double inclinometer methods of measuring lumbar flexion and extension. *Phys Ther.* 1993;73:26–37.

67. Rose MJ. The statistical analysis of the intra-observer repeatability of four clinical measurement techniques. *Physiotherapy.* 1991;77: 89–91.

68. Newton M, Waddell G. Reliability and validity of clinical measurement of lumbar spine in patients with chronic low back pain. *Physiotherapy.* 1991;77:796–800.

69. Lee CN, Robbins DP, Roberts HJ, et al. Reliability and validity of single inclinometer measurements for thoracic spine range of motion. *Physiotherapy Canada.* 2003;55: 73–78.

70. Samo DG, Chen SC, Crampton A, et al. Validity of three lumbar sagittal motion measurement methods: surface inclinometers compared with radiographs. *J Occup Environmental Med.* 1997;39:209–216.

71. Saur PM, Ensink F-B M, Frese K, et al. Lumbar range of motion: reliability and validity of the inclinometer technique in the clinical measurement of trunk flexibility. *Spine.* 1996;21:1332–1338.

72. Williams RM, Goldsmith CH, Minuk T. Validity of the double inclinometer method for measuring lumbar flexion. *Physiotherapy Canada.* 1998;Spring:147–152.

73. Mayer TG, Tencer AF, Kristoferson S, Mooney V. Use of noninvasive techniques for quantification of spinal range-of-motion in normal subjects and chronic low-back dysfunction patients. *Spine.* 1984;9:588–595.

74. Loebl WY. Measurement of spinal posture and range of spinal movement. *Ann Phys Med.* 1967;9:103–110.

75. Reynolds PMG. Measurement of spinal mobility: a comparison of three methods. *Rheumatol Rehab.* 1975;14:180–185.

76. Nitschke JE, Nattrass CL, Disler PB, et al. Reliability of the American Medical Association Guides' model for measuring spinal range of motion. *Spine.* 1999;24:262–268.

77. Mellin G. Measurement of thoracolumbar posture and mobility with a Myrin inclinometer. *Spine.* 1986;11: 759–762.

78. Mellin G, Kiiski R, Weckström A. Effects of subject position on measurements of flexion, extension, and lateral flexion of the spine. *Spine.*1991;16:1108–1110.

79. Rondinelli R, Murphy J, Esler A, et al. Estimation of normal lumbar flexion with surface inclinometry. *Am J Phys Med Rehabil.* 1992;71:219–224.

80. Mayer RS, Chen I-H, Lavender SA, et al. Variance in the measurement of sagittal lumbar spine range of motion among examiners, subjects, and instruments. *Spine.* 1995;20:1489–1493.

81. Patel RS. Intratester and intertester reliability of the inclinometer in measuring true lumbar flexion. *Phys Ther.* 1992;72:S44.

82. Ng JK-F, Kippers V, Richardson C, Parnianpour M. Range of motion and lordosis of the lumbar spine. *Spine.* 2001;26: 53–60.

83. Keeley J, Mayer TG, Cox R, et al. Quantification of lumbar function Part 5: reliability of range-of-motion measures in the sagittal plane and an in vivo rotation measurement technique. *Spine.* 1986;11:31–35.

84. Neblett R, Mayer TG, Gatchel RJ, et al. Quantifying the lumbar flexion-relaxation phenomenon. *Spine.* 2003;28: 1435–1446.

85. Chen SC, Samo DG, Chen EH, et al. Reliability of three lumbar sagittal motion measurement methods: surface inclinometers. *J Occupational Environmental Med.* 1997;39: 217–223.

86. Boline PD, Keating JC, Haas M, Anderson AV. Interexaminer reliability and discriminant validity of inclinometric measurement of lumbar rotation in chronic low-back pain patients and subjects without low-back pain. *Spine.* 1992; 17:335–338.

87. Performance Attainment Associates, 958 Lydia Drive, Roseville, MN 55113.

88. Breum J, Wiberg J, Bolton JE. Reliability and concurrent validity of the BROMII for measuring lumbar mobility. *J Manip Physiol Ther.* 1995;18:497–502.

89. Madson TJ, Youdas JW, Suman VJ. Reproducibility of lumbar spine range of motion measurements using the back range of motion device. *JOSPT.* 1999;29:470–477.

90. Smith LK, Weiss EL, Lemkuhl LD. *Brunnstrom's Clinical Kinesiology.* 5th ed. Philadelphia: FA Davis; 1996.

91. Lindh M. Biomechanics of the lumbar spine. In: Nordin M, Frankel VH. *Basic Biomechanics of the Musculoskeletal System.* 2nd ed. Philadelphia: Lea & Febiger; 1989.

92. Cailliet R. *Neck and Arm Pain.* 3rd ed. Philadelphia: FA Davis; 1991.

93. Hutton JT, Shapiro I, Christians B. Functional significance of restricted gaze. *Arch Phys Med Rehabil.* 1982;63:617–619.

94. Muñoz M. Congenital absence of the inferior rectus muscle. *Am J Ophthalmol.* 1992;121:327–329.

95. Pemberton PL, Calder I, O'Sullivan C, Crockard HA. The champagne angle. *Anaesthesia.* 2002;57:402–403.

96. MacConaill MA, Basmajian JV. *Muscles and Movements: A Basis for Human Kinesiology.* Huntington, NY: RE Krieger; 1977.

97. Cailliet R. *Low Back Pain Syndrome.* 5th ed. Philadelphia: FA Davis; 1995.

98. Hsieh CJ, Pringle RK. Range of motion of the lumbar spine required for four activities of daily living. *J Manipulative Physiol Therap.* 1994;17:353–358.

EXERCISES AND QUESTIONS

See the Answer Guide in Appendix F for suggested answers to the following exercises and questions.

1. PALPATION

A. For each of the spinal movements listed below:
—Identify the anatomic landmarks used to measure the spinal ROM using a tape measure
—Palpate these landmarks on a partner
—Identify other spinal movements that also use all of the same anatomic landmarks to evaluate the spinal ROM.
   i. Neck flexion
   ii. Neck lateral flexion
   iii. Thoracolumbar spine extension
   iv. Lumbar spine flexion
   v. Trunk rotation

B. For each of the spinal movements listed below:
—Identify the anatomic landmarks used to measure the spinal ROM using inclinometers
—Palpate these landmarks on a partner
—Identify other spinal movements that use all of the same anatomic landmarks to evaluate the spinal ROM.
   i. Neck extension
   ii. Thoracolumbar spine extension
   iii. Lumbar spine flexion
   iv. Trunk lateral flexion
   v. Thoracic spine rotation

C. Identify the surface anatomy locations the therapist would use when using the CROM to assess neck ROM.

2. ASSESSMENT AND MEASUREMENT OF AROM

For each of the movements listed below, demonstrate measurement of the AROM on a partner *using a tape measure* and answer the question(s) that follow. Have a third partner evaluate your performance using the appropriate practical test form in Appendix E. Record your findings on the recording form on page 274.

TMJ Movements
   i. Identify the jaw movements that occur at the TMJs
   ii. Describe the articular surfaces that make up the TMJs
   iii. Identify the TMJ movements that can be measured using a ruler; demonstrate the measurement of these movements
   iv. Describe how functional ROM can be determined for mouth opening.

Neck Extension
If the mouth is open when measuring neck extension using a tape measure, what effect will this have on the ROM measurement?

Neck Left Lateral Flexion
What substitute movements should be avoided when assessing neck lateral flexion?

Neck Right Rotation
   i. If a therapist measures neck rotation using inclinometry, what is the start position for the measurement?
   ii. Where would the therapist position the inclinometer(s) to take the measurement for neck rotation?

Thoracolumbar Spine Flexion
Can thoracolumbar spine flexion be measured using inclinometers? If so, identify the inclinometer placements used to take the measurement.

Lumbar Spine Flexion
Identify other lumbar spine ROM that can be measured using a tape measure and the same anatomical landmarks.

Thoracolumbar Spine Extension (Prone Press-Up)
Identify factors that may result in inaccurate ROM measurements when measuring thoracolumbar spine extension ROM using the prone press-up position and a tape measure.

Thoracolumbar Spine Rotation
Identify the anatomic landmarks used to position the tape measure for the measurement of thoracolumbar spine rotation AROM

Thoracolumbar Spine Lateral Flexion
   i. What substitute movements should be avoided when assessing thoracolumbar spine lateral flexion?
   ii. Demonstrate a second method to assess thoracolumbar spine lateral flexion using a tape measure.
   iii. Can thoracolumbar spine lateral flexion AROM be measured using inclinometers? If so, identify where the inclinometers would be placed to take the measurement.

AROM RECORDING FORM

Patient's Name _____   Therapist _____

Left Side					Right Side			
	*		*	**Date of Measurement**	*		*	
				Head, Neck and Trunk				
				Mandible: Depression				
				Protrusion				
				Lateral deviation				
				Neck: Flexion (0–45°)				
				Extension (0–45°)				
				Lateral flexion (0–45°)				
				Rotation (0–60°)				
				Trunk: Flexion (0–80°, 10 cm)				
				Extension (0–20–30°)				
				Lateral flexion (0–35°)				
				Rotation (0–45°)				
				Hypermobility:				
				Comments:				

3. MUSCLE LENGTH ASSESSSMENT AND MEASUREMENT

Toe-Touch Test
  i.   The toe-touch test measures only hamstring muscle length. True or false?
  ii. The toe-touch test measures only spinal ROM. True or false?
  iii. The toe-touch test provides a composite measure of hip, spine, and shoulder girdle ROM. True or false?

4. FUNCTIONAL ROM AT THE HEAD, NECK AND TRUNK

A. For each spinal motion listed below, identify three daily activities that require the specified movement:
  i.   thoracolumbar flexion
  ii. thoracolumbar extension
  iii. cervical spine rotation
  iv. cervical spine lateral flexion.
B. Sit and keep your head in the anatomical position. Move your eyes to look up, down, and side to side. Note the range of your field of vision. If you could not move your neck, what strategies would you use to increase your field of vision?
C. Identify the TMJ, cervical, thoracic, and/or lumbar spine motion(s) required to perform the following activities:
  i.   sitting and tying a shoe with the foot flat on the floor
  ii. combing the hair on the back of the head
  iii. brushing one's teeth
  iv. reaching for a wallet in a back pocket.

SECTION III

Sample Numerical Recording Form: Range of Motion Measurement

Patient's Name _____

Diagnosis _____

Therapist _____

Date of Birth/Age _____

Date of Onset _____

AROM ☐   PROM ☐

Recording:

1. The Neutral Zero Method defined by the American Academy of Orthopaedic Surgeons[1] is used for measurement and recording.

2. Average ranges defined by the American Academy of Orthopaedic Surgeons,[1] are provided in parentheses.

3. The columns designated with asterisks are used for indicating limitation of range of motion and referencing for summarization.

4. Space is left at the end of each section to record hypermobile ranges and comments regarding positioning of the patient or body part, measuring instrument, edema, pain, and/or end feel.

Patient's Name _____   Therapist _____

Left Side				Date of Measurement	Right Side			
	*		*		*		*	
				Head, Neck, and Trunk				
				Mandible: Depression				
				Protrusion				
				Lateral deviation				
				Neck: Flexion (0–45°)				
				Extension (0–45°)				
				Lateral flexion (0–45°)				
				Rotation (0–60°)				
				Trunk: Flexion (0–80°, 10 cm)				
				Extension (0–20–30°)				
				Lateral flexion (0–35°)				
				Rotation (0–45°)				
				Hypermobility:				
				Comments:				
				Scapula				
				Elevation				
				Depression				
				Abduction				
				Adduction				
				Shoulder Complex				
				Elevation through Flexion (0–180°)				
				Elevation through Abduction (0–180°)				

Patient's Name ______________________________ Therapist ____________________________

Left Side						Right Side		
	*		*	**Date of Measurement**	*		*	
				Shoulder (Glenohumeral) Joint				
				Flexion (0–120°)[2]				
				Abduction (0–90° to 120°)[2]				
				Extension (0–60°)				
				Horizontal abduction (0–45°)				
				Horizontal adduction (0–135°)				
				Internal rotation (0–70°)				
				External rotation (0–90°)				
				Hypermobility: Comments:				
				Elbow and Forearm				
				Flexion (0–150°)				
				Supination (0–80°)				
				Pronation (0–80°)				
				Hypermobility: Comments:				
				Wrist				
				Flexion (0–80°)				
				Extension (0–70°)				
				Ulnar deviation (0–30°)				
				Radial deviation (0–20°)				
				Hypermobility: Comments:				

Patient's Name _____   Therapist _____

	*		*	Date of Measurement	*		*	
				Thumb				
				CM flexion (0–15°)				
				CM extension (0–20°)				
				abduction (0–70°)				
				MCP flexion (0–50°)				
				IP flexion (0–80°)				
				Opposition				
				Hypermobility:				
				Comments:				
				Fingers				
				MCP digit 2 flexion (0–90°)				
				extension (0–45°)				
				abduction				
				adduction				
				MCP digit 3 flexion (0–90°)				
				extension (0–45°)				
				abduction (radial)				
				adduction (ulnar)				
				MCP digit 4 flexion (0–90°)				
				extension (0–45°)				
				abduction				
				adduction				
				MCP digit 5 flexion (0–90°)				
				extension (0–45°)				
				abduction				
				adduction				
				PIP digit 2 flexion (0–100°)				
				3 flexion (0–100°)				
				4 flexion (0–100°)				
				5 flexion (0–100°)				

Patient's Name _____   Therapist _____

	*		*	Date of Measurement	*		*	
				DIP digit 2 flexion (0–90°)				
				3 flexion (0–90°)				
				4 flexion (0–90°)				
				5 flexion (0–90°)				
				Composite finger abduction/thumb extension—Distance between:				
				Thumb–digit 2				
				Digit 2–digit 3				
				Digit 3–digit 4				
				Digit 4–digit 5				
				Composite flexion—Distance between:				
				Finger pulp-distal palmar crease				
				Finger pulp-proximal palmar crease				
				Hypermobility:				
				Comments:				
				Hip				
				Flexion (0–120°)				
				Extension (0–30°)				
				Abduction (0–45°)				
				Adduction (0–30°)				
				Internal rotation (0–45°)				
				External rotation (0–45°)				
				Hypermobility:				
				Comments:				
				Knee				
				Flexion (0–135°)				
				Tibial rotation				
				Patellar mobility—Distal glide				
				Patellar mobility—Medial-lateral glide				
				Hypermobility:				
				Comments:				

Left Side · Right Side

Patient's Name _____   Therapist _____

	Left Side					Right Side			
	*		*	**Date of Measurement**		*		*	
				Ankle					
				Dorsiflexion (0–20°)					
				Plantarflexion (0–50°)					
				Inversion (0–35°)					
				Eversion (0–15°)					
				Hypermobility:					
				Comments:					
				Toes					
				MTP great toe flexion (0–45°)					
				extension (0–70°)					
				abduction					
				MTP digit 2 flexion (0–40°)					
				extension (0–40°)					
				MTP digit 3 flexion (0–40°)					
				extension (0–40°)					
				MTP digit 4 flexion (0–40°)					
				extension (0–40°)					
				MTP digit 5 flexion (0–40°)					
				extension (0–40°)					
				IP great toe flexion (0–90°)					
				PIP digit 2 flexion (0–35°)					
				PIP digit 3 flexion (0–35°)					
				PIP digit 4 flexion (0–35°)					
				PIP digit 5 flexion (0–35°)					
				Hypermobility:					
				Comments:					

Summary of Limitation:

Additional Comments:

[1]American Academy of Orthopaedic Surgeons: *Joint Motion: Method of Measuring and Recording*. Chicago: AAOS; 1965.
[2]Levangie PK, Norkin CC. *Joint Structure and Function: A Comprehensive Analysis*. 3rd ed. Philadelphia: FA Davis; 2001.

Validity and Reliability of Selected Instruments Used to Measure Joint Range of Motion

Instruments Used to Measure TMJ AROM

Ruler

Walker and colleagues (1) evaluated the construct validity of using a ruler to measure active range of motion (AROM) of the temporomandibular joints (TMJs) for mandibular depression and lateral deviation and protrusion. They suggested that the measurement techniques using a ruler would exhibit construct validity if ruler measurements made it possible to discriminate among 15 subjects (2 males and 13 females; mean age 35.2 years) with TMJ disorders and 15 subjects (3 males and 12 females; mean age 42.9 years) without TMJ disorders. The measurement of mouth opening was the only measure that showed construct validity for identifying TMJ pathology. Therefore, the authors concluded that mouth opening measured by ruler might be a way of documenting and monitoring the status of patients with TMJ disorders.

These same investigators (1) studied the intra- and intertester reliability of assessing active mandibular depression, lateral deviation, and protrusion using a ruler. Two physical therapists skilled at measuring the active TMJ movements used standardized procedures and completed three measurement sessions with a week between sessions. At each measurement session, the therapists each measured the TMJ movements of 30 subjects (15 subjects with TMJ disorders and 15 healthy subjects). Results showed acceptable intratester reliability and good to excellent intertester reliability using a ruler to assess the TMJ AROM.

Dijkstra and coworkers (2) compared four methods (radiographs, goniometry, and linear methods) of assessing TMJ mobility for mouth opening with 28 healthy subjects (15 males and 13 females; mean age 29.6 years) presenting with no TMJ disorder and a symmetrical mouth-opening pattern. They concluded that using a ruler to measure the distance between the central incisors in maximal mouth opening is a reliable and accurate measure of TMJ mobility when evaluating progress within a subject over time. However, mandibular length may influence how much the mouth can be opened. Therefore, when comparing different subjects with the same linear mouth opening, one cannot conclude similar TMJ mobility.

Higbie and associates (3) examined the intra- and intertester reliability of using a ruler to measure mouth opening of 40 healthy subjects (20 males and 20 females; ages 18–54 years). Mouth opening was measured with the subject's neck in the protracted, neutral, and retracted position. Two experienced physical therapists were trained in the measurement procedures. One therapist measured mouth opening in each head position. The second therapist repeated the same sequence of measurements after a 5-minute rest period was given to the subject. The therapists repeated the measurements on 10 subjects 7 days later to assess the day-to-day reliability of measurements. To measure mouth opening, the researchers found high intra- and interrater and day-to-day reliability using a ruler and specific and accurate client instructions for head and neck position.

Dworkin and colleagues (4) evaluated the intertester reliability of using a ruler to measure the TMJ AROM of 64 subjects. The subjects, mainly women between 20 and 40 years of age, included healthy volunteers and patients with occlusal problems and TMJ disorders. Three experienced dental hygienists were trained in standardized procedures to measure TMJ AROM using a ruler, and four experienced clinical TMD (specialist) dentists were not trained in the standardized procedures. Results showed extremely high intertester reliability for mouth opening and less than desirable intertester reliability for lateral deviation and protrusion measurements. Examiners trained in the standardized procedure had better intertester reliability than the untrained examiners, supporting the importance of using standardized procedures for reliable clinical measurement of TMJ AROM.

Instruments Used to Measure Cervical Spine AROM

Tape Measure

In reviewing the literature, no studies were found that examined the validity of measuring cervical spine ROM using a tape measure. Several studies (5–8) assessed the reliability of using the tape measure to assess cervical spine ROM. The reliability of the tape measure was evaluated measuring healthy subjects in two of the studies and patients with ankylosing spondylitis in the other studies.

Hsieh and Yeung (5) examined the intratester reliability of an experienced and an inexperienced tester when using a tape measure to assess the AROM of the cervical spine of 34 healthy subjects (27 males and 7 women; mean age 18.2 years). The inexperienced tester had prior instruction and supervised practice in the measurement method. The experienced tester measured 17 subjects and the inexperienced tester measured 17 different subjects. Each tester measured the AROM for cervical flexion, extension, right and left lateral flexion, and right and left rotation. Immediately following the first set of measurements, each tester performed a second set of measurements. Using the tape measure to assess cervical spine AROM produced good intratester reliability, with measurements taken on the same day by either an experienced or an inexperienced tester, although the experienced tester had less variation in repeated measurements. The researchers recommended the clinical use of the tape measure to assess neck ROM and pointed out that the tape measure is a tool that is easily available, convenient to use, and inexpensive.

Balogun and coworkers (6) assessed the intra- and intertester reliability of measuring neck AROM using the tape measure and the "Myrin" gravity-referenced goniometer. In this study, three experienced physical therapists practiced a standardized measurement procedure for cervical AROM using the tape measure. Three therapists each assessed 21 healthy undergraduate physical therapy students (none were of the endomorphic somatotype) on two occasions with 4 to 110 days (mean of 19.8 days) between the two test occasions. The authors found the intratester reliability for both the tape measure and the "Myrin" goniometer to be moderately high for all measures except flexion, which was poor. The authors suggested that redefining anatomical landmarks and testing instructions for flexion measurements might improve reliability. Intertester reliability was slightly higher for the tape measure than the "Myrin" goniometer. The researchers recommended the simple, low-cost tape measure for wider clinical use.

Pile and associates (7) had five experienced testers measure the cervical lateral flexion of 10 patients with ankylosing spondylitis (5 males, median age 41 years; 5 females, median age 35 years) using a tape measure and a universal goniometer. Despite results that showed what appeared to be good intertester reliability for both the tape measure and universal goniometer, the authors recommended the use of the universal goniometer because it was easier to use.

Viitanen and colleagues (8) studied the intra- and intertester reliability of a tape measure for cervical flexion, lateral flexion, and rotation AROM. Two physical therapists each repeated measurements of the cervical AROM of 52 male subjects with idiopathic ankylosing spondylitis on 2 successive days, at the same time of day on each occasion. The researchers assessed intratester reliability using measures from one of the therapists. Little detail was provided

on the reliability results, but all measurements using a tape measure were reported to show good reliability.

Jordan (9) assessed the literature on the reliability of tools used to measure cervical spine ROM in clinical settings and could give "no strong recommendation for any tool" but suggested the tape measure may be the preferred clinical option. The tape measure is inexpensive, portable, and clinically acceptable, but Jordan (9) found that it needs more support in the literature.

Inclinometry

Most of the research on the validity of measuring cervical spine ROM using inclinometry studied the CROM, which is described in the next section. The research pertaining to the validity of other types of inclinometers for measuring cervical spine ROM is described in this section.

Bush and associates (10) assessed the validity of measuring cervical spine AROM using single and double inclinometry techniques and a single inclinometry stabilization technique. Thirty-four physical therapists each performed inclinometric measurements on the same three healthy subjects. One subject performed cervical spine flexion and extension, another performed right and left lateral flexion AROM, and a third performed right and left cervical rotation ROM for each of the 34 therapists. The inclinometry measurements were compared to radiological measurements of sagittal and frontal plane motions and computed tomography scan measurements of transverse plane motions of the cervical spine. The inclinometry and radiographic/tomographic measurements were performed separately. On the basis of the criteria used by the researchers, the only valid methods of measurement were single inclinometry for flexion and extension, double inclinometry for flexion, and the single inclinometry stabilization measurement of extension.

Herrmann (11) compared radiographic measurements and inclinometric measurements of the total neck flexion and extension PROM of 11 subjects. The inclinometer was strapped to the lateral aspect of the head just above the ears to measure neck PROM. The radiographic measurements matched the inclinometer measurements. The investigator concluded the inclinometer could be used as a valid tool for measuring passive head and neck motion in the sagittal plane.

Hole and colleagues (12) evaluated the concurrent validity of the CROM and the single inclinometer. Two final-year chiropractic students, practiced in the use of the two instruments, evaluated the cervical spine AROM of 30 healthy young adults. Each tester took two sets of cervical spine AROM measurements on each subject with each instrument. The CROM and the single inclinometer showed good agreement (i.e., concurrent validity) for measurements taken in the vertical planes (i.e., flexion, extension and lateral flexion) but not for transverse plane motion (i.e., rotation). The researchers suggested the different subject positioning used for each instrument when assessing rotation could be the reason for the lack of concurrent validity for the rotation ROM.

Studies conducted to determine the intra- and intertester reliability of the inclinometer for measuring cervical spine ROM included only healthy subjects. These studies, using different types of inclinometers, in most instances showed the inclinometer to be a reliable tool for measuring cervical spine AROM.

Ålund and Larsson (13) compared electrogoniometric measures of neck AROM with simultaneous measurements using a conventional gravity goniometer (inclinometer) to assess flexion, extension, and lateral flexion ROM and a compass goniometer to assess rotation ROM. The inclinometers were applied using a Velcro strap to the lateral and dorsal aspects of the head. The compass goniometer was mounted on top of the head, above the component of the electrogoniometer used to measure rotation. The investigator examined each of 10 healthy subjects (6 men, 4 women, mean age 32 years) twice, with 1 week between examinations. The results showed that the inclinometers gave reproducible results fully comparable to the electrogoniometric measures; however, the compass goniometer results were not reproducible.

As part of a larger study of the relationship between subjective reports of neck pain and cervical spine mobility, Hagen and associates (14) examined the intratester reliability of the OB goniometer. One examiner assessed the cervical spine AROM of 11 healthy subjects (6 men, 5 women) on two occasions within a 2- to 4-day period. The researchers found the OB goniometer to have fair to high intratester reliability for measurements of active cervical spine flexion, extension, and lateral flexion using the inclinometer, and cervical spine rotation using the compass goniometer.

Balogun and coworkers (6) assessed the intra- and intertester reliability of the tape measure and the "Myrin" gravity-referenced goniometer to measure cervical spine AROM. Three physical therapists each assessed the 21 healthy subjects using the tape measure and the OB goniometer on two occasions with 4 to 110 days (mean 19.8 days) between occasions. They found the intratester reliability for both the tape measure and the "Myrin" goniometer to be moderately high for all measures except flexion, which was poor. The authors suggested redefining anatomical landmarks and testing instructions for flexion measurements to improve reliability. Intertester reliability was slightly higher for the tape measure than the "Myrin" goniometer. The researchers recommended the low-cost, simple-to-use tape measure for wider clinical use.

The intertester reliability of measuring cervical spine flexion, extension, lateral flexion, and rotation AROM was examined by Bush and associates (10) comparing the measurements performed by 34 physical therapists on three healthy subjects. The therapists used three methods of employing the inclinometer to measure the cervical ROM in the sagittal and frontal planes: single inclinometry, double inclinometry, and a single inclinometry stabilization technique. The inclinometers were positioned with one inclinometer over the superior aspect of the head and the second inclinometer over T1 to measure flexion and lateral flexion and over the spine of the scapula to measure cervical extension. Using the single inclinometry stabilization method, one inclinometer was placed over the superior aspect of the head and the subject flexed or abducted one upper limb 90° and with the hand at this level held onto a stable surface to stabilize the thoracic spine. The therapists measured rotation using the single inclinometer technique only, with the subject in supine. One subject performed cervical spine flexion and extension, another performed right and left lateral flexion AROM, and a third performed right and left cervical rotation ROM for each of the 34 therapists for each measurement method. All measurements were found to be reliable between testers for all three measurement methods.

Zachman and coworkers (15) had two chiropractors measure the cervical spine flexion, extension, and lateral flexion AROM of 24 healthy subjects (12 men, 12 women; ages 6–51 years) using the rangiometer and the universal goniometer. The rangiometer partly consists of an inclinometer attached to a headpiece for measuring cervical spine movements in the sagittal and frontal planes. The researchers assessed intertester reliability for both instruments. They concluded that the inclinometer was moderately reliable and the universal goniometer was less reliable than the inclinometer. They also noted that the inclinometer does not require the therapist to locate as many landmarks and appears to be quicker and easier to use compared to the universal goniometer.

In a study by Alaranta and colleagues (16), the total active movement in each of the sagittal and frontal planes (i.e., flexion plus extension; right plus left lateral flexion, respectively) was assessed on 24 healthy subjects using a liquid inclinometer attached to a "cloth helmet." The investigators also evaluated the total (i.e., right plus left) cervical rotation AROM with the subjects in supine using a gravitational inclinometer attached to a "cloth helmet." The study results showed "overall good" intertester reliability for the liquid and gravitational inclinometers.

Tucci and associates (17) assessed the intertester reliability of an inclinometer mounted on a headgear (i.e., a wooden block with an arch to fit the head, secured to the head with an elastic strap) and the universal goniometer. One experienced and one inexperienced tester measured the cervical spine ROM of 11 healthy subjects using the inclinometer. Two experienced examiners measured the cervical ROM of 10 healthy subjects using the universal goniometer. The authors also assessed the intratester reliability of the universal goniometer and the inclinometer with one experienced tester measuring the cervical ROM of 10 healthy subjects. The researchers concluded that the tested inclinometer is a simple, reliable, and quick way to measure cervical spine ROM and has a high degree of intertester reliability even with inexperienced examiners.

A unique inclinometer for measuring cervical spine AROM was examined for intra- and intertester reliability by Defibaugh (18). The device consisted of a pendulum goniometer held in the mouth with a mouthpiece attachment. In this study, the subject performed cervical flexion, extension, and lateral flexion in the sitting position and cervical rotation in the supine position. One tester evaluated the cervical AROM of 15 male subjects on two occasions with 1 to 7 days between measures. Results showed moderate to high intratester reliability. To assess intertester reliability, the investigator and one of seven other physical therapists with varied experience levels measured cervical spine AROM within 2 hours of each other in another set of 15 male subjects. Results showed good intertester reliability.

Hole and colleagues (12) evaluated the intra- and intertester reliability of the CROM and single inclinometer using two final-year chiropractic students who were practiced in the use of these two instruments to evaluate cervical spine AROM. With each instrument, each student took two sets of cervical spine AROM measurements on 30 healthy young adults. Almost perfect levels of intratester reliability were found for both instruments. Intertester reliability for the CROM was almost perfect; for the single inclinometer, the reliability was substantial. The authors concluded the CROM would be the method of choice for measuring cervical spine ROM.

CROM

Analyzing the normative cervical ROM literature, Chen and colleagues (19) concluded that the reliability of radiography for measuring cervical spine movement has not been proven, and that radiography requires more careful assessment before being adopted as a gold standard. Owing to the lack of a gold standard for cervical spine ROM, true validity cannot be tested; the best that can be done is to assess concurrent agreement between instruments and procedures (19). Four studies (12,20–22) examined the validity of the CROM.

Ordway and coworkers (20) compared measures of the cervical flexion and extension of 20 asymptomatic volunteers using the CROM, radiographs, and the 3-Space (a computerized tracking system). The flexion and extension measures from the CROM correlated well with the gravity-referenced measures from the radiographs. The authors concluded that the CROM is reliable for measuring flexion and extension, even though it cannot measure isolated movement of the cervical spine from that of the upper thoracic spine. Therefore, it is necessary to standardize patient positioning when assessing flexion and extension using the CROM to minimize the contribution of upper thoracic spine motion from the measurement.

Tousignant and associates (21) evaluated the criterion validity of the CROM for measuring cervical spine flexion and extension in 31 healthy adults. In a subsequent study Tousignant and coworkers (22) assessed the criterion validity of the CROM to measure cervical lateral flexion in 42 patients with neck pain. In both studies, the measurements of neck positions from the CROM were compared to those from conventional radiographs. The CROM was found to be a valid tool for measuring flexion and extension in healthy subjects (21) and lateral flexion in patients with neck dysfunction (22).

Hole and colleagues (12) evaluated the concurrent validity of the CROM and the single inclinometer. Two final-year chiropractic students, practiced in the use of the two instruments, evaluated the cervical spine AROM of 30 healthy young adults. Each tester took two sets of cervical spine AROM measurements on each subject with each instrument. The measurements of the CROM and the single inclinometer were consistent with each other for flexion, extension, and lateral flexion but not for rotation. However, the different positions used to assess rotation with each instrument could be the reason for the lack of concurrent validity.

Several studies examined the reliability of the CROM for measuring the cervical spine flexion, extension, lateral flexion, and rotation AROM of subjects with cervical spine pathology (23,24) and healthy subjects (12,25–27). "Reliability of the cervical range of motion device has been well established" (22, p. 812).

Youdas and colleagues (23) evaluated and compared the intratester reliability of the CROM and the universal goniometer and the intertester reliability of the CROM, the universal goniometer, and visual estimation. Sixty patients with orthopaedic pathology of the cervical spine participated in this study. While both the CROM and universal goniometer showed good to high reliability when the same therapist used either instrument to measure the patient repeatedly, the authors found that the CROM and the universal goniometer should not be used interchangeably when performing repeated measurements on the same patient due to the poor between-device reliability. The CROM, with good to high intertester reliability, proved to be the more reliable method of assessing the cervical spine ROM when different therapists measured the same patient.

Rheault and associates (24) evaluated only intertester reliability of the CROM, with two testers measuring the AROM of 22 subjects with a history of cervical spine pathology. They concluded that the CROM is a reliable instrument for measuring cervical spine ROM between testers and reported small mean differences between the testers' measures (0.5° to 3.6°).

Peolsson and associates (25) assessed the intra- and intertester reliability of the CROM and the cervical measurement system (CMS) (a plastic framed helmet that includes two gravity inclinometers, a compass, and two spirit levels). Two physical therapists measured the cervical AROM of 30 healthy subjects, taking three measurements with each instrument on two different occasions within a 1-week period. While both the CROM and the CMS were shown to be reliable instruments, the CROM showed higher reliability overall.

Capuano-Pucci and colleagues (26) had two testers evaluate the cervical spine AROM of 20 healthy subjects with no cervical spine pathology. Each tester, using the CROM, measured each cervical spine motion twice on two different occasions, days apart. They concluded that the CROM has acceptable intra- and intertester reliability.

Youdas and coworkers (27) conducted two pilot studies to examine the intra- and intertester reliability of the CROM to assess cervical spine AROM before determining normal values of cervical spine AROM using the CROM in 337 healthy subjects. Each of five testers measured the cervical spine AROM of six healthy subjects selected from a pool of 30 subjects. These five testers each took two sets of cervical spine AROM measurements to assess intratester reliability. To evaluate intertester reliability, three testers measured the cervical spine AROM of 20 healthy subjects, with measurements of each subject being made by the testers within minutes of each other. They concluded that the CROM device showed good intra- and interrater reliability.

Hole and colleagues (12) evaluated the intra- and intertester reliability of the CROM and single inclinometer. Two final-year chiropractic students were practiced in the use of these two instruments to evaluate cervical spine AROM. With each instrument, each student took two sets of cervical spine AROM measurements on 30 healthy young adults. Almost perfect levels of intratester reliability were found for both instruments (although levels for the single inclinometer were slightly less than for the CROM). Intertester reliability for the CROM was almost perfect; for the single inclinometer, the reliability was substantial. The authors concluded that the CROM, as opposed to the single inclinometer, would be the method of choice for measuring cervical spine ROM.

Jordan (9) reviewed the literature to assess the reliability of tools to measure cervical spine ROM in clinical settings. Jordan identified the CROM to be the most reliable tool, but added that the CROM may not be the most practical tool in the clinical setting due to cost, portability, and specificity for use in measuring only cervical spine ROM. Jordan (9) concluded that reliability appears to be good for a population of mixed pathologic conditions, but more research is needed using normal subjects and those with specific neck pathology.

Universal Goniometer

Pile and associates (7) had five experienced testers measure the cervical lateral flexion of 10 patients with ankylosing spondylitis (5 men, median age 41 years; 5 women, median age 35 years) using a tape measure and a universal goniometer. Despite results that showed what appeared to be good intertester reliability for both the tape measure and universal goniometer, the authors recommended the use of the universal goniometer because it was easier to use.

Zachman and coworkers (15) had two chiropractors measure the cervical spine flexion, extension, and lateral flexion AROM of 24 healthy subjects (12 males, 12 females, ages 6–51 years) using the rangiometer and the universal goniometer. The rangiometer partly consists of an inclinometer attached to a headpiece for measuring cervical spine movements in the sagittal and frontal planes. The researchers assessed intertester reliability for both instruments. They found the inclinometer to be moderately reliable and the universal goniometer to be less reliable than the inclinometer. They also noted that the inclinometer does not require the therapist to locate as many landmarks and appears to be quicker and easier to use compared to the universal goniometer.

Tucci and associates (17) assessed the intertester reliability of an inclinometer mounted on a headgear (i.e., a wooden block with an arch to fit the head, secured to the head with an elastic strap) and the universal goniometer. One experienced and one inexperienced tester measured the cervical spine ROM of 11 healthy subjects using the inclinometer. Two experienced examiners measured the cervical ROM of 10 healthy subjects using the universal goniometer. The authors also assessed the intratester reliability of the universal goniometer and the inclinometer with one experienced tester measuring the cervical ROM

of 10 healthy subjects. One experienced examiner assessed cervical ROM using the inclinometer and the universal goniometer. The researchers found better reliability for measures of cervical spine ROM using the inclinometer with an inexperienced and experienced examiner than when cervical ROM was measured using the universal goniometer and two experienced examiners.

Youdas and colleagues (23) evaluated and compared the intratester reliability of the CROM and the universal goniometer and the intertester reliability of the CROM, the universal goniometer, and visual estimation. Sixty patients with orthopaedic pathology of the cervical spine participated in this study. While both the CROM and universal goniometer showed good to high reliability when the same therapist used either instrument to measure the patient repeatedly, the authors cautioned that the CROM and the universal goniometer should not be used interchangeably when performing repeated measurements on the same patient due to the poor between-device reliability. The CROM, with good to high intertester reliability, proved to be the more reliable method of assessing the cervical spine ROM when different therapists measured the same patient.

Instruments Used to Measure Thoracic Spine and Lumbar Spine AROM

Tape Measure/Ruler

Little research has been conducted to determine the validity of the tape measure to measure thoracic and/or lumbar spine ROM. Two research teams (28,29) investigated the validity of using the tape measure to evaluate lumbar spine flexion AROM by comparing tape measurements with measures obtained by radiography. Macrae and Wright (29) used the Schöber and modified Schöber methods to measure lumbar flexion ROM; Portek and colleagues (28) used only the modified Schöber method.

To measure lumbar flexion AROM using a tape measure and the Schöber or modified Schöber method, the subject is in standing position. For the Schöber method, the skin is marked over the spine at the level of the lumbosacral junction and a point 10 cm superior to the lumbosacral junction. For the modified Schöber method, the skin is marked in the midline at points 5 cm inferior and 10 cm superior to the lumbosacral junction. At the end of the forward flexion ROM, distances are remeasured between the superior and inferior marks for each method. The increase in distance between the marks at the end of the ROM (i.e., the increase from 10 cm for the Schöber method and from 15 cm for the modified Schöber method) represents the lumbar flexion AROM.

Portek and colleagues (28) assessed 11 healthy male subjects and found little correlation between the tape measurements using the modified Schöber method and the x-ray measurements. The authors concluded that the modified Schöber method gives only a linear index of movement and does not reflect true spinal movement. Assessing subjects with and without spinal disease,

Macrae and Wright (29) found a linear relationship between the lumbar flexion measurements obtained using the Schöber and modified Schöber methods and the x-ray measurements. However, using the modified Schöber method, the accuracy of the measurement of lumbar flexion was superior.

Research conducted to establish the reliability of using the tape measure for thoracic and/or lumbar spine AROM measurement is presented by the spinal region and motion assessed.

Thoracolumbar Extension

PSIS to C7 Method (see Figs. 9-58 and 9-60). Frost and colleagues (30) examined the intra- and intertester reliability of measuring thoracolumbar spine extension AROM using a tape measure. Three physical therapists each measured trunk extension ROM in 24 healthy subjects (12 men, 12 women; mean age 33.8 years). The therapists measured the distance between the points at the midline at the level of the PSIS and the C7 spinous process with the subject in standing and at the end position for trunk extension. The difference between the start and end measures represented the trunk extension ROM. The results showed poor intra- and intertester measurement reliability. They suggested that more accurate palpation of bony landmarks would lessen the amount of error.

Prone Press-Up (see Figs. 9-65 and 9-66). Bandy and Reese (39) assessed the intra- and intertester reliability of using the tape measure to quantify the range of lumbar spine extension using the prone press-up position. Two experienced and two inexperienced examiners each used the tape measure to assess lumbar extension ROM by measuring the distance between the sternal notch and the plinth. Each group of examiners measured the ROM of all 63 healthy subjects (20 men, 43 women; mean age 25.95 years) with the pelvis stabilized with a strap and without external stabilization, on two separate occasions 1 day apart. The researchers found the tape measure to be reliable for measuring lumbar extension using the prone press-up, with and without the use of the pelvic stabilization strap, for both experienced and inexperienced examiners. However, the ROM values were found to be greater when the subject's pelvis was stabilized with the strap. Therefore, these two methods of assessing lumbar spine extension ROM should not be used interchangeably. In addition, with the pelvis unstrapped, the researchers noted the subjects were concerned with keeping the pelvis against the plinth and therefore were unable "to attain full range of lumbar extension."

Lumbar Flexion/Extension

Schöber Method. The intertester reliability of measuring lumbar flexion AROM using the Schöber method and thoracolumbar extension and right and left lateral flexion ROM using the universal goniometer was investigated by Fitzgerald and associates (31). All four spinal movements, as measured by two testers on each of 17 healthy subjects, showed substantial intertester reliability. The Schöber method in particular showed high intertester reliability.

Modified Schöber Method. Several researchers examined the intratester (28,32,33) and/or intertester (28,33–35) reliability of measuring lumbar flexion AROM using the tape measure and the modified Schöber method.

Gill and coworkers (32) examined the intratester reliability of the modified Schöber, the fingertip-to-floor, and the double inclinometer methods of assessing ROM in standing. For each measurement method, one tester measured spinal flexion and extension movements twice, with a 10-minute rest between measurements, for each of 10 healthy adult subjects (five males, five females). Reliability for the double inclinometer method was good; that for the fingertip-to-floor method was poor. The most reliable method was the modified Schöber method, and the researchers recommended it for routine clinical evaluation of lumbar spine ROM.

Portek and colleagues (28) assessed the intra- and intertester reliability of using the modified Schöber method to measure lumbar spine flexion AROM. For intratester reliability, one tester took 10 measurements on one male subject at the same time of day on 10 different days. To evaluate intertester reliability two testers measured the same 14 patients admitted for minor orthopaedic surgery who were not taking drugs and had no low back pain. A significant difference between the results of different testers was reported; it was thought to be due to the movement of the skin over the bony landmarks causing movement of the marks relative to one another as the measurements were taken. The authors concluded that the measurement of spinal flexion using the modified Schöber method must be made by the same tester for the measurement to have validity.

Hyytiäinen and colleagues (33) had three therapists use the modified Schöber method to measure the lumbar spine flexion ROM of 30 male shipyard employees. These researchers found the method to be easy and quick to perform; intratester reliability was strong, but intertester reliability needed improvement.

Oksanen and Salminen (34) assessed the intertester reliability of several methods of measuring spinal mobility, including the modified Schöber method. Two experienced physical therapists performed lumbar spine flexion ROM measurements of 30 school children (15 years of age) using the modified Schöber method. Fifteen of the children had recurrent or continuous low back pain and 15 had no low back pain. The two therapists performed the ROM measurements consecutively during the same session. The modified Schöber method exhibited high intertester reliability in measuring the lumbar flexion ROM in this group of school children.

Burdett and associates (35) assessed the intertester reliability of the measurement of spinal flexion using a modification of the modified Schöber method. The researchers replaced the standard 5-cm mark placed inferior to the level of the PSIS with a mark 3 cm inferior to the level of the PSIS. To establish intertester reliability, two physical therapists, practiced in the measurement technique, assessed the lumbar spine flexion ROM of 23 healthy subjects. Using the criteria selected by the authors, they reported a "relatively low" reliability of the tape measure in the measurement of lumbar flexion.

The modified Schöber method can also be used to measure the lumbar spine extension ROM by recording the decrease in the 15-cm distance between the landmarks at the end of the lumbar extension ROM. This method of measuring lumbar spine extension is the called the modified Schöber attraction method. Gill and coworkers (32) and Beattie and associates (36) assessed the reliability of measuring lumbar spine extension using this method.

Gill and coworkers (32) examined the intratester reliability of the modified Schöber attraction method. One tester measured lumbar extension AROM twice, with a 10-minute rest between measurements, for each of 10 healthy adult subjects (five males, five females). The modified Schöber attraction method of measuring lumbar spine extension was repeatable, and the researchers recommended the method for routine clinical evaluation of lumbar spine ROM.

Beattie and associates (36) examined the intra- and intertester reliability of the modified Schöber attraction method for measuring lumbar spine extension with 100 subjects (50 men, 50 women; mean age 37.6 years) with "significant" limiting low back pain and 100 subjects (37 men, 63 women; mean age 32.4 years) without "significant" limiting low back pain. To assess intratester reliability, one physical therapist measured each subject twice within a short time span. A second therapist subsequently measured 11 subjects from the group without "significant" low back pain to assess intertester reliability. The modified Schöber attraction method showed good intratester reliability for both subject groups. Intertester reliability was high for the small subject group assessed. Beattie and associates (36) concluded that the modified Schöber attraction method of assessing lumbar spine extension appears reliable.

Modified-Modified Schöber Method (see Figs. 9-67 through 9-70). To measure lumbar flexion or extension AROM using the modified-modified Schöber method, the subject is in standing position. The skin is marked over the spine at the level of the PSIS and at a point 15 cm superior to the level of the PSIS. A tape measure is used at the end of the lumbar flexion or extension ROM to measure the increase or decrease, respectively, in the distance between the marks at the level of the PSIS and 15 cm superior. The change in distance represents the lumbar flexion or extension AROM.

Van Adrichem and van der Korst (37) tested the reproducibility of measuring the lumbar flexion AROM using a mark placed in the midline between the PSIS and marks placed 5, 10, 15, and 20 cm superior to the level of the PSIS. To test the reliability of the measurements, five healthy young men were measured seven times at 1-week intervals. The researchers concluded that a mark 15 cm superior seemed to best represent the true length of the lumbar spine, and their findings showed that "a simple reliable clinical assessment of lumbar flexibility can be made by measuring the increasing distance between two skin marks 15 cm apart" (37, p. 90) during lumbar flexion.

Williams and coworkers (38) assessed the intra- and intertester reliability of measuring active lumbar flexion and extension using the modified-modified Schöber and double inclinometer methods. Three physical therapists with similar training in the standardized measurement protocols assessed 15 subjects (7 men, 8 women; mean age 35.7 years) with chronic low back pain. The therapists measured lumbar flexion and extension ROM using these two methods in two separate sessions, with 2 days between sessions. The therapists positioned the inclinometers in the midline at the same spinal levels marked for the modified-modified Schöber method. The results indicated that the modified-modified Schöber method had moderate reliability and the double inclinometer method had questionable reliability. The researchers concluded that the modified-modified Schöber method is a reliable and time-efficient method to use for measuring lumbar flexion and extension ROM.

Thoracolumbar Lateral Flexion

Lateral Flexion: Fingertip-to-Floor Measurement Method (see Figs. 9-75 and 9-76). Frost and colleagues (30) evaluated the intra- and intertester reliability of trunk lateral flexion AROM by measuring the distance between the middle fingertip and the floor at the end of the lateral flexion ROM. Three physical therapists measured the right lateral flexion of 24 healthy subjects (12 men, 12 women; mean age 33.8 years) using the fingertip-to-floor method. Each therapist assessed each subject on two separate occasions at the same time of day 1 week apart. On each occasion, the therapist measured right lateral flexion three times in succession. This method of measuring lateral trunk flexion showed good intra- and intertester measurement reliability.

Lateral Flexion: Thigh Measurement Method (see Figs. 9-77 through 9-79). Several studies (16,33,34,40,41) assessed healthy subjects to evaluate the reliability of measuring lateral trunk flexion using a tape measure to measure the distance between marks placed on the lateral thigh at the level of the tip of the middle finger at the start and end of trunk lateral flexion AROM. These studies reported good to strong intra- and/or intertester reliability for the thigh measurement method for healthy subjects. Rose (40) studied the intratester reliability of this measurement technique. In this study, one physical therapist measured the trunk lateral flexion ROM of 18 physical therapy students (3 men and 15 women; mean age 19.5 years) with no history of low back pain. The therapist measured each subject twice with a 3-week interval between measures. Rose concluded the intratester reliability was poor, but noted that error may have been introduced into the study by several subjects having taken part in an exercise class between measures.

Mellin (41) and Hyytiäinen and coworkers (33) assessed the intra- and intertester reliability of the thigh measurement method to determine trunk lateral flexion ROM. In the study by Mellin (41), two physical therapists performed the measurements of lateral flexion using a tape measure for 39 healthy subjects. Mellin found the intra- and intertester reliabilities for this method of assessing trunk lateral flexion ROM to be good and "acceptable for most purposes." (41, p. 87) Hyytiäinen and coworkers (33) had three therapists measure the range of lateral flexion for 30 male shipyard employees.

Intra- and intertester reliability was strong and the researchers noted that as well as being reproducible, the method was quick and easy to perform.

Oksanen and Salminen (34) evaluated the intertester reliability of measuring trunk lateral flexion ROM using the thigh measurement method. Two experienced physical therapists performed the measurements of trunk lateral flexion ROM consecutively in the same session. The therapists performed the measurements on 30 schoolchildren (15 years of age). The study results for the thigh measurement method for determining lateral flexion ROM of the spine showed high intertester reliability.

Alaranta and colleagues (16) had two trained physical therapists use the thigh measurement method to measure the trunk lateral flexion of 17 healthy subjects. Unlike other studies, in which the measurements recorded and evaluated were of right and left lateral flexion, the measurement recorded by Alaranta and colleagues was the mean of the distances assessed for right and left trunk lateral flexion. These researchers found a high intertester reliability when using the tape measure to assess lateral trunk flexion.

Thoracolumbar Rotation (see Figs. 9-84 and 9-85)

Only one study (30) was found that examined a method of measurement for trunk rotation AROM using a tape measure. With the subject sitting and the tape placed over the posterior aspect of the trunk, the distance was measured between the tip of the acromion process and the greater trochanter at the end of the trunk rotation ROM. Frost and colleagues (30) evaluated the intra- and intertester reliability of this method of measuring trunk rotation ROM. They reported poor reliability for the measurements performed with 24 healthy subjects and suggested that the bony landmarks selected and inaccurate palpation of bony landmarks may have affected the measurement accuracy and reliability.

Toe-Touch Test (see Figs. 9-90 and 9-91). The toe-touch test or fingertip-to-floor method of assessing ROM provides a composite measure of hip, spine, and shoulder girdle ROM. The majority of studies (30,33,34,42) that examined the intra- and/or intertester reliability of the toe-touch test reported good to strong reliability for this assessment method.

Gill and coworkers (32) examined the intratester reliability of the fingertip-to-floor method. The tester measured the fingertip-to-floor distance twice for each of 10 healthy subjects (five men, five women), with a 10-minute rest between measurements. The fingertip-to-floor method showed poor repeatability; the investigators suggested that this was probably due to the measurement being less specific to lumbar vertebral movement, as it includes movement of other parts of the spine and joints of the upper extremity.

Three physical therapists measured the fingertip-to-floor distance of 24 healthy subjects (12 men, 12 women; mean age 33.8 years), and Frost and colleagues (30) evaluated the intra- and intertester reliability of the measurements. Each therapist assessed each subject on two separate occasions at the same time of day 1 week apart. On each occasion, the therapist measured fingertip-to-floor distance three times in succession. The results showed good intra- and intertester measurement reliability.

Hyytiäinen and colleagues (33) had three therapists use a meter board to measure the forward bending ROM for 30 male shipyard employees. There was strong intra- and intertester reliability, and the researchers noted that as well as being reproducible, the method proved to be quick and easy to perform.

Oksanen and Salminen (34) examined the intertester reliability of measuring finger-to-floor distance using a meter board. Two experienced physical therapists assessed the finger-to-floor distance measurements of 30 school children (aged 15 years). The therapists performed the measurements consecutively in the same session. The intertester reliability was high for the finger-to-floor distance measurements.

Newton and Waddell (42) had an orthopaedic consultant and a research physical therapist assess 20 subjects with low back pain to examine the intertester reliability of the fingertip-to-floor method. The researchers found the fingertip-to-floor method to be reliable.

Inclinometry

The work by Lee and colleagues (43) was the only study found in the literature that examined the validity of measuring thoracic spine ROM using inclinometry. These researchers compared single inclinometer measures with radiographic measures of thoracic spine left (14 subjects) and right (15 subjects) lateral flexion. The researchers reported poor to moderate validity for the measurement of thoracic spine lateral flexion by single inclinometry and concluded that because of the low validity, the usefulness of the technique in the clinic should be "minimized" until further research establishes validity.

Studies (28,35,44–47) conducted to determine the validity of measuring lumbar spine AROM using inclinometry examined lumbar flexion and extension. These studies compared the inclinometer measurements to x-ray measurements. The study findings were mixed, with three research groups (28,35,44) reporting low validity and an equal number (45–47) finding inclinometry to be a valid means of assessing the lumbar spine AROM.

Portek and colleagues (28) assessed the validity of the double inclinometer method (with inclinometers placed over S1 and L1) of measuring active lumbar spine flexion in sitting and active lumbar extension in prone. The investigators compared the double inclinometer measurements with those of active lumbar flexion and extension assessed by x-rays with the subject in standing. There was little correlation between the double inclinometer and the x-ray results of the healthy male subjects assessed. The authors concluded that the inclinometer method gives only a linear index of movement but does not reflect true spinal movement.

Samo and coworkers (44) assessed the validity of three different inclinometers (including one computerized inclinometer) by comparison with radiographic measures. Thirty subjects positioned in a fixed frame performed lumbar flexion and extension ROM to predetermined angles. The x-rays of each position were taken immediately after the three measures were made with each type of inclinometer (with inclinometers positioned at S1 and T12) while the subject held the same position. The results showed a poor relationship between the x-ray measurements and the measurements from each of the three inclinometers. The researchers concluded that the three inclinometers were not valid for measuring lumbar flexion and extension.

In a study by Burdett and associates (35), one therapist used the inclinometer to measure the lumbar curve and sacral angle of 10 subjects in upright relaxed stance, 6 subjects in trunk flexion, and 11 subjects in trunk extension. The researchers compared the inclinometer measurements with sagittal plane x-rays of the low back taken with the subjects in the same positions. They found the validity of the inclinometer to be low compared with the x-ray measurements.

Saur and colleagues (45) studied the validity of assessing lumbar spine ROM using the double inclinometer technique with the inclinometers positioned at S1 and T12. The researchers took simultaneous measurements of the lumbar spine AROM (i.e., flexion, extension, and total flexion and extension ROM) of 54 patients with chronic low back pain using double inclinometry and dynamic radiography. The inclinometer technique was valid based on the high correlation between the measures obtained with the inclinometer and the x-rays. The authors concluded the "inclinometer technique is clinically suitable for measuring lumbar motion" (45, p. 1337) for flexion, extension, and total flexion-extension.

Williams and coworkers (46) examined 18 subjects with chronic low back pain (10 men, 8 women; mean age of 41.2 years) to assess the validity of the double inclinometer technique. A radiologist took x-ray measurements of lumbar flexion ROM. The double inclinometry measures were taken immediately after the x-rays while the subject maintained the test position. A physical therapist performed the double inclinometer measurements with the subjects standing and the inclinometers positioned at the level of the PSIS and 15 cm superior to the level of the PSIS. Comparison of the x-ray and double inclinometry measurements indicated the double inclinometry technique to be a valid method for measuring lumbar flexion ROM.

As part of a larger study, Mayer and colleagues (47) compared the x-ray and double inclinometry (with inclinometers placed over the sacrum and at T12–L1) measurements of lumbar spine flexion and extension AROM of 12 patients with chronic lumbar spine pain. There was no significant difference between the measures taken by x-ray and those taken using the double inclinometry method. The researchers concluded that inclinometry is a "simple, effective quantitative technique to assessing disability and measuring progress in rehabilitation" (47, p. 594).

Many researchers have employed various types of inclinometers to determine the reliability of using the inclinometer to measure thoracolumbar and lumbar spine ROM. Only one research group (43) studied the reliability of using the inclinometer to measure thoracic spine ROM. The research on the reliability of inclinometry is presented according to spinal region and motion(s).

Thoracic Flexion/Extension/Lateral Flexion

Lee and colleagues (43) examined the intra- and intertester reliability of measuring thoracic spine ROM using single inclinometry. On separate days, two physical therapy master's students used the single inclinometer method to measure the thoracic spine flexion, extension, and lateral flexion ROM of 31 healthy subjects (18 men, 13 women; 18–35 years of age). The testers positioned the inclinometer over the spine of T1 and then T12 to take the measurements. The authors interpreted the intra- and intertester reliability to be generally good, but noted that the usefulness of the single inclinometer in the clinical setting is minimal owing to the low validity reported in this study.

Thoracolumbar Flexion/Extension/Lateral Flexion

In the late sixties, Loebl provided a descriptive report of "a new, simple method for accurate clinical measurement of spinal posture and movements" (48, p. 103) using the inclinometer. The inclinometer was placed on the vertebral spines of S1, T12, T1, and a point midway between T1 and T12 to measure the spinal AROM of nine normal subjects. Loebl concluded that the inclinometer method was quick and accurate to within 10% of the total ROM for the majority of subjects.

Reynolds (49) assessed the intra- and intertester reliabilities for measuring spinal mobility using the inclinometer, the skin distraction method, and the spondylometer. Two inexperienced testers used the three measurement methods to assess thoracolumbar flexion, extension, total sagittal, and lateral flexion ROM and lumbar lateral flexion ROM. One tester performed 10 measurements of one subject on different occasions to assess the intratester reliability. The intratester reliability of the inclinometer was acceptable for thoracolumbar spine flexion, total sagittal ROM, and lateral flexion measurements, while lumbar lateral flexion and thoracolumbar extension were not as reproducible. Intertester reliability, based on the measurements of the two testers on two subjects, was acceptable for all measurements using the inclinometer. In comparing the three measurement techniques, Reynolds concluded the inclinometer was "the most versatile and of acceptable accuracy" (49, p. 180).

Nitschke and coworkers (50) researched the intra- and intertester reliability of using a universal goniometer and an electronic dual inclinometer to measure flexion, extension, and lateral flexion ROM of the thoracolumbar and lumbar spinal regions, according to the guidelines set out by the AMA Guides to the Evaluation of Permanent Impairment. Two physicians, trained in the ROM assessment techniques, performed all measurements. Thirty-four subjects (13 men, mean age 47.7 years; 21 women, mean age 40.1 years) with chronic low back pain took part in the study. To assess intratester reliability, one examiner measured 23 of the subjects on two occasions. For intertester reliability, one examiner measured the ROM using the goniometer and the inclinometer before the second examiner repeated the ROM measurements on the same day. The researchers concluded that the universal goniometer and double inclinometer methods of measuring low back ROM for patients with chronic low back pain have poor intra- and intertester reliability.

The reliability of measuring spinal ROM using the OB "Myrin" inclinometer was studied by Mellin (51) and Mellin and colleagues (52). Mellin (51) examined the intra- and intertester reliability for measurements of thoracolumbar flexion, extension, and lateral flexion. Two physical therapists performed the ROM measurements on 25 healthy subjects (9 men, 16 women; mean age 31.3 years). For positioning of the OB inclinometer, the therapists placed marks at the level of the PSIS, 20 cm superior to the PSIS, and at T1. To examine intratester reliability, the therapist measured 10 subjects two times on 2 consecutive days and one subject 10 times. For intertester reliability, the two therapists measured 15 subjects on consecutive days. The reproducibility of measurements of lateral flexion was poorer than for measurements of flexion and extension. However, Mellin noted the "reproducibility of the measurements proved to be acceptable" and the "accuracy of the methods described makes them useful for measurements of thoracolumbar mobility in the sagittal and frontal planes. However, training is needed in the methods, manipulation of the instruments, and instructions to give the subjects before the measurements can be considered reliable" (51, p. 761).

In a later study by Mellin and colleagues (52), two physical therapists used the OB inclinometer to measure the thoracolumbar spine flexion, extension, and lateral flexion ROM of 27 healthy subjects (10 men, 17 women; mean age 30.6 years). The researchers examined the intratester reliability of the measurements and the effect of subject position on measurements (i.e., measuring three different positions each for flexion and lateral flexion and two different positions for extension). In general, repeatability of spinal measurements was not affected to any extent by subject position, and the authors reported that repeatability corresponded with the earlier measurements by Mellin (51).

Lumbar Flexion/Extension/Lateral Flexion

Gill and coworkers (32) examined the intratester reliability of the double inclinometer (with the inclinometers positioned over the sacrum and T12–L1 spinous processes), modified Schöber, and fingertip-to-floor methods of assessing ROM in standing. For each measurement method, spinal flexion and extension movements were measured twice for each of 10 healthy subjects (five men, five women), with a 10-minute rest between measurements. Repeatability for the double inclinometer method was good.

Ng and associates (53) evaluated the intratester reliability of the inclinometer (positioned at L5–S1 and T12–L1 interspinous spaces) to measure lumbar flexion, extension, and lateral flexion. The ROM carried out on 12 healthy male subjects was measured with the subjects standing in a pelvic stabilization frame. The intratester reliability was good for all lumbar spine measures.

To assess intertester reliability, Saur and colleagues (45) had a physician and physical therapist use the double inclinometer technique (with the inclinometers placed at S1 and T12) to measure the active lumbar flexion, extension, and total flexion and extension ROM in standing of 48

patients with chronic low back pain. The testers took the measurements with a maximum of 2 days between measures. Results showed high intertester reliability for lumbar flexion and total flexion and extension ROM but poor intertester reliability for lumbar extension ROM.

Burdett and associates (35) assessed the intertester reliability for measuring lumbar flexion and extension using the inclinometer placed over the sacrum and at the thoracolumbar junction. Two therapists measured the lumbar flexion ROM of 23 healthy subjects. Using the criteria selected by the researchers the measures were considered highly reliable for lumbar flexion but relatively low for measurement of lumbar extension.

Alaranta and colleagues (16) assessed the intertester reliability of the double inclinometer for measuring lumbar flexion and extension ROM. Two physical therapists measured the ROM of 17 healthy subjects with the inclinometers placed at the level of the PSIS and at T12. The intertester reliability was reported to be "fairly good."

Portek and colleagues (28) assessed the intra- and intertester reliability of the inclinometer method of measuring lumbar spine flexion and extension AROM. For intratester reliability, one tester performed 10 measurements on one male subject at the same time of day on 10 different days. To assess the intertester reliability, two testers measured the same 14 patients admitted for minor orthopaedic surgery who were not taking drugs and had no low back pain. The results indicated that the inclinometer measurements of spinal mobility are reproducible by different testers using a closely monitored technique.

Chen and colleagues (54) had 30 volunteers stand in a fixed frame and perform lumbar flexion and extension to predetermined angles. To assess the reliability of three different inclinometers (including one computerized inclinometer), three occupational health professionals independently performed inclinometer measurements of lumbar sagittal motion. The authors judged the intra- and intertester reliabilities of the inclinometers to be "mostly clinically undesirable" and "poor," respectively, for measuring lumbar sagittal motion.

Williams and coworkers (38) employed the double inclinometer and modified-modified Schöber methods to assess the intra- and intertester reliability of using these techniques to measure lumbar flexion and extension AROM. Three physical therapists with similar training in the standardized measurement protocols assessed 15 subjects (7 men, 8 women; mean age 35.7 years) with chronic low back pain. In two separate sessions, the therapists measured lumbar flexion and extension ROM using the modified-modified Schöber and double inclinometer methods, with 2 days between sessions. The therapists placed the inclinometers over the midline at the level of the PSIS and at a mark 15 cm superior. The results showed that the modified-modified Schöber method has moderate reliability and the double inclinometer method has questionable reliability. The researchers concluded that the double inclinometer technique requires improvement.

In a study by Rondinelli and associates (55), two physical therapists examined the lumbar flexion ROM of eight healthy subjects between the ages of 18 and 30 years using standardized single and double inclinometry techniques.

The therapists positioned the inclinometers at the sacral midpoint and T12 according to the AMA guidelines (1990). Each therapist measured the lumbar flexion ROM three times on each subject in one day. The intratester reliability for the single inclinometer measurements was high and acceptable, whereas the double inclinometer results showed only moderate intratester reliability. The intertester reliability for both inclinometry techniques was low and therefore unacceptable. The authors concluded that the findings of this study do not bode well for the ability of the clinician to use inclinometry reliably to assess spinal mobility for the purposes of determining impairment.

Keeley and colleagues (56) reported a "high degree" of intra- and intertester reliability for measuring lumbar flexion and extension AROM using the double inclinometer technique with the inclinometers positioned over the sacrum and T12–L1. In this study, two physical therapists measured 11 healthy subjects (4 men, 7 women; mean ages of 28.3 and 30.1 years, respectively) and 9 subjects with chronic low back pain (2 men, 7 women; mean ages of 35 and 39.4 years, respectively).

Patel (57) evaluated the intra- and intertester reliability of measuring lumbar flexion using inclinometers positioned at the levels of the L1 and S1 spinous processes. The lumbar AROM was measured on 25 healthy subjects between 21 and 37 years of age. When one therapist performed the lumbar flexion measurement twice on the same patient, Patel found the double inclinometer method to be reliable. However, when the lumbar flexion measurements performed by a second therapist were compared to those of the other therapist, Patel found the intertester reliability to be moderate.

Mayer and associates (58) compared the intra- and intertester reliability of measurements made by 14 and 11 testers, respectively, using the fluid-filled inclinometer, electronic inclinometer, and kyphometer. The testers measured the lumbar spine flexion ROM of 18 healthy subjects (9 men and 9 women; 18–49 years of age) with each instrument aligned over the sacrum and the interspace between T12 and L1. There was good intratester reliability for all three instruments, but intertester reliability was poor, possibly owing to the inability of the testers to locate the bony landmarks necessary for instrument placement.

As part of a larger study examining lumbar spine function, Neblett and associates (59) examined the intra- and intertester reliability of two physical therapists using the dual inclinometer method to measure the lumbar flexion of 10 healthy subjects. The inclinometers were positioned at the level of the sacrum and T12 for the measurements. With the subject standing, lumbar flexion ROM was performed at a regulated speed and the motion was stopped and measured when surface EMG signals indicated relaxation of the lumbar muscles. These researchers found excellent intra- and intertester reliability using dual inclinometry to measure the lumbar flexion ROM under the prescribed conditions.

Thoracic and Lumbar Spine Rotation

Alaranta and colleagues (16) assessed the intertester reliability of measuring total right and left trunk rotation ROM with the subjects in sitting, using the OB "Myrin" goniometer. The physical therapist positioned the OB goniometer at the inferior level of the scapulae. Two physical therapists measured 17 healthy subjects' trunk rotation ROM. The results showed good intertester reliability for the measurement of total trunk rotation using the OB goniometer.

Boline and associates (60) examined the intertester reliability of the inclinometer, positioned at the T12–L1 level, to measure lumbar rotation with subjects forward flexed to face the floor in the standing position. In this study, two chiropractors measured the lumbar rotation ROM of 25 subjects with chronic low back pain and 25 healthy subjects (28 men, 22 women; age range 28–38 years). Each subject was measured by the one chiropractor and immediately measured again by the second chiropractor. The authors found intertester reliability to be moderate to good for measuring lumbar rotation using the inclinometer.

Universal Goniometer

Thoracolumbar Flexion/Extension/Lateral Flexion

The intertester reliability of measuring lumbar flexion AROM using the Schöber method and thoracolumbar extension and right and left lateral flexion ROM using the universal goniometer was investigated by Fitzgerald and associates (31). All four spinal movements as measured by two testers on each of 17 healthy subjects showed substantial intertester reliability.

Nitschke and coworkers (50) researched the intra- and intertester reliability of using a universal goniometer and an electronic dual inclinometer to measure flexion, extension, and lateral flexion ROM of the thoracolumbar and lumbar spinal regions, according to the guidelines set out by the AMA Guides to the Evaluation of Permanent Impairment. Two physicians, trained in the ROM assessment techniques, performed all measurements. Thirty-four subjects (13 men, mean age 47.7 years; 21 women, mean age 40.1 years) with chronic low back pain took part in the study. To assess intratester reliability, one examiner measured 23 of the subjects on two occasions. For intertester reliability, one examiner measured the ROM using the goniometer and the inclinometer before the second examiner repeated the ROM measurements on the same day. The researchers concluded that the universal goniometer and double inclinometer methods of measuring low back ROM for patients with chronic low back pain have poor intra- and intertester reliability.

Back Range-of-Motion Instrument

The Back Range-of-Motion Instrument (BROM II; Performance Attainment Associates, Roseville, MN) (61) is a relatively new tool designed to measure AROM of the lumbar spine. The BROM II consists of two units for the measurement of back ROM. The first, a frame that contains a protractor scale, is positioned over S1 and held in place using Velcro straps. An L-shaped extension arm slides into the frame, and this device is used to measure lumbar flexion and extension ROM. The second, a frame that holds two inclinometers, is positioned horizontally over the T12 spinous process and held in place by the therapist during the measurement of lateral flexion and rotation. One inclinometer lies in the frontal plane with a gravity-dependent needle for measurement of lateral flexion; a second, oriented in the transverse plane, contains a compass needle that reacts to Earth's magnetic field for measurement of rotation. A magnetic yoke is positioned around the pelvis to eliminate substitute pelvic motion from the rotation measurement.

Studies (55,62,63) assessing the reliability of the BROM II were carried out using healthy young subjects. Breum and colleagues (62), assessing the intra- and intertester reliability of the BROM II, found it to be reliable for measuring active flexion and lateral flexion, but reliability for extension and rotation was considered unacceptable.

Rondinelli and associates (55) used two testers to examine eight subjects and obtain reliability estimates of lumbar flexion AROM using the BROM II, single inclinometry, and double inclinometry. For the BROM II, the intratester reliability was reported to be acceptable and intertester reliability unacceptable for lumbar flexion. The BROM II had a median range of measurement error of 16°, compared to 8.5° for single inclinometry and 10.5° for double inclinometry.

Intratester reliability of the BROM II was also studied by Madson and coworkers (63), who found the instrument to be reliable for measuring active lateral flexion and rotation. However, intratester reliability of lumbar spine flexion and extension AROM was reported to be poor and fair, respectively. The authors suggested that because of the high reliability of tape measure measurements, the tape measure should be preferred over the BROM II for flexion and extension ROM measurement.

The BROM II is relatively expensive, and from the research to date, it does not appear to be superior to other means of measuring AROM of the lumbar spine. For this reason, the BROM II is not used to demonstrate ROM assessment in this text.

References

1. Walker N, Bohannon RW, Cameron D. Discriminant validity of temporomandibular joint range of motion measurements obtained with a ruler. *JOSPT*. 2000;30:484–492.
2. Dijkstra PU, De Bont LGM, Stegenga B, Boering G. Temporomandibular joint mobility assessment: a comparison between four methods. *J Oral Rehab*. 1995;22:439–444.
3. Higbie EJ, Seidel-Cobb D, Taylor LF, Cummings GS. Effect of head position on vertical mandibular opening. *JOSPT*. 1999;29:127–130.
4. Dworkin SF, LeResche L, DeRouen T, VonKorff M. Assessing clinical signs of temporomandibular disorders: reliability of clinical examiners. *J Prosthet Dent*. 1990;63:574–579.
5. Hsieh C-Y, Yeung BW. Active neck motion measurements with a tape measure. *JOSPT*. 1986;8:88–92.
6. Balogun JA, Abereoje OK, Olaogun MO, Obajuluwa VA. Inter- and intratester reliability of measuring neck motions with tape measure and Myrin gravity-reference goniometer. *JOSPT*. 1989;10:248–253.
7. Pile KD, Laurent MR, Salmond CE, et al. Clinical assessment of ankylosing spondylitis: a study of observer variation in spinal measurements. *Br J Rheumatol*. 1991;30:29–34.
8. Viitanen JV, Kokko M-L, Heikkilä S, Kautiainen H. Neck mobility assessment in ankylosing spondylitis: a clinical study of nine measurements including new tape methods for cervical rotation and lateral flexion. *Br J Rheumatol*. 1998;37:377–381.
9. Jordan K. Assessment of published reliability studies for cervical range-of-motion measurement tools. *J Manipulative Physiol Ther*. 2000;23:180–195.
10. Bush KW, Collins N, Portman L, Tillett N. Validity and intertester reliability of cervical range of motion using inclinometer measurements. *J Manipulative Ther*. 2000;8:52–61.
11. Herrmann DB. Validity study of head and neck flexion-extension motion comparing measurements of a pendulum goniometer and roentgenograms. *JOSPT*. 1990;11:414–418.
12. Hole DE, Cook JM, Bolton JE. Reliability and concurrent validity of two instruments for measuring cervical range of motion: effects of age and gender. *Man Ther*. 1995;1:36–42.
13. Ålund M, Larsson S-E. Three-dimensional analysis of neck motion: a clinical method. *Spine*. 1990;15:87–91.
14. Hagen KB, Harms-Ringdahl K, Enger NO, et al. Relationship between subjective neck disorders and cervical spine mobility and motion-related pain in male machine operators. *Spine*. 1997;22:1501–1507.
15. Zachman ZJ, Traina AD, Keating JC Jr., et al. Interexaminer reliability and concurrent validity of two instruments for the measurement of cervical ranges of motion. *J Manipulative Physiol Ther*. 1989;12:205–210.
16. Alaranta H, Hurri H, Heliövaara M, et al. Flexibility of the spine: normative values of goniometric and tape measurements. *Scand J Rehab Med*. 1994;26:147–154.
17. Tucci SM, Hicks JE, Gross EG, et al. Cervical motion assessment: a new, simple and accurate method. *Arch Phys Med Rehabil*. 1986;67:225–230.
18. Defibaugh JJ. Part II: An experimental study of head motion in adult males. *Phys Ther*. 1964;44:163–168.
19. Chen J, Solinger AB, Poncet JF, Lantz CA. Meta-analysis of normative cervical motion. *Spine*. 1999;24:1571–1578.
20. Ordway N, Seymour R, Donelson RG, et al. Cervical sagittal range-of-motion analysis using three methods. *Spine*. 1997;22:501–508.
21. Tousignant M, de Bellefeuille L, O'Donoughue S, Grahovac S. Criterion validity of the cervical range of motion (CROM) goniometer for cervical flexion and extension. *Spine*. 2000;25:324–330.
22. Tousignant M, Duclos E, Lafleche S, et al. Validity study for the cervical range of motion device used for lateral flexion in patients with neck pain. *Spine*. 2002;27:812–817.
23. Youdas JW, Carey JR, Garrett TR. Reliability of measurements of cervical spine range of motion: comparison of three methods. *Phys Ther*. 1991;71:23–29.
24. Rheault W, Albright B, Byers C, et al. Inter-tester reliability of the cervical range of motion device. *JOSPT*. 1992;15:147–150.
25. Peolsson A, Hedlund R, Ertzgaard S, Oberg B. Intra- and inter-tester reliability and range of motion of the neck. *Physiother Can*. 2000; Summer:233–242.
26. Capuano-Pucci D, Rheault W, Aukai J, et al. Intra-tester and inter-tester reliability of the cervical range of motion device. *Arch Phys Med Rehabil*. 1991;72:338–340.
27. Youdas JW, Garrett TR, Suman VJ, et al. Normal range of motion of the cervical spine: an initial goniometric study. *Phys Ther*. 1992;72:770–780.
28. Portek I, Pearcy MJ, Reader GP, Mowat AG. Correlation between radiographic and clinical measurement of lumbar spine movement. *Br J Rheumatol*. 1983;22:197–205.
29. Macrae IF, Wright V. Measurement of back movement. *Ann Rheum Dis*. 1969;28:584–589.
30. Frost M, Stuckey S, Smalley LA, Dorman G. Reliability of measuring trunk motions in centimeters. *Phys Ther*. 1982;62:1431–1437.

31. Fitzgerald GK, Wynveen KJ, Rheault W, Rothschild B. Objective assessment with establishment of normal values for lumbar spinal range of motion. *Phys Ther.* 1983;63; 11:1776–1781.

32. Gill K, Krag MH, Hohnson GB, et al. Repeatability of four clinical methods for assessment of lumbar spinal motion. *Spine.* 1968;13:50–53.

33. Hyytiäinen K, Salminen JJ, Suvitie T, et al. Reproducibility of nine tests to measure spinal mobility and trunk muscle strength. *Scand J Rehab Med.* 1991;23:3–10.

34. Oksanen A, Salminen JJ. Tests of spinal mobility and muscle strength in the young: reliability and normative values. *Physiother Theor Pract.* 1996;12:151–160.

35. Burdett RG, Brown KE, Fall MP. Reliability and validity of four instruments for measuring lumbar spine and pelvic motions. *Phys Ther.* 1986;66:677–684.

36. Beattie P, Rothstein JM, Lamb RL. Reliability of the attraction method for measuring lumbar spine backward bending. *Phys Ther.* 1987;67:364–369.

37. van Adrichem JAM, van der Korst JK. Assessment of the flexibility of the lumbar spine. *Scand J Rheumatol.* 1973;2:87–91.

38. Williams R, Binkley J, Bloch R, et al. Reliability of the modified-modified Schöber and double inclinometer methods of measuring lumbar flexion and extension. *Phys Ther.* 1993; 73:26–37.

39. Bandy WD, Reese NB. Strapped versus unstrapped techniques of the prone press-up for measurement of lumbar extension using a tape measure: differences in magnitude and reliability of measurements. *Arch Phys Med Rehab.* 2004;85:99–103.

40. Rose MJ. The statistical analysis of the intra-observer repeatability of four clinical measurement techniques. *Physiotherapy.* 1991;77: 89–91.

41. Mellin GP. Accuracy of measuring lateral flexion of the spine with a tape. *Clin Biomech.* 1986;1:85–89.

42. Newton M, Waddell G. Reliability and validity of clinical measurement of lumbar spine in patients with chronic low back pain. *Physiotherapy.* 1991;77:796–800.

43. Lee CN, Robbins DP, Roberts HJ, et al. Reliability and validity of single inclinometer measurements for thoracic spine range of motion. *Physiother Can.* 2003;55:73–78.

44. Samo DG, Chen SC, Crampton A, et al. Validity of three lumbar sagittal motion measurement methods: surface inclinometers compared with radiographs. *J Occup Environ Med.* 1997;39:209–216.

45. Saur PM, Ensink F-BM, Frese K, et al. Lumbar range of motion: reliability and validity of the inclinometer technique in the clinical measurement of trunk flexibility. *Spine.* 1996;21:1332–1338.

46. Williams RM, Goldsmith CH, Minuk T. Validity of the double inclinometer method for measuring lumbar flexion. *Physiother Can.* 1998;Spring:147–152.

47. Mayer TG, Tencer AF, Kristoferson S, Mooney V. Use of non-invasive techniques for quantification of spinal range-of-motion in normal subjects and chronic low-back dysfunction patients. *Spine.* 1984;9:588–595.

48. Loebl WY. Measurement of spinal posture and range of spinal movement. *Ann Phys Med.* 1967;9:103–110.

49. Reynolds PMG. Measurement of spinal mobility: a comparison of three methods. *Rheumatol Rehab.* 1975;14:180–185.

50. Nitschke JE, Nattrass CL, Disler PB, et al. Reliability of the American Medical Association Guides' model for measuring spinal range of motion. *Spine.* 1999;24:262–268.

51. Mellin G. Measurement of thoracolumbar posture and mobility with a Myrin inclinometer. *Spine.* 1986;11:759–762.

52. Mellin G, Kiiski R, Weckström A. Effects of subject position on measurements of flexion, extension, and lateral flexion of the spine. *Spine.* 1991;16:1108–1110.

53. Ng JK-F, Kippers V, Richardson C, Parnianpour M. Range of motion and lordosis of the lumbar spine. *Spine.* 2001;26: 53–60.

54. Chen SC, Samo DG, Chen EH, et al. Reliability of three lumbar sagittal motion measurement methods: surface inclinometers. *J Occup Environ Med.* 1997;39:217–223.

55. Rondinelli R, Murphy J, Esler A, et al. Estimation of normal lumbar flexion with surface inclinometry. *Am J Phys Med Rehabil.* 1992;71:219–224.

56. Keeley J, Mayer TG, Cox R, et al. Quantification of lumbar function, Part 5: Reliability of range-of-motion measures in the sagittal plane and an in vivo rotation measurement technique. *Spine.* 1986;11:31–35.

57. Patel RS. Intratester and intertester reliability of the inclinometer in measuring true lumbar flexion. *Phys Ther.* 1992;72:S44.

58. Mayer RS, Chen I-H, Lavender SA, et al. Variance in the measurement of sagittal lumbar spine range of motion among examiners, subjects, and instruments. *Spine.* 1995;20: 1489–1493.

59. Neblett R, Mayer TG, Gatchel RJ, et al. Quantifying the lumbar flexion-relaxation phenomenon. *Spine.* 2003;28: 1435–1446.

60. Boline PD, Keating JC, Haas M, Anderson AV. Interexaminer reliability and discriminant validity of inclinometric measurement of lumbar rotation in chronic low-back pain patients and subjects without low-back pain. *Spine.* 1992;17: 335–338.

61. Performance Attainment Associates, 958 Lydia Drive, Roseville, MN 55113.

62. Breum J, Wiberg J, Bolton JE. Reliability and concurrent validity of the BROMII for measuring lumbar mobility. *J Manipulative Physiol Ther.* 1995;18:497–502.

63. Madson TJ, Youdas JW, Suman VJ. Reproducibility of lumbar spine range of motion measurements using the back range of motion device. *JOSPT.* 1999;29:470–477.

Summary of Patient Positioning for the Assessment and Measurement of Joint Range of Motion and Muscle Length

The assessment and measurement of joint range of motion (ROM) and muscle length presented in this textbook first shows the optimal *start position* that could be used to test the joint movement on the basis of the position that offers the best stabilization. In some instances, other positions could be used to assess or measure the joint motion or position. These positions are termed *alternate start positions* and are documented if they are common in clinical practice or if the preferred start position is impractical or contraindicated for some patients.

The following chart summarizes the *preferred (P)* and *alternate (A)* start positions used by the therapist when assessing and measuring active and passive joint ROM. This summary provides the reader with the knowledge essential to perform an organized and efficient assessment and measurement of joint ROM and muscle length that avoids unnecessary patient position changes and fatigue.

Joint Motion	Sitting	Supine	Prone
Shoulder			
Elevation through flexion	A	P	
Extension	A		P
Elevation through abduction	A	P	
Adduction	A	P	
Horizontal adduction	P	A	
Horizontal abduction	P	A	
Internal rotation	A		P
External rotation	A	P	
Pectoralis major length		P	
Pectoralis minor length		P	
Elbow			
Flexion	A	P	
Extension	A	P	
Forearm			
Supination	P		

Joint Motion	Sitting	Supine	Prone
Pronation	P		
Biceps brachii length		P	
Triceps length	P	A	
Wrist			
Flexion	P		
Extension	P		
Radial deviation	P		
Ulnar deviation	P		
Hand			
Finger/thumb movements	P		
Long finger flexors length	P		
Long finger extensors length	P		
Lumbricales length	P		

Joint Motion	Sitting	Supine	Prone	Side-lying	Standing
Hip					
Flexion		P			
Extension			P		
Abduction		P			
Adduction		P			
Internal rotation	P	A	A		
External rotation	P	A	A		
Hip flexors length		P			
Tensor fascia latae length			P	A	
Adductors length		P			
Knee					
Flexion		P			
Extension		P			
Tibial rotation	P				
Rectus femoris length		A	P		
Hamstrings length	A	P			

Joint Motion	Sitting	Supine	Prone	Side-lying	Standing
Ankle					
Dorsiflexion	A	P			
Plantarflexion	A	P			
Gastrocnemius length		A			P
Soleus length					P
Subtalar joint					
Inversion		P	A		
Eversion		P	A		
Foot					
Toe movements		P			
Spine					
Flexion					P
Extension			P		A
Rotation	P				
Side flexion					P
Neck					
Flexion	P				
Extension	P				
Side flexion	P				
Rotation	P				
TMJ					
Elevation	P				
Depression	P				

Gait

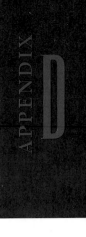
The gait cycle consists of a series of motions that occur between consecutive initial contacts of one leg (1). The gait cycle is divided into two phases: the stance phase, when the foot is in contact with the ground and the body advances over the weight-bearing limb, and the swing phase, when the limb is unweighted and advanced forward in preparation for the next stance phase. Each phase is further subdivided into a total of eight instants (1) or freeze frames. Five instants occur in the stance phase and three occur in the swing phase of the gait cycle. The description of the normal gait pattern is provided so that the implications of the findings on assessment of joint range of motion and manual muscle strength can be understood in relation to gait. The average positions and the motions of the joints during the gait cycle that are reported in this appendix were adapted from the Rancho Los Amigos gait analysis forms as cited in Levangie and Norkin (2). The right leg is used to illustrate the joint positions and motions of the lower limb throughout the gait cycle.

Stance Phase

The lower limb is advanced in front of the body during the swing phase and the stance phase begins at initial contact (Fig. D-1) when the heel makes the first contact between the foot and the ground. At initial contact the pelvis is rotated forward and the trunk is rotated backward on the stance side. The rotation of the pelvis counteracts the trunk rotation to prevent excessive trunk motion. On the opposite sides the upper extremity is flexed at the shoulder. As the body advances over the supporting limb through the stance phase, the pelvis rotates backward and the trunk rotates forward on the swing side. As the weight-bearing leg extends at the hip, the upper limb on the opposite side extends. The average joint positions and the motions of the right lower limb in the sagittal plane are described and illustrated.

Motion from *A* to *B* (Figs. D-1 and D-2): *hip:* extension (from 30 to 25° flexion); *knee:* flexion (from 0 to 15° flexion); *ankle:* plantarflexion (from 0 to 15° plantarflexion); *MTP joints of toes:* 0°.

Motion from *B* to *C* (Figs. D-2 and D-3): *hip:* extension (from 25 to 0° flexion); *knee:* extension (from 15 to 5° flexion); *ankle:* dorsiflexion (from 15° plantarflexion to 5 to 10° dorsiflexion); *MTP joints of toes:* remain at 0°.

Motion from *C* to *D* (Figs. D-3 and D-4): *hip:* extension (from 0° flexion to 10 to 20° extension); *knee:* extension (from 5° flexion to 0°); *ankle:* dorsiflexion (from 5 to 10° dorsiflexion to 0° dorsiflexion); *MTP joints of toes:* extension (from 0 to 20° extension).

Motion from *D* to *E* (Figs. D-4 and D-5): *hip:* flexion (from 10 to 20° extension to 0°); *knee:* flexion (from 0 to 30° flexion); *ankle:* plantarflexion (from 0 to 20° plantarflexion); *MTP joints of toes:* extension (from 30° extension to 50 to 60° extension).

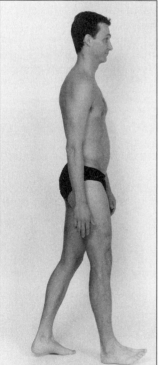

Figure D-1 Initial contact (*A*).

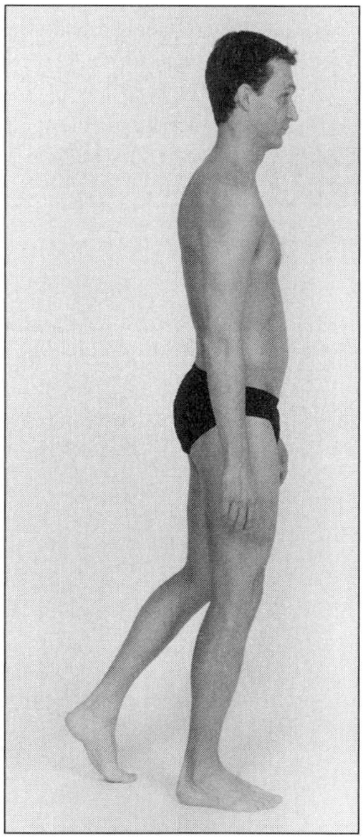

Figure D-2 Loading response (*B*).

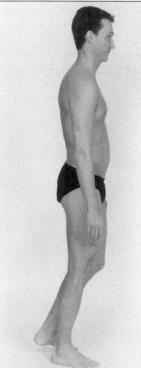

Figure D-3 Midstance (*C*).

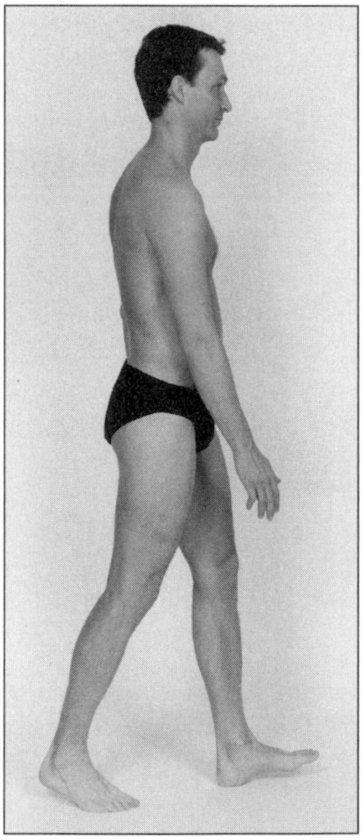

Figure D-4 Terminal stance (*D*).

Swing Phase

The swing phase begins after preswing when the foot leaves the ground and is advanced forward in the line of progression in preparation for initial contact. The positions and motions of the right lower limb are described and illustrated.

Motion from *E* to *F* (Figs. D-5 and D-6): *hip:* flexion (from 0 to 20° flexion); *knee:* flexion (from 30° flexion to 60° flexion); *ankle:* dorsiflexion (from 20° plantarflexion to 10° plantarflexion).

Motion from *F* to *G* (Figs. D-6 and D-7): *hip:* flexion (from 20° flexion to 30° flexion); *knee:* extension (from 60° flexion to 30° flexion); *ankle:* dorsiflexion (from 10° plantarflexion to 0°).

Motion from *G* to *H* (Figs. D-7 and D-8): *hip:* remains flexed at 30°; *knee:* extension (from 30° flexion to 0°); *ankle:* remains at 0°.

Motion from *H* to *A* (Figs. D-8 and D-1): *hip:* remains flexed at 30°; *knee:* remains extended at 0°; *ankle:* remains at 0°.

REFERENCES

1. Koerner I. *Observation of Human Gait.* Edmonton, Alberta: Health Sciences Media Services and Development, University of Alberta; 1986.
2. Levangie PK, Norkin CC. *Joint Structure & Function: A Comprehensive Analysis.* 3rd ed. Philadelphia: FA Davis; 2001.

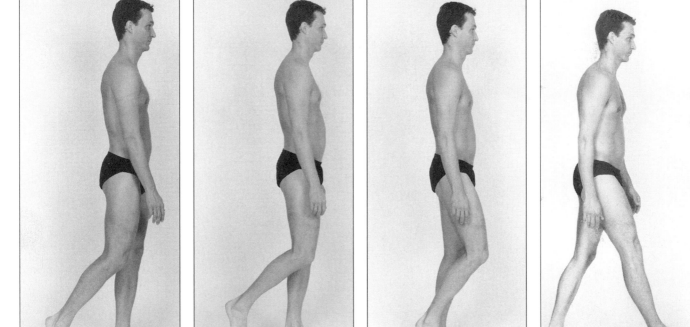

Figure D-5 Preswing (*E*).   **Figure D-6** Initial Swing (*F*).   **Figure D-7** Midswing (*G*).   **Fugire D-8** Terminal swing (*H*).

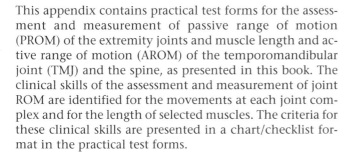

Practical Testing Evaluation Forms

This appendix contains practical test forms for the assessment and measurement of passive range of motion (PROM) of the extremity joints and muscle length and active range of motion (AROM) of the temporomandibular joint (TMJ) and the spine, as presented in this book. The clinical skills of the assessment and measurement of joint ROM are identified for the movements at each joint complex and for the length of selected muscles. The criteria for these clinical skills are presented in a chart/checklist format in the practical test forms.

Purpose of the Practical Test Forms

To become proficient in the clinical skills of assessment and measurement of joint ROM requires knowledge, attention to detail, and practice—the same requirements that apply to becoming proficient at playing an instrument or sport. When practicing the joint ROM assessment and measurement skills, the practical test forms are helpful in evaluating proficiency.

Use of the Practical Test Forms

These practical test forms are designed to be used by a group of three persons. One person serves as the "educator/evaluator" and selects a specific joint PROM or muscle length test or a movement of the TMJ or spine from the "List of Practical Test Items" provided in this appendix. A second person, the "therapist," demonstrates the assessment and measurement for the selected test item with a partner, who plays the role of the "patient." The "educator/evaluator" evaluates the "therapist's" performance using the appropriate practical test form.

Recording Performance

A clear overhead projection or transparency film is placed over the practical test form, and an overhead transparency marker is used by the "educator/evaluator" to write on the clear film when recording the "therapist's" performance. The transparency film is wiped off and reused for subsequent testing. Alternatively, the appropriate practical test form can be accessed on the website and printed by instructors for classroom use.

As the "therapist" performs the assessment and measurement of a specific joint ROM, the "educator/evaluator" places a check mark opposite each item that is correctly performed and an "X" beside each item incorrectly performed or omitted. When test criteria do not apply to the test situation, a dash is marked opposite the item. These notations are marked in the space provided at the right side of the column containing the list of criteria. Other comments regarding the "therapist's" performance are written in the space provided.

The "Sample Numeric Recording Form: ROM Measurement" in Appendix A is used by the "therapist" to record the "patient's" joint AROM, PROM, end feel, and/or muscle length. The form can be accessed on the website and printed by instructors for classroom use.

Post-Test Discussion and Feedback

The three members of the group discuss the "therapist's" performance following each test. It may be useful for the "therapist" to perform a self-evaluation before the other two group members provide their feedback. A practical test form can be used for this purpose. Patient feedback may include comments related to the "therapist's" interpersonal skills, the "patient's" emotional and physical comfort (e.g., general body comfort and warmth, therapist's grip, and support of body parts) during the test, perceived confidence level of the therapist, and the ability of the "patient" to clearly understand explanations and instructions given by the "therapist" verbally or through demonstration. This post-test discussion and feedback should be presented with sensitivity and in a positive manner to promote a positive learning experience.

Practical Test Items

PROM Assessment and Measurement Testing: Shoulder Complex

Scapular elevation
Scapular depression
Scapular abduction
Scapular adduction
Shoulder elevation through flexion
Glenohumeral joint flexion
Shoulder extension
Shoulder elevation through abduction
Glenohumeral joint abduction
Shoulder horizontal abduction
Shoulder horizontal adduction
Shoulder internal rotation
Shoulder external rotation

Muscle Length Assessment and Measurement Testing: Shoulder Complex

Pectoralis minor
Pectoralis major

PROM Assessment and Measurement Testing: Elbow and Forearm

Elbow flexion
Elbow extension/hyperextension
Forearm supination
Forearm pronation

Muscle Length Assessment and Measurement Testing: Elbow and Forearm

Biceps brachii
Triceps brachii

PROM Assessment and Measurement Testing: Wrist and Hand

Wrist flexion
Wrist extension
Wrist ulnar deviation
Wrist radial deviation
Finger MCP flexion
Finger MCP extension
Finger MCP abduction
Finger MCP adduction
Finger IP flexion
Finger IP extension
Thumb CM flexion
Thumb CM extension
Thumb MCP flexion
Thumb MCP extension
Thumb IP flexion
Thumb IP extension
Thumb CM abduction
Thumb and fifth finger opposition

Muscle Length Assessment and Measurement Testing: Wrist and Hand

Finger flexors
Finger extensors
Lumbricales

PROM Assessment and Measurement Testing: Hip

Hip flexion
Hip extension
Hip abduction
Hip adduction
Hip internal rotation
Hip external rotation

Muscle Length Assessment and Measurement Testing: Hip

Hamstrings (SLR)
Hamstrings passive knee extension (PKE)
Hip flexors (Thomas test)
Hip adductors
Tensor fascia latae (iliotibial band) (Ober's test)
Tensor fascia latae (iliotibial band) (Ober's test: trunk prone)

PROM Assessment and Measurement Testing: Knee

Knee flexion

Knee extension/hyperextension

Patellar distal glide

Patellar medial-lateral glide

Tibial rotation

Muscle Length Assessment and Measurement Testing: Knee

Hamstrings

Rectus femoris

PROM Assessment and Measurement Testing: Ankle and Foot

Ankle dorsiflexion

Ankle plantarflexion

Subtalar inversion

Subtalar eversion

Great toe MTP joint flexion

Great toe MTP joint extension

Great toe MTP joint abduction

Great toe MTP joint adduction

Great toe IP joint flexion

Great toe IP joint extension

Muscle Length Assessment and Measurement Testing: Ankle and Foot

Gastrocnemius

AROM Assessment and Measurement Testing: Head, Neck, and Trunk

TMJ: occlusion and depression of the mandible

TMJ: protrusion of the mandible

TMJ: lateral deviation of the mandible

Neck flexion

Neck extension

Neck lateral flexion

Neck rotation

Trunk flexion—thoracolumbar spine

Trunk extension—thoracolumbar spine

Trunk extension—thoracolumbar spine (prone press-up)

Trunk flexion—lumbar spine

Trunk extension—lumbar spine

Trunk lateral flexion—thoracolumbar spine

Trunk rotation—thoracolumbar spine

Chest expansion

Muscle Length Assessment and Measurement Testing: Trunk and Hamstrings

Trunk extensors and hamstrings (toe-touch test)

PROM Assessment and Measurement Testing: Shoulder Complex

Movement	Start Position	Stabilization	Therapist's Hand Placement	End Position	Recording	Instructions	Handling/ Comments
SCAPULAR ELEVATION	1. Side-ly, hips and knees flexed ☐ 2. Head supported on pillow ☐ 3. Arm at side ☐	1. Trunk stabilized ☐	1. One hand: on superior aspect of shoulder girdle ☐ 2. Other hand: cups inferior angle of scapula, while forearm supports patient's upper extremity ☐	1. Therapist elevates scapula to limit of motion ☐ 2. Full PROM achieved ☐ 3. Trunk stabilized ☐	1. Full PROM ☐ 2. End feel ☐	1. Verbal (clear/concise) ☐ 2. Demonstration (clear) ☐	1. Adequate support of limb/limb segment ☐ 2. Comfortable grip ☐ 3. Safe body mechanics of therapist ☐ Comments:
SCAPULAR DEPRESSION	1. Side-ly, hips and knees flexed ☐ 2. Head supported on pillow ☐ 3. Arm at side ☐	1. Trunk stabilized ☐	1. One hand: on superior aspect of shoulder girdle ☐ 2. Other hand: cups inferior angle of scapula, while forearm supports patient's upper extremity ☐	1. Therapist depresses scapula to limit of motion ☐ 2. Full PROM achieved ☐ 3. Trunk stabilized ☐	1. Full PROM ☐ 2. End feel ☐	1. Verbal (clear/concise) ☐ 2. Demonstration (clear) ☐	1. Adequate support of limb/limb segment ☐ 2. Comfortable grip ☐ 3. Safe body mechanics of therapist ☐ Comments:
SCAPULAR ABDUCTION	1. Side-ly, hips and knees flexed ☐ 2. Head supported on pillow ☐ 3. Arm at side ☐	1. Trunk stabilized ☐	1. One hand: on superior aspect of shoulder girdle ☐ 2. Other hand: grasps vertebral border and inferior angle of scapula, while forearm supports patient's upper extremity ☐	1. Therapist abducts scapula to limit of motion ☐ 2. Full PROM achieved ☐ 3. Trunk stabilized ☐	1. Full PROM ☐ 2. End feel ☐	1. Verbal (clear/concise) ☐ 2. Demonstration (clear) ☐	1. Adequate support of limb/limb segment ☐ 2. Comfortable grip ☐ 3. Safe body mechanics of therapist ☐ Comments:
SCAPULAR ADDUCTION	1. Side-ly, hips and knees flexed ☐ 2. Head supported on pillow ☐ 3. Arm at side ☐	1. Trunk stabilized ☐	1. One hand: on superior aspect of shoulder girdle ☐ 2. Other hand: grasps axillary border and inferior angle of scapula, while forearm supports patient's upper extremity ☐	1. Therapist adducts scapula to limit of motion ☐ 2. Full PROM achieved ☐ 3. Trunk stabilized ☐	1. Full PROM ☐ 2. End feel ☐	1. Verbal (clear/concise) ☐ 2. Demonstration (clear) ☐	1. Adequate support of limb/limb segment ☐ 2. Comfortable grip ☐ 3. Safe body mechanics of therapist ☐ Comments:

— STEP 1 — | — STEP 2 —

PROM Measurement: Using a Universal Goniometer

Movement	PROM Assessment of End Feel	Start Position	Axis	Stationary Arm	End Position	Movable Arm	Recording	Instructions	Handling/Comments
SHOULDER ELEVATION THROUGH FLEXION	1. Start position 2. Stabilized 3. Therapist distal hand placement 4. Slight traction 5. End position (Full PROM achieved) 6. End Feel	1. Crook ly 2. Arm at side, palm faces medially 3. Trunk stabilized	1. Lateral aspect center humeral head	1. Parallel lateral midline of trunk 2. Position maintained for start position 3. Position maintained for end position	1. Humerus moved anteriorly and upward to limit of motion 2. Scapular and glenohumeral motion 3. Full PROM achieved 4. Trunk stabilized	1. Parallel long axis of humerus 2. Position maintained for start position 3. Position maintained for end position	1. Full PROM 2. End feel	1. Verbal (clear/concise) 2. Demonstration (clear)	1. Adequate support of limb/limb segment 2. Comfortable grip 3. Safe body mechanics of therapist Comments:
GLENO-HUMERAL JOINT FLEXION	1. Start position 2. Stabilized 3. Therapist distal hand placement 4. Slight traction 5. End position (Full PROM achieved) 6. End Feel	1. Crook ly 2. Arm at side, palm faces medially 3. Trunk stabilized 4. Scapula stabilized	1. Lateral aspect center humeral head	1. Parallel lateral midline of trunk 2. Position maintained for start position 3. Position maintained for end position	1. Humerus moved anteriorly and upward to limit of motion 2. Glenohumeral joint motion only 3. Full PROM achieved 4. Trunk stabilized 5. Scapula stabilized	1. Parallel long axis of humerus 2. Position maintained for start position 3. Position maintained for end position	1. Full PROM 2. End feel	1. Verbal (clear/concise) 2. Demonstration (clear)	1. Adequate support of limb/limb segment 2. Comfortable grip 3. Safe body mechanics of therapist Comments:
SHOULDER EXTENSION	1. Start position 2. Stabilized 3. Therapist distal hand placement 4. Slight traction 5. End position (Full PROM achieved) 6. End Feel	1. Prone 2. Arm at side, palm faces medially 3. Scapula stabilized	1. Lateral aspect center humeral head	1. Parallel lateral midline of trunk 2. Position maintained for start position 3. Position maintained for end position	1. Humerus moved posteriorly to limit of glenohumeral joint motion 2. Full PROM achieved 3. Scapula stabilized	1. Parallel long axis of humerus, pointing to lateral epicondyle of humerus 2. Position maintained for start position 3. Position maintained for end position	1. Full PROM 2. End feel	1. Verbal (clear/concise) 2. Demonstration (clear)	1. Adequate support of limb/limb segment 2. Comfortable grip 3. Safe body mechanics of therapist Comments:

(continues)

PROM Assessment and Measurement Testing: Shoulder Complex (continued)

	STEP 1		STEP 2							
			PROM Measurement: Using a Universal Goniometer							
Movement	PROM Assessment of End Feel	Start Position	Axis	Stationary Arm	End Position	Movable Arm	Recording	Instructions	Handling/Comments	
SHOULDER ABDUCTION THROUGH ELEVATION	1. Start position ☐☐ 2. Stabilized ☐☐ 3. Therapist distal hand placement ☐ 4. Slight traction ☐ 5. End position (Full PROM achieved) ☐☐ 6. End Feel ☐☐	1. Supine ☐ 2. Arm at side, in adduction and external rotation ☐ 3. Trunk stabilized ☐	1. Midpoint anterior aspect gleno-humeral joint, about 1.3 cm inferior and lateral to coracoid process ☐	1. Parallel sternum ☐ 2. Position maintained for start position ☐ 3. Position maintained for end position ☐	1. Humerus moved laterally and upward to limit of motion ☐ 2. Scapular and gleno-humeral motion ☐ 3. Full PROM achieved ☐ 4. Trunk stabilized ☐	1. Parallel long axis of humerus ☐ 2. Position maintained for start position ☐ 3. Position maintained for end position ☐	1. Full PROM ☐☐ 2. End feel ☐	1. Verbal (clear/concise) ☐ 2. Demonstration (clear) ☐	1. Adequate support of limb/limb segment ☐ 2. Comfortable grip ☐ 3. Safe body mechanics of therapist ☐ Comments:	
GLENO-HUMERAL JOINT ABDUCTION	1. Start position ☐☐ 2. Stabilized ☐☐ 3. Therapist distal hand placement ☐ 4. Slight traction ☐ 5. End position (Full PROM achieved) ☐☐ 6. End feel ☐☐	1. Supine ☐ 2. Arm at side, elbow flexed to 90° ☐ 3. Trunk stabilized ☐ 4. Scapula and clavicle stabilized ☐	1. Midpoint anterior aspect gleno-humeral joint, about 1.3 cm inferior and lateral to coracoid process ☐	1. Parallel sternum ☐ 2. Position maintained for start position ☐ 3. Position maintained for end position ☐	1. Humerus moved laterally and upward to limit of motion ☐ 2. Glenohumeral joint motion only ☐ 3. Full PROM achieved ☐ 4. Trunk stabilized ☐ 5. Scapula and clavicle stabilized ☐	1. Parallel long axis of humerus ☐ 2. Position maintained for start position ☐ 3. Position maintained for end position ☐	1. Full PROM ☐☐ 2. End feel ☐	1. Verbal (clear/concise) ☐ 2. Demonstration (clear) ☐	1. Adequate support of limb/limb segment ☐ 2. Comfortable grip ☐ 3. Safe body mechanics of therapist ☐ Comments:	
SHOULDER HORIZONTAL ABDUCTION	1. Start position ☐☐ 2. Stabilized ☐☐ 3. Therapist distal hand placement ☐ 4. Slight traction ☐ 5. End position (full PROM achieved) ☐☐ 6. End feel ☐☐	1. Sitting ☐ 2. Shoulder abducted or flexed to 90° and neutral rotation ☐ 3. Elbow flexed, forearm midposition ☐ 4. Trunk stabilized ☐ 5. Scapula stabilized ☐	1. On top of acromion process ☐	1. Perpen-dicular to trunk ☐ 2. Position maintained for start position ☐ 3. Position maintained for end position ☐	1. Arm supported in abduction or flexion ☐ 2. Humerus moved posteriorly to limit of motion ☐ 3. Full PROM achieved ☐ 4. Trunk stabilized ☐ 5. Scapula stabilized ☐	1. Parallel long axis of humerus ☐ 2. Position maintained for start position ☐ 3. Position maintained for end position ☐	1. Full PROM ☐☐ 2. End feel ☐ 3. Start position recorded: shoulder 90° abduction ☐	1. Verbal (clear/concise) ☐ 2. Demonstration (clear) ☐	1. Adequate support of limb/limb segment ☐ 2. Comfortable grip ☐ 3. Safe body mechanics of therapist ☐ Comments:	

SHOULDER HORIZONTAL ADDUCTION

1. Start position ☐ ☐
2. Stabilized ☐
3. Therapist distal hand placement ☐
4. Slight traction ☐
5. End position (Full PROM achieved) ☐ ☐
6. End Feel ☐

1. Sitting ☐	1. On top of acromion process ☐
2. Shoulder abducted or flexed to 90° and neutral rotation ☐	
3. Elbow flexed, forearm midposition ☐	
4. Trunk stabilized ☐	
5. Scapula stabilized ☐	

1. Perpendicular to trunk ☐
2. Position maintained for start position ☐
3. Position maintained for end position ☐ achieved ☐
4. Trunk stabilized ☐
5. Scapula stabilized ☐

1. Arm supported in abduction or flexion ☐
2. Humerus moved anteriorly across chest to limit of motion ☐
3. Full PROM ☐

1. Parallel long axis of humerus ☐
2. Position maintained for start position ☐
3. Position maintained for end position ☐

1. Full PROM ☐
2. End feel ☐
3. Start position recorded: shoulder 90° abduction ☐

1. Verbal (clear/concise) ☐
2. Demonstration (clear) ☐

1. Adequate support of limb/limb segment ☐
2. Comfortable grip ☐
3. Safe body mechanics of therapist ☐
Comments:

SHOULDER INTERNAL ROTATION

1. Start position ☐ ☐
2. Stabilized ☐
3. Therapist distal hand placement ☐
4. Slight traction ☐
5. End position (Full PROM achieved) ☐ ☐
6. End Feel ☐

1. Prone ☐	1. On olecranon process of ulna ☐
2. Shoulder abducted 90°, elbow flexed 90°, forearm midposition ☐	
3. Pad under humerus ☐	
4. Scapula stabilized ☐	
5. Position of humerus maintained ☐	

1. Perpendicular to floor ☐
2. Position maintained for start position ☐
3. Position maintained for end position of humerus maintained ☐

1. Palm of hand moved toward ceiling to limit of motion ☐
2. Full PROM achieved ☐
3. Scapula stabilized ☐
4. Position for end position ☐

1. Parallel long axis of ulna, pointing to ulnar styloid process ☐
2. Position maintained for start position ☐
3. Position maintained ☐

1. Full PROM ☐
2. End feel ☐

1. Verbal (clear/concise) ☐
2. Demonstration (clear) ☐

1. Adequate support of limb/limb segment ☐
2. Comfortable grip ☐
3. Safe body mechanics of therapist ☐
Comments:

SHOULDER EXTERNAL ROTATION

1. Start position ☐ ☐
2. Stabilized ☐
3. Therapist distal hand placement ☐
4. Slight traction ☐
5. End position (Full PROM achieved) ☐ ☐
6. End Feel ☐

1. Supine ☐	1. On olecranon process of ulna ☐
2. Shoulder abducted 90°, elbow flexed 90°, forearm midposition ☐	
3. Pad under humerus ☐	
4. Scapula stabilized ☐	

1. Perpendicular to floor ☐
2. Position maintained for start position ☐
3. Position maintained for end position ☐

1. Dorsum of hand moved toward floor to limit of motion ☐
2. Full PROM achieved ☐
3. Scapula stabilized ☐

1. Parallel long axis of ulna, pointing to ulnar styloid process ☐
2. Position maintained for start position ☐
3. Position maintained for end position ☐

1. Full PROM ☐
2. End feel ☐

1. Verbal (clear/concise) ☐
2. Demonstration (clear) ☐

1. Adequate support of limb/limb segment ☐
2. Comfortable grip ☐
3. Safe body mechanics of therapist ☐
Comments:

Muscle Length Assessment and Measurement Testing: Shoulder Complex

Muscle	Start Position	Stabilization	End Position	Measurement of Joint Position Using Universal Goniometer	Recording	Instructions	Handling/Comments
PECTORALIS MAJOR	1. Supine ☐ 2. Shoulder external rotation, 90° elevation through plane midway between flexion and abduction, elbow flexed 90° ☐	1. Therapist's hand on contralateral shoulder to stabilize trunk ☐	1. Shoulder moved to limit of horizontal abduction ☐ 2. Full PROM achieved ☐ 3. Trunk stabilized ☐	Shoulder horizontal abduction 1. Axis: on top of acromion process ☐ 2. Stationary arm: perpendicular to trunk ☐ 3. Movable arm: parallel long axis of humerus ☐	1. Full PROM ☐ 2. End feel ☐	1. Verbal (clear/concise) ☐ 2. Demonstration (clear) ☐	1. Adequate support of limb/limb segment ☐ 2. Comfortable grip ☐ 3. Safe body mechanics of therapist ☐ Comments:
PECTORALIS MINOR	1. Supine ☐ 2. Scapula over side of plinth ☐ 3. Shoulder external rotation, 80° flexion, elbow flexed ☐	1. Trunk stabilized ☐	1. Therapist applies force through long axis of shaft of humerus to move shoulder girdle to limit of scapular retraction ☐ 2. Scapula moved to limit of retraction ☐ 3. Full PROM achieved ☐ 4. Trunk stabilized ☐		1. Full PROM ☐ 2. End feel ☐	1. Verbal (clear/concise) ☐ 2. Demonstration (clear) ☐	1. Adequate support of limb/limb segment ☐ 2. Comfortable grip ☐ 3. Safe body mechanics of therapist ☐ Comments:

PROM Assessment and Measurement Testing: Elbow and Forearm

	STEP 1		STEP 2 — PROM Measurement: Using a Universal Goniometer						
Movement	PROM Assessment of End Feel	Start Position	Axis	Stationary Arm	End Position	Movable Arm	Recording	Instructions	Handling/ Comments
ELBOW FLEXION	1. Start position ☐ 2. Stabilized ☐ 3. Therapist distal hand placemen ☐ 4. Slight traction ☐ 5. End position (full PROM achieved) ☐ 6. End feel ☐	1. Supine ☐ 2. Shoulder and elbow in anatomical position ☐ 3. Towel under distal humerus ☐ 4. Humerus stabilized ☐	1. Over lateral epicondyle of humerus ☐	1. Parallel long axis humerus, pointing toward tip of acromion process ☐ 2. Position maintained for start position ☐ 3. Position maintained for end position ☐	1. Forearm moved anteriorly to limit of elbow flexion ☐ 2. Full PROM achieved ☐ 3. Humerus stabilized ☐	1. Parallel long axis of radius, pointing toward styloid process of radius ☐ 2. Position maintained for start position ☐ 3. Position maintained for end position ☐	1. Full PROM ☐ 2. End feel ☐	1. Verbal (clear/ concise) ☐ 2. Demonstration (clear) ☐	1. Adequate support of limb/limb segment ☐ 2. Comfortable grip ☐ 3. Safe body mechanics of therapist ☐ Comments:
ELBOW EXTENSION/ HYPER-EXTENSION	1. Start position ☐ 2. Stabilized ☐ 3. Therapist distal hand placement ☐ 4. Slight traction ☐ 5. End position (full PROM achieved) ☐ 6. End feel ☐	1. Supine ☐ 2. Shoulder and elbow in anatomical position ☐ 3. Towel under distal humerus ☐ 4. Humerus stabilized ☐	1. Over lateral epicondyle of humerus ☐	1. Parallel long axis humerus, pointing toward tip of acromion process ☐ 2. Position maintained for start position ☐ 3. Position maintained for end position ☐	1. Forearm moved posteriorly to limit of elbow extension/ hyperextension ☐ 2. Full PROM achieved ☐ 3. Humerus stabilized ☐	1. Parallel long axis of radius, pointing toward styloid process of radius ☐ 2. Position maintained for start position ☐ 3. Position maintained for end position ☐	1. Full PROM ☐ 2. End feel ☐	1. Verbal (clear/ concise) ☐ 2. Demonstration (clear) ☐	1. Adequate support of limb/limb segment ☐ 2. Comfortable grip ☐ 3. Safe body mechanics of therapist ☐ Comments:

(continues)

PROM Assessment and Measurement Testing: Elbow and Forearm (continued)

	STEP 1	STEP 2							
		PROM Measurement: Using a Universal Goniometer							
Movement	PROM Assessment of End Feel	Start Position	Axis	Stationary Arm	End Position	Movable Arm	Recording	Instructions	Handling/Comments
FOREARM SUPINATION	1. Start position ☐☐ 2. Stabilized ☐☐ 3. Therapist distal hand placement ☐ 4. Slight traction ☐ 5. End position (full PROM achieved) ☐☐ 6. End feel ☐☐	1. Sitting ☐ 2. Arm at side, elbow flexed 90° ☐ 3. Forearm midposition ☐ 4. Pencil held tightly in hand, wrist in neutral position ☐ 5. Humerus stabilized ☐	1. Over head of third metacarpal ☐	1. Perpendicular to floor ☐ 2. Position maintained for start position ☐ 3. Position maintained for end position ☐	1. Forearm rotated so palm faces up toward ceiling ☐ 2. Full PROM achieved ☐ 3. Humerus stabilized ☐ 4. Position of pencil maintained ☐	1. Parallel to pencil ☐ 2. Position maintained for start position ☐ 3. Position maintained for end position ☐	1. Full PROM ☐ 2. End feel ☐	1. Verbal (clear/concise) ☐ 2. Demonstration (clear) ☐	1. Adequate support of limb/limb segment ☐ 2. Comfortable grip ☐ 3. Safe body mechanics of therapist ☐ Comments:
FOREARM PRONATION	1. Start position ☐☐ 2. Stabilized ☐☐ 3. Therapist distal hand placement ☐ 4. Slight traction ☐ 5. End position (full PROM achieved) ☐☐ 6. End feel ☐☐	1. Sitting ☐ 2. Arm at side, elbow flexed 90° ☐ 3. Forearm midposition ☐ 4. Pencil held tightly in hand, wrist in neutral position ☐ 5. Humerus stabilized ☐	1. Over head of third metacarpal ☐	1. Perpendicular to floor ☐ 2. Position maintained for start position ☐ 3. Position maintained for end position ☐	1. Forearm rotated so palm faces down toward floor ☐ 2. Full PROM achieved ☐ 3. Humerus stabilized ☐ 4. Position of pencil maintained ☐	1. Parallel to pencil ☐ 2. Position maintained for start position ☐ 3. Position maintained for end position ☐	1. Full PROM ☐ 2. End feel ☐	1. Verbal (clear/concise) ☐ 2. Demonstration (clear) ☐	1. Adequate support of limb/limb segment ☐ 2. Comfortable grip ☐ 3. Safe body mechanics of therapist ☐ Comments:

Muscle Length Assessment and Measurement Testing: Elbow and Forearm

Muscle	Start Position	Stabilization	End Position	Measurement of Joint Position Using Universal Goniometer	Recording	Instructions	Handling/Comments
BICEPS BRACHII	1. Supine ☐ 2. Shoulder in extension over edge of plinth ☐ 3. Elbow flexed, forearm pronated ☐	1. Humerus stabilized ☐	1. Elbow extended ☐ 2. Elbow moved to limit of extension ☐ 3. Full PROM achieved ☐ 4. Humerus stabilized ☐	Elbow extension 1. Axis: over lateral epicondyle of humerus ☐ 2. Stationary arm: parallel long axis humerus pointing toward tip of acromion process ☐ 3. Movable arm: parallel long axis of radius, pointing toward styloid process of radius ☐	1. Full PROM ☐ 2. End feel ☐	1. Verbal (clear/concise) ☐ 2. Demonstration (clear) ☐	1. Adequate support of limb/limb segment ☐ 2. Comfortable grip ☐ 3. Safe body mechanics of therapist ☐ Comments:
TRICEPS BRACHII	1. Sitting ☐ 2. Full shoulder elevation through flexion, and shoulder external rotation ☐ 3. Elbow in anatomical position, forearm supinated ☐	1. Humerus stabilized ☐	1. Elbow flexed ☐ 2. Elbow moved to limit of flexion ☐ 3. Full PROM achieved ☐ 4. Humerus stabilized ☐	Elbow Flexion 1. Axis: over lateral epicondyle of humerus ☐ 2. Stationary arm: parallel long axis humerus pointing toward tip of acromion process ☐ 3. Movable arm: parallel long axis of radius, pointing toward styloid process of radius ☐	1. Full PROM ☐ 2. End feel ☐	1. Verbal (clear/concise) ☐ 2. Demonstration (clear) ☐	1. Adequate support of limb/limb segment ☐ 2. Comfortable grip ☐ 3. Safe body mechanics of therapist ☐ Comments:

PROM Assessment and Measurement Testing: Wrist and Hand

	STEP 1			STEP 2 — PROM Measurement: Using a Universal Goniometer					
Movement	PROM Assessment of End Feel	Start Position	Axis	Stationary Arm	End Position	Movable Arm	Recording	Instructions	Handling/Comments
WRIST FLEXION	1. Start position ☐ 2. Stabilized ☐ 3. Therapist distal hand placement ☐ 4. Slight traction ☐ 5. End position (full PROM achieved) ☐ 6. End feel ☐	1. Sitting ☐ 2. Elbow flexed, forearm pronated, wrist in anatomical position, fingers slightly extended ☐ 3. Forearm stabilized ☐	1. Lateral aspect of wrist at level of ulnar styloid process ☐	1. Parallel long axis of ulna ☐ 2. Position maintained for start position ☐ 3. Position maintained for end position ☐	1. Wrist moved in anterior direction to limit of motion ☐ 2. Full PROM achieved ☐ 3. Forearm stabilized position ☐	1. Parallel long axis of fifth metacarpal ☐ 2. Position maintained for start position ☐ 3. Position maintained for end ☐	1. Full PROM ☐ 2. End feel ☐	1. Verbal (clear/concise) ☐ 2. Demonstration (clear) ☐	1. Adequate support of limb/limb segment ☐ 2. Comfortable grip ☐ 3. Safe body mechanics of therapist ☐ Comments:
WRIST EXTENSION	1. Start position ☐ 2. Stabilized ☐ 3. Therapist distal hand placement ☐ 4. Slight traction ☐ 5. End position (full PROM achieved) ☐ 6. End feel ☐	1. Sitting ☐ 2. Elbow flexed, forearm pronated, wrist in anatomical position, fingers slightly flexed ☐ 3. Forearm stabilized ☐	1. Lateral aspect of wrist at level of ulnar styloid process ☐	1. Parallel long axis of ulna ☐ 2. Position maintained for start position ☐ 3. Position maintained for end position ☐	1. Wrist moved in posterior direction to limit of motion ☐ 2. Full PROM achieved ☐ 3. Forearm stabilized position ☐	1. Parallel long axis of fifth metacarpal ☐ 2. Position maintained for start position ☐ 3. Position maintained for end ☐	1. Full PROM ☐ 2. End feel ☐	1. Verbal (clear/concise) ☐ 2. Demonstration (clear) ☐	1. Adequate support of limb/limb segment ☐ 2. Comfortable grip ☐ 3. Safe body mechanics of therapist ☐ Comments:
WRIST ULNAR DEVIATION	1. Start position ☐ 2. Stabilized ☐ 3. Therapist distal hand placement ☐ 4. Slight traction ☐ 5. End position (full PROM achieved) ☐ 6. End feel ☐	1. Sitting ☐ 2. Elbow flexed, forearm pronated, palm of hand rests lightly on table ☐ 3. Wrist and fingers in anatomical position ☐ 4. Forearm stabilized ☐	1. Posterior aspect wrist over capitate ☐	1. Along midline of forearm ☐ 2. Position maintained for start position ☐ 3. Position maintained for end position ☐	1. Wrist adducted to ulnar side to limit of motion ☐ 2. Full PROM achieved ☐ 3. Forearm stabilized ☐	1. Parallel long axis shaft of third metacarpal ☐ 2. Position maintained for start position ☐ 3. Position maintained for end position ☐	1. Full PROM ☐ 2. End feel ☐	1. Verbal (clear/concise) ☐ 2. Demonstration (clear) ☐	1. Adequate support of limb/limb segment ☐ 2. Comfortable grip ☐ 3. Safe body mechanics of therapist ☐ Comments:

WRIST RADIAL DEVIATION

1. Start position ☐
2. Stabilized ☐
3. Therapist distal hand placement ☐
4. Slight traction ☐
5. End position (full PROM achieved) ☐
6. End feel ☐

- 1. Sitting ☐
- 2. Elbow flexed, forearm pronated, palm of hand rests lightly on table ☐
- 3. Wrist and fingers in anatomical position ☐
- 4. Forearm stabilized ☐

- 1. Posterior aspect of wrist over capitate ☐

- 1. Along midline of forearm ☐
- 2. Position maintained for start position ☐
- 3. Position maintained for end position ☐

- 1. Wrist abducted to radial side to limit of motion ☐
- 2. Full PROM achieved ☐
- 3. Forearm stabilized ☐

- 1. Parallel long axis shaft of third metacarpal ☐
- 2. Position maintained for start position ☐
- 3. Position maintained for end position ☐

- 1. Full PROM ☐
- 2. End feel ☐

- 1. Verbal (clear/concise) ☐
- 2. Demonstration (clear) ☐

- 1. Adequate support of limb/limb segment ☐
- 2. Comfortable grip ☐
- 3. Safe body mechanics of therapist ☐
- Comments:

FINGER MCP FLEXION

1. Start position ☐
2. Stabilized ☐
3. Therapist distal hand placement ☐
4. Slight traction ☐
5. End position (full PROM achieved) ☐
6. End feel ☐

- 1. Sitting ☐
- 2. Elbow flexed, forearm rests on table, wrist slightly extended, MCP joint of finger in anatomical position ☐
- 3. Metacarpal stabilized ☐

- 1. On posterior aspect of MCP joint ☐

- 1. Parallel long axis shaft of metacarpal ☐
- 2. Position maintained for start position ☐
- 3. Position maintained for end position ☐

- 1. Proximal phalanx moved toward palm to limit of flexion ☐
- 2. IP joints allowed to extend ☐
- 3. Full PROM achieved ☐
- 4. Metacarpal stabilized ☐

- 1. Parallel long axis of proximal phalanx ☐
- 2. Position maintained for start position ☐
- 3. Position maintained for end position ☐

- 1. Full PROM ☐
- 2. End feel ☐

- 1. Verbal (clear/concise) ☐
- 2. Demonstration (clear) ☐

- 1. Adequate support of limb/limb segment ☐
- 2. Comfortable grip ☐
- 3. Safe body mechanics of therapist ☐
- Comments:

FINGER MCP EXTENSION

1. Start position ☐
2. Stabilized ☐
3. Therapist distal hand placement ☐
4. Slight traction ☐
5. End position (full PROM achieved) ☐
6. End feel ☐

- 1. Sitting ☐
- 2. Elbow flexed, forearm rests on table, wrist slightly flexed, MCP joint of finger in anatomical position ☐
- 3. Metacarpal stabilized ☐

- 1. On anterior aspect of MCP joint ☐

- 1. Parallel long axis shaft of metacarpal ☐
- 2. Position maintained for start position ☐
- 3. Position maintained for end position ☐

- 1. Proximal phalanx moved in posterior direction to limit of extension ☐
- 2. IP joints allowed to flex ☐
- 3. Full PROM achieved ☐
- 4. Metacarpal stabilized ☐

- 1. Parallel long axis of proximal phalanx ☐
- 2. Position maintained for start position ☐
- 3. Position maintained for end position ☐

- 1. Full PROM ☐
- 2. End feel ☐

- 1. Verbal (clear/concise) ☐
- 2. Demonstration (clear) ☐

- 1. Adequate support of limb/limb segment ☐
- 2. Comfortable grip ☐
- 3. Safe body mechanics of therapist ☐
- Comments:

(continues)

PROM Assessment and Measurement Testing: Wrist and Hand

	STEP 1	STEP 2							
	PROM Assessment of End Feel	PROM Measurement: Using a Universal Goniometer							
Movement		Start Position	Axis	Stationary Arm	End Position	Movable Arm	Recording	Instructions	Handling/Comments
FINGER MCP ABDUCTION	1. Start position ☐ 2. Stabilized ☐ 3. Therapist distal hand placement ☐ 4. Slight traction ☐ 5. End position (Full PROM achieved) ☐ 6. End Feel ☐	1. Sitting ☐ 2. Elbow flexed, forearm pronated and palm of hand rests on table ☐ 3. Wrist and fingers in anatomical position ☐ 4. Metacarpals stabilized ☐	1. On posterior surface of MCP joint ☐	1. Parallel long axis of metacarpal ☐ 2. Position maintained for start position ☐ 3. Position maintained for end position ☐	1. Finger is moved away from midline of hand to limit of MCP abduction ☐ 2. Full PROM achieved ☐ 3. Metacarpals stabilized ☐	1. Parallel long axis of proximal phalanx ☐ 2. Position maintained for start position ☐ 3. Position maintained for end position ☐	1. Full PROM ☐ 2. End feel ☐	1. Verbal (clear/concise) ☐ 2. Demonstration (clear) ☐	1. Adequate support of limb/limb segment ☐ 2. Comfortable grip ☐ 3. Safe body mechanics of therapist ☐ Comments:
FINGER MCP ADDUCTION	1. Start position ☐ 2. Stabilized ☐ 3. Therapist distal hand placement ☐ 4. Slight traction ☐ 5. End position (Full PROM achieved) ☐ 6. End Feel ☐	1. Sitting ☐ 2. Elbow flexed, forearm pronated and palm of hand rests on table ☐ 3. Wrist and finger in anatomical position ☐ 4. Nontest fingers out of way ☐ 5. Metacarpals stabilized ☐	1. On posterior surface of MCP joint ☐	1. Parallel long axis of metacarpal ☐ 2. Position maintained for start position ☐ 3. Position maintained for end position ☐	1. Finger is moved toward midline of hand to limit of MCP adduction ☐ 2. Full PROM achieved ☐ 3. Metacarpals stabilized ☐	1. Parallel long axis of proximal phalanx ☐ 2. Position maintained for start position ☐ 3. Position maintained for end position ☐	1. Full PROM ☐ 2. End feel ☐	1. Verbal (clear/concise) ☐ 2. Demonstration (clear) ☐	1. Adequate support of limb/limb segment ☐ 2. Comfortable grip ☐ 3. Safe body mechanics of therapist ☐ Comments:
FINGER IP FLEXION	1. Start position ☐ 2. Stabilized ☐ 3. Therapist distal hand placement ☐ 4. Slight traction ☐ 5. End position (Full PROM achieved) ☐ 6. End Feel ☐	1. Sitting ☐ 2. Forearm rests on table, wrist and fingers in anatomical position ☐ 3. PIP joint: proximal phalanx stabilized ☐ DIP joint: Middle phalanx stabilized ☐	1. Over posterior surface of IP joint ☐	1. Parallel long axis of: PIP joint: proximal phalanx ☐ DIP joint: middle phalanx ☐ 2. Position maintained for start position ☐ 3. Position maintained for end position ☐	1. PIP or DIP joint flexed to limit of motion ☐ 2. Full PROM achieved ☐ 3. PIP joint: proximal phalanx stabilized ☐ DIP joint: middle phalanx stabilized ☐	1. Parallel long axis of: middle PIP joint: phalanx distal DIP joint: phalanx ☐ 2. Position maintained for start position ☐ 3. Position maintained for end position ☐	1. Full PROM ☐ 2. End feel ☐	1. Verbal (clear/concise) ☐ 2. Demon stration (clear) ☐	1. Adequate support of limb/limb segment ☐ 2. Comfortable grip ☐ 3. Safe body mechanics of therapist ☐ Comments:

FINGER IP EXTENSION

1. Start position ☐
2. Stabilized ☐
3. Therapist distal hand placement ☐
4. Slight traction ☐
5. End position (full PROM achieved) ☐
6. End feel ☐

- 1. Sitting ☐
- 2. Forearm rests on table, wrist and fingers in anatomical position ☐
- 3. PIP joint: proximal phalanx stabilized DIP joint: middle phalanx stabilized ☐

- 1. Over anterior surface of IP joint ☐

- 1. Parallel long axis of: PIP joint: phalanx DIP joint: middle phalanx ☐
- 2. Position maintained for start position ☐
- 3. Position maintained for end position ☐

- 1. PIP or DIP joint extended to limit of motion ☐
- 2. Full PROM achieved ☐
- 3. PIP joint: Proximal phalanx stabilize DIP joint: middle phalanx stabilized ☐

- 1. Parallel long axis of: PIP joint: middle phalanx DIP joint: distal phalanx ☐
- 2. Position maintained for start position ☐
- 3. Position maintained for end position ☐

- 1. Full PROM ☐
- 2. End feel (clear) ☐

- 1. Verbal (clear/concise) ☐
- 2. Demonstration ☐

- 1. Adequate support of limb/limb segment ☐
- 2. Comfortable grip ☐
- 3. Safe body mechanics of therapist ☐
- Comments:

THUMB CM FLEXION

1. Start position ☐
2. Stabilized ☐
3. Therapist distal hand placement ☐
4. Slight traction ☐
5. End position (full PROM achieved) ☐
6. End feel ☐

- 1. Sitting ☐
- 2. Elbow flexed, forearm in mid-position, wrist neutral position ☐
- 3. Thumb MCP and IP joints in anatomical position ☐
- 4. Trapezium, wrist, and forearm stabilized ☐

- 1. Over anterior aspect first CM joint ☐

- 1. Parallel long axis of radius ☐
- 2. Position maintained for start position ☐
- 3. Position maintained for end position ☐

- 1. Thumb CM joint flexed to limit of motion ☐
- 2. Full PROM achieved ☐
- 3. Trapezium, wrist, and forearm stabilized ☐

- 1. Parallel long axis thumb meta-carpal ☐
- 2. Position maintained for start position ☐
- 3. Position maintained for end position ☐

- 1. Full PROM ☐
- 2. End feel ☐

- 1. Verbal (clear/concise) ☐
- 2. Demonstration (clear) ☐

- 1. Adequate support of limb/limb segment ☐
- 2. Comfortable grip ☐
- 3. Safe body mechanics of therapist ☐
- Comments:

THUMB CM EXTENSION

1. Start position ☐
2. Stabilized ☐
3. Therapist distal hand placement ☐
4. Slight traction ☐
5. End position (full PROM achieved) ☐
6. End feel ☐

- 1. Sitting ☐
- 2. Elbow flexed, forearm in midposition, wrist neutral position ☐
- 3. Thumb MCP and IP joints in anatomical position ☐
- 4. Trapezium, wrist, and forearm stabilized ☐

- 1. Over anterior aspect first CM joint ☐

- 1. Parallel long axis of radius ☐
- 2. Position maintained for start position ☐
- 3. Position maintained for end position ☐

- 1. Thumb CM joint extended to limit of motion ☐
- 2. Full PROM achieved ☐
- 3. Trapezium, wrist, and forearm stabilized ☐

- 1. Parallel long axis thumb metacarpal ☐
- 2. Position maintained for start position ☐
- 3. Position maintained for end position ☐

- 1. Full PROM ☐
- 2. End feel ☐

- 1. Verbal (clear/concise) ☐
- 2. Demonstration (clear) ☐

- 1. Adequate support of limb/limb segment ☐
- 2. Comfortable grip ☐
- 3. Safe body mechanics of therapist ☐
- Comments:

(continues)

PROM Assessment and Measurement Testing: Wrist and Hand (continued)

STEP 1 — **STEP 2**

Movement	PROM Assessment of End Feel	PROM Measurement: Using a Universal Goniometer							
		Start Position	Axis	Stationary Arm	End Position	Movable Arm	Recording	Instructions	Handling/Comments
THUMB MCP FLEXION	1. Start position ☐ 2. Stabilized ☐ 3. Therapist distal hand placement ☐ 4. Slight traction ☐ 5. End position (full PROM achieved) ☐ 6. End feel ☐	1. Sitting 2. Elbow flexed, forearm rests on table in midposition, wrist, thumb and fingers in anatomical position ☐ 3. First metacarpal stabilized ☐	1. Over posterior or lateral aspect of MCP joint of thumb ☐	1. Parallel long axis of first metacarpal 2. Position maintained for start position ☐ 3. Position maintained for end position ☐	1. Proximal phalanx moved across palm to limit of MCP joint flexion ☐ 2. Full PROM achieved ☐ 3. First metacarpal stabilized ☐	1. Parallel long axis of proximal phalanx ☐ 2. Position maintained for start position ☐ 3. Position maintained for end position ☐	1. Full PROM ☐ 2. End feel ☐	1. Verbal (clear/concise) ☐ 2. Demonstration (clear) ☐	1. Adequate support of limb/limb segment ☐ 2. Comfortable grip ☐ 3. Safe body mechanics of therapist ☐ Comments:
THUMB MCP EXTENSION	1. Start position ☐ 2. Stabilized ☐ 3. Therapist distal hand placement ☐ 4. Slight traction ☐ 5. End position (full PROM achieved) ☐ 6. End feel ☐	1. Sitting 2. Elbow flexed, forearm rests on table in midposition, wrist, thumb and fingers in anatomical position ☐ 3. First metacarpal stabilized ☐	1. Over anterior or lateral aspect of MCP joint of thumb ☐	1. Parallel long axis of first metacarpal 2. Position maintained for start position ☐ 3. Position maintained for end position ☐	1. Proximal phalanx moved to limit of MCP joint extension ☐ 2. Full PROM achieved ☐ 3. First metacarpal stabilized ☐	1. Parallel long axis of proximal phalanx ☐ 2. Position maintained for start position ☐ 3. Position maintained for end position ☐	1. Full PROM ☐ 2. End feel ☐	1. Verbal (clear/concise) ☐ 2. Demonstration (clear) ☐	1. Adequate support of limb/limb segment ☐ 2. Comfortable grip ☐ 3. Safe body mechanics of therapist ☐ Comments:
THUMB IP FLEXION	1. Start position ☐ 2. Stabilized ☐ 3. Therapist distal hand placement ☐ 4. Slight traction ☐ 5. End position (full PROM achieved) ☐ 6. End feel ☐	1. Sitting 2. Elbow flexed, forearm rests on table in midposition, wrist, thumb and fingers in anatomical position ☐ 3. Proximal phalanx stabilized ☐	1. Over posterior or lateral aspect of IP joint of thumb ☐	1. Parallel long axis proximal phalanx of thumb 2. Position maintained for start position ☐ 3. Position maintained for end position ☐	1. IP joint flexed to limit of motion ☐ 2. Full PROM achieved ☐ 3. Proximal phalanx stabilized ☐	1. Parallel long axis of distal phalanx ☐ 2. Position maintained for start position ☐ 3. Position maintained for end position ☐	1. Full PROM ☐ 2. End feel ☐	1. Verbal (clear/concise) ☐ 2. Demonstration (clear) ☐	1. Adequate support of limb/limb segment ☐ 2. Comfortable grip ☐ 3. Safe body mechanics of therapist ☐ Comments:

PROM and AROM Assessment and Measurement Testing: Wrist and Hand

	STEP 1						STEP 2		
				PROM Measurement: Using a Universal Goniometer and Ruler					
Movement	**PROM Assessment of End Feel**	**Start Position**	**Axis**	**End Position**	**Stationary Arm**	**Movable Arm**	**Recording**	**Instructions**	**Handling/Comments**
THUMB IP EXTENSION	1. Start position □ 2. Stabilized □ 3. Therapist distal hand placement □ 4. Slight traction □ 5. End position (full PROM achieved) □ 6. End feel □	1. Sitting □ 2. Elbow flexed, forearm rests on table in midposition, wrist, thumb and fingers in anatomical position □ 3. Proximal phalanx stabilized □	1. Over anterior or lateral aspect of IP joint of thumb □	1. IP joint extended to limit of motion □ 2. Full PROM achieved □ 3. Proximal phalanx stabilized □	1. Parallel long axis of proximal phalanx of thumb □ 2. Position maintained for start position □ 3. Position maintained for end position □	1. Parallel long axis of distal phalanx □ 2. Position maintained for start position □ 3. Position maintained for end position □	1. Full PROM □ 2. End feel □	1. Verbal (clear/concise) □ 2. Demonstration (clear) □	1. Adequate support of limb/limb segment □ 2. Comfortable grip □ 3. Safe body mechanics of therapist □ Comments:
THUMB CM ABDUCTION	1. Start position □ 2. Stabilized □ 3. Therapist distal hand placement □ 4. Slight traction □ 5. End position (full PROM achieved) □ 6. End feel □	1. Sitting □ 2. Elbow flexed, forearm in midposition, wrist and fingers in anatomical position □ 3. Thumb in contact along side of index finger □ 4. Second metacarpal stabilized □	1. Posterior aspect, junction at bases of first and second metacarpals □	1. Thumb moved in plane perpendicular to palm to limit of abduction □ 2. Full PROM achieved □ 3. Second metacarpal stabilized □	1. Parallel long axis second metacarpal □ 2. Position maintained for start position □ 3. Position maintained for end position □	1. Parallel long axis first metacarpal □ 2. Position maintained for start position □ 3. Position maintained for end position □	1. Full PROM □ 2. End feel □	1. Verbal (clear/concise) □ 2. Demonstration (clear) □	1. Adequate support of limb/limb segment □ 2. Comfortable grip □ 3. Safe body mechanics of therapist □ Comments:
THUMB AND FIFTH FINGER OPPOSITION	1. Start position □ 2. Stabilized □ 3. Therapist distal hand placement □ 4. Slight traction □ 5. End position (full PROM achieved) □ 6. End feel □	1. Sitting □ 2. Elbow flexed forearm supinated, wrist in anatomical position □ 3. Fingers and thumb relaxed □ 4. Forearm stabilized □		1. Active thumb and fifth finger opposition to limit of motion (so pads of thumb and finger in same plane) □ 2. Forearm stabilized □		1. Linear measurement between center tip of thumb pad and center tip of fifth finger pad □	1. Full AROM □	1. Verbal (clear/concise) □ 2. Demonstration (clear) □	1. Adequate support of limb/limb segment □ 2. Comfortable grip □ 3. Safe body mechanics of therapist □ Comments:

Muscle Length Assessment and Measurement Testing: Wrist and Hand

Muscle	Start Position	Stabilization	End Position	Measurement of Joint Position Using Universal Goniometer	Recording	Instructions	Handling/Comments
FINGER FLEXORS	1. Supine 2. Elbow extended, forearm supinated, wrist in anatomical position, fingers extended □	1. Humerus stabilized □ 2. Radius and ulna stabilized □	1. With fingers held in extension, wrist moved to limit of extension □ 2. Full PROM achieved □ 3. Humerus stabilized □ 4. Radius and ulna stabilized □	Wrist extension 1. Axis: lateral aspect wrist at level of ulnar styloid process □ 2. Stationary arm: parallel long axis of ulna □ 3. Movable arm: parallel long axis of fifth metacarpal □	1. Full PROM □ 2. End feel □	1. Verbal (clear/concise) □ 2. Demonstration (clear □	1. Adequate support of limb/limb segment □ 2. Comfortable grip □ 3. Safe body mechanics of therapist □ Comments:
FINGER EXTENSORS	1. Sitting 2. Elbow extended, forearm pronated, wrist in anatomical position, fingers flexed □	1. Radius and ulna stabilized □	1. With fingers held in flexion, wrist moved to limit of flexion □ 2. Full PROM achieved □ 3. Radius and ulna stabilized □	Wrist flexion 1. Axis: lateral aspect of wrist at level of ulnar styloid process □ 2. Stationary arm: parallel long axis of ulna □ 3. Movable arm: parallel long axis of fifth metacarpal □	1. Full PROM □ 2. End feel □	1. Verbal (clear/concise) □ 2. Demonstration (clear) □	1. Adequate support of limb/limb segment □ 2. Comfortable grip □ 3. Safe body mechanics of therapist □ Comments:
LUMBRICALES	1. Sitting 2. Elbow flexed, forearm in midposition or supinated, wrist extended, IP joints of fingers flexed □	1. Metacarpals stabilized □	1. With IP joints held in flexion, MCP joints moved to limit of extension □ 2. Full PROM achieved □ 3. Metacarpals stabilized □	MCP joint extension 1. Axis: lateral to MCP joint of index finger or medial to MCP joint of little finger □ 2. Stationary arm: parallel long axis of metacarpal □ 3. Movable arm: parallel long axis of proximal phalanx □	1. Full PROM □ 2. End feel □	1. Verbal (clear/concise) □ 2. Demonstration (clear) □	1. Adequate support of limb/limb segment □ 2. Comfortable grip □ 3. Safe body mechanics of therapist □ Comments:

PROM Assessment and Measurement Testing: Hip

	STEP 1		STEP 2						
Movement	PROM Assessment of End Feel	Start Position	PROM Measurement: Using A Universal Goniometer						
			Axis	Stationary Arm	End Position	Movable Arm	Recording	Instructions	Handling/ Comments
HIP FLEXION	1. Start position ☐☐ 2. Stabilized ☐ 3. Therapist distal hand placement☐ 4. Slight traction ☐ 5. End position (full PROM achieved) ☐☐ 6. End feel ☐	1. Supine ☐ 2. Test side hip and knee in anatomical position ☐ 3. Nontest side hip and knee flexed or extended ☐ 4. Pelvis in neutral position☐ 5. Trunk and pelvis stabilized ☐	1. Over greater trochanter ☐	1. Parallel midaxillary line of trunk ☐ 2. Position maintained for start position ☐ 3. Position maintained for end position ☐	1. With knee flexed, hip is flexed to limit of motion ☐ 2. Full PROM achieved ☐ 3. Pelvis stabilized ☐	1. Parallel long axis of femur, pointing toward lateral epicondyle ☐ 2. Position maintained for start position ☐ 3. Position maintained for end position ☐	1. Full PROM ☐ 2. End feel ☐	1. Verbal (clear/ concise) ☐ 2. Demonstration (clear) ☐	1. Adequate support of limb/limb segment ☐ 2. Comfortable grip ☐ 3. Safe body mechanics of therapist ☐ Comments
HIP EXTENSION	1. Start position ☐ 2. Stabilized ☐ 3. Therapist distal hand placement☐ 4. Slight traction ☐ 5. End position (full PROM achieved) ☐ 6. End feel ☐	1. Prone ☐ 2. Hips and knees in anatomical position ☐ 3. Feet over end of plinth ☐ 4. Pelvis stabilized with strap or by second therapist ☐	1. Over greater trochanter ☐	1. Parallel midaxillary line of trunk ☐ 2. Position maintained for start position ☐ 3. Position maintained for end position ☐	1. With knee extended, hip is extended to limit of motion ☐ 2. Full PROM achieved ☐ 3. Pelvis stabilized maintained for end position ☐	1. Parallel long axis of femur, pointing toward lateral epicondyle ☐ 2. Position maintained for start position ☐ 3. Position ☐	1. Full PROM ☐ 2. End feel ☐	1. Verbal (clear/ concise) ☐ 2. Demonstration (clear) ☐	1. Adequate support of limb/limb segment ☐ 2. Comfortable grip ☐ 3. Safe body mechanics of therapist ☐ Comments:
HIP ABDUCTION	1. Start position ☐ 2. Stabilized ☐ 3. Therapist distal hand placement☐ 4. Slight traction ☐ 5. End position (full PROM achieved) ☐ 6. End feel ☐	1. Supine ☐ 2. Hip and knee in anatomical position ☐ 3. Pelvis is level ☐ 4. Pelvis stabilized ☐	1. Over ipsilateral ASIS ☐	1. Along line joining the two ASISs ☐ 2. Position maintained for start position ☐ 3. Position maintained for end position ☐	1. Hip is abducted to limit of motion ☐ 2. Full PROM achieved ☐ 3. Pelvis stabilized ☐	1. Parallel long axis of femur pointing to midline of patella ☐ 2. Position maintained for start position ☐ 3. Position maintained for end position ☐	1. Full PROM ☐ 2. End feel ☐	1. Verbal (clear/ concise) ☐ 2. Demonstration (clear) ☐	1. Adequate support of limb/limb segment ☐ 2. Comfortable grip ☐ 3. Safe body mechanics of therapist ☐ Comments:

(continues)

PROM Assessment and Measurement Testing: Hip (continued)

Movement	STEP 1 — PROM Assessment of End Feel	STEP 2 — PROM Measurement: Using A Universal Goniometer							
		Start Position	Axis	Stationary Arm	End Position	Movable Arm	Recording	Instructions	Handling/Comments
HIP ADDUCTION	1. Start position 2. Stabilized 3. Therapist distal hand placement 4. Slight traction 5. End position (full PROM achieved) 6. End feel	1. Supine 2. Hip and knee in anatomical position 3. Pelvis is level 4. Contralateral hip abducted 5. Pelvis stabilized	1. Over ipsilateral ASIS	1. Along line joining the two ASISs 2. Position maintained for start position 3. Position maintained for end position	1. Hip adducted to limit of motion 2. Full PROM achieved 3. Pelvis stabilized	1. Parallel long axis of femur pointing to midline of patella 2. Position maintained for start position 3. Position maintained for end position	1. Full PROM 2. End feel	1. Verbal (clear/concise) 2. Demonstration (clear)	1. Adequate support of limb/limb segment 2. Comfortable grip 3. Safe body mechanics of therapist Comments:
HIP INTERNAL ROTATION	1. Start position 2. Stabilized 3. Therapist distal hand placement 4. Slight traction 5. End position (full PROM achieved) 6. End feel	1. Sitting grasping edge of plinth 2. Pad is placed under thigh to keep thigh horizontal 3. Contralateral hip abducted and foot supported 4. Pelvis and femur stabilized	1. Over midpoint of patella	1. Perpendicular to floor 2. Position maintained for start position 3. Position maintained for end position	1. Hip internally rotated to limit of motion 2. Full PROM achieved 3. Pelvis and femur stabilized	1. Parallel anterior midline of tibia 2. Position maintained for start position 3. Position maintained for end position	1. Full PROM 2. End feel	1. Verbal (clear/concise) 2. Demonstration (clear)	1. Adequate support of limb/limb segment 2. Comfortable grip 3. Safe body mechanics of therapist Comments:
HIP EXTERNAL ROTATION	1. Start position 2. Stabilized 3. Therapist distal hand placement 4. Slight traction 5. End position (full PROM achieved) 6. End feel	1. Sitting grasping edge of plinth 2. Pad is placed under thigh to keep thigh horizontal 3. Contralateral hip abducted and foot supported 4. Pelvis and femur stabilized	1. Over midpoint of patella	1. Perpendicular to floor 2. Position maintained for start position 3. Position maintained for end position	1. Hip externally rotated to limit of motion 2. Full PROM achieved 3. Pelvis and femur stabilized	1. Parallel anterior midline of tibia 2. Position maintained for start position 3. Position maintained for end position	1. Full PROM 2. End feel	1. Verbal (clear/concise) 2. Demonstration (clear)	1. Adequate support of limb/limb segment 2. Comfortable grip 3. Safe body mechanics of therapist Comments:

Muscle Length Assessment and Measurement Testing: Hip

Muscle	Start Position	Stabilization	End Position	Measurement of Joint Position Using Universal Goniometer	Recording	Instructions	Handling/Comments
HAMSTRINGS (SLR)	1. Supine ☐ 2. Low back and sacrum flat on plinth ☐ 3. Ankle relaxed in plantarflexion ☐	1. Nontest thigh stabilized on plinth ☐ 2. Excessive anterior or posterior pelvic tilt avoided ☐	1. Hip flexed to limit of motion ☐ 2. Knee maintained in extension ☐ 3. Ankle relaxed in plantarflexion ☐ 4. Full PROM achieved ☐ 5. Nontest thigh stabilized on plinth ☐ 6. Excessive pelvic tilt avoided ☐	Hip flexion 1. Axis: over greater trochanter ☐ 2. Stationary arm: parallel midaxillary line of trunk ☐ 3. Movable arm: parallel long axis of femur, pointing toward lateral epicondyle ☐	1. Full PROM ☐ 2. End feel ☐	1. Verbal (clear/concise) ☐ 2. Demonstration (clear) ☐	1. Adequate support of limb/limb segment ☐ 2. Comfortable grip ☐ 3. Safe body mechanics of therapist ☐ Comments:
HAMSTRINGS PASSIVE KNEE EXTENSION (PKE)	1. Supine ☐ 2. Hip flexed 90°, patient holds distal thigh to maintain position ☐ 3. Knee flexed ☐ 4. Ankle relaxed in plantarflexion ☐	1. Thigh stabilized in 90° hip flexion ☐ 2. Posterior pelvic tilt avoided ☐ 3. If necessary nontest thigh stabilized on plinth ☐	1. Knee extended to limit of motion ☐ 2. Ankle relaxed in plantarflexion ☐ 3. Full PROM achieved ☐ 4. Thigh stabilized ☐ 5. Posterior pelvic tilt avoided ☐	Knee flexion 1. Axis: over the lateral epicondyle of the femur ☐ 2. Stationary arm: parallel longitudinal axis of femur, pointing toward greater trochanter ☐ 3. Movable arm: parallel long axis of fibula, pointing toward lateral malleolus ☐	1. Full PROM ☐ 2. End feel ☐	1. Verbal (clear/concise) ☐ 2. Demonstration (clear) ☐	1. Adequate support of limb/limb segment ☐ 2. Comfortable grip ☐ 3. Safe body mechanics of therapist ☐ Comments:
HIP FLEXORS (Thomas Test)	1. Sitting, with edge of plinth at midthigh level ☐ 2. Patient assisted into supine ☐ 3. Nontest hip held in flexion ☐ 4. Sacrum and lumbar spine flat on plinth ☐	1. Pelvis and lumbar spine stabilized ☐ 2. Anterior pelvic tilt avoided ☐	1. Leg falls toward plinth in neutral rotation ☐ 2. Hip is extended to limit of motion ☐ 3. Knee free to extend ☐ 4. Full PROM achieved ☐ 5. Pelvis and lumbar spine stabilized ☐ 6. Anterior pelvic tilt avoided ☐	Hip extension 1. Axis: over greater trochanter ☐ 2. Stationary arm: parallel midaxillary line of trunk ☐ 3. Movable arm: parallel long axis of femur, pointing toward lateral epicondyle ☐	1. Full PROM ☐ 2. End feel ☐	1. Verbal (clear/concise) ☐ 2. Demonstration (clear) ☐	1. Adequate support of limb/limb segment ☐ 2. Comfortable grip ☐ 3. Safe body mechanics of therapist ☐ Comments:

(continues)

Muscle Length Assessment and Measurement Testing: Hip (continued)

Muscle	Start Position	Stabilization	End Position	Measurement of Joint Position Using Universal Goniometer	Recording	Instructions	Handling/Comments
HIP ADDUCTORS	1. Supine ☐ 2. Hip and knee in anatomical position ☐ 3. Nontest hip abducted, knee flexed, and foot rests on stool beside plinth ☐ 4. Pelvis is level ☐	1. Pelvis stabilized ☐	1. Hip is abducted to limit of motion ☐ 2. Full PROM achieved ☐ 3. Pelvis stabilized ☐	Hip abduction 1. Axis: over ipsilateral ASIS ☐ 2. Stationary arm: Along line joining the two ASISs ☐ 3. Movable arm: parallel along axis of femur, pointing to midline of patella ☐	1. Full ☐ PROM ☐ 2. End feel ☐	1. Verbal (clear/ concise) ☐ 2. Demonstration (clear) ☐	1. Adequate support of limb/limb segment ☐ 2. Comfortable grip ☐ 3. Safe body mechanics of therapist ☐ Comments:
TENSOR FASCIA LATAE (ILIOTIBIAL BAND) (OBER'S TEST)	1. Sidely on nontest side ☐ 2. Patient holds nontest hip and knee in flexion ☐ 3. Hip abducted and extended, in neutral rotation, knee flexed 90° ☐	1. Therapist stands against buttocks ☐ 2. Pelvis stabilized downward at iliac crest ☐	1. Leg allowed to fall toward plinth ☐ 2. Hip is adducted to limit of motion ☐ 3. Full PROM achieved ☐ 4. Pelvis stabilized ☐ 5. Hip maintained in extension and neutral rotation ☐	Hip adduction Second therapist instructed to measure joint position: 1. Axis: over ipsilateral ASIS ☐ 2. Stationary arm: Along line joining the two ASISs ☐ 3. Movable arm: parallel long axis of femur, pointing to midline of patella ☐	1. Full ☐ PROM ☐ 2. End feel ☐	1. Verbal (clear/ concise) ☐ 2. Demonstration (clear) ☐	1. Adequate support of limb/limb segment ☐ 2. Comfortable grip ☐ 3. Safe body mechanics of therapist ☐ Comments:
TENSOR FASCIA LATAE (ILIOTIBIAL BAND) (OBER'S TEST: TRUNK PRONE)	1. Prone over end of plinth with nontest hip and knee flexed, foot on floor under plinth ☐ 2. Arms overhead grasp plinth ☐ 3. Hip abducted and extended, in neutral rotation, knee flexed 90° ☐	1. Therapist stabilizes pelvis ☐	1. Hip is adducted to limit of motion ☐ 2. Full PROM achieved ☐ 3. Pelvis stabilized ☐	Hip adduction Second therapist instructed to measure joint position: 1. Axis: posterior aspect of pelvis over projected location of ipsilateral ASIS ☐ 2. Stationary arm: Along line joining the two ASISs projected to posterior aspect of pelvis ☐ 3. Movable arm: parallel long axis of femur ☐	1. Full ☐ PROM ☐ 2. End feel ☐	1. Verbal (clear/ concise) ☐ 2. Demonstration (clear) ☐	1. Adequate support of limb/limb segment ☐ 2. Comfortable grip ☐ 3. Safe body mechanics of therapist ☐ Comments:

PROM Assessment and Measurement Testing: Knee

STEP 1 ———— **STEP 2**

PROM Measurement: Using A Universal Goniometer

Movement	PROM Assessment of End Feel	Start Position	Axis	Stationary Arm	End Position	Movable Arm	Recording	Instructions	Handling/Comments
KNEE FLEXION	1. Start position ☐ 2. Stabilized ☐ 3. Therapist distal hand placement ☐ 4. Slight traction ☐ 5. End position (full PROM achieved) ☐ 6. End feel ☐	1. Supine ☐ 2. Hip and knee in anatomical position ☐ 3. Towel under distal thigh ☐ 4. Pelvis and femur stabilized ☐	1. Over lateral epicondyle of femur ☐	1. Parallel longitudinal axis of femur, pointing toward greater trochanter ☐ 2. Position maintained for start position ☐ 3. Position maintained for end position ☐	1. Hip and knee flexed ☐ 2. Heel moved toward buttock to limit of knee flexion ☐ 3. Full PROM achieved ☐ 4. Pelvis and femur stabilized ☐	1. Parallel long axis of fibula, pointing toward the lateral malleolus ☐ 2. Position maintained for start position ☐ 3. Position maintained for end position ☐	1. Full PROM ☐ 2. End feel ☐	1. Verbal (clear/concise) ☐ 2. Demonstration (clear) ☐	1. Adequate support of limb/limb segment ☐ 2. Comfortable grip ☐ 3. Safe body mechanics of therapist ☐ Comments:
KNEE EXTENSION/ HYPER-EXTENSION	1. Start position ☐ 2. Stabilized ☐ 3. Therapist distal hand placement ☐ 4. Slight traction ☐ 5. End position (full PROM achieved) ☐ 6. End feel ☐	1. Supine ☐ 2. Hip and knee in anatomical position ☐ 3. Towel under distal thigh ☐ 4. Femur stabilized ☐	1. Over lateral epicondyle of femur ☐	1. Parallel longitudinal axis of femur, pointing toward greater trochanter ☐ 2. Position maintained for start position ☐ 3. Position maintained for end position ☐	1. Knee extended/hyper-extended to limit of motion ☐ 2. Full PROM achieved ☐ 3. Femur stabilized ☐	1. Parallel long axis of fibula, pointing toward the lateral malleolus ☐ 2. Position maintained for start position ☐ 3. Position maintained for end position ☐	1. Full PROM ☐ 2. End feel ☐	1. Verbal (clear/concise) ☐ 2. Demonstration (clear) ☐	1. Adequate support of limb/limb segment ☐ 2. Comfortable grip ☐ 3. Safe body mechanics of therapist ☐ Comments:

(continues)

PROM Assessment and Measurement Testing: Shoulder Complex

Movement	Start Position	Stabilization	Hand Placement	Therapist's End Position	Recording	Instructions	Handling/Comments
PATELLAR DISTAL GLIDE	1. Supine 2. Roll supports knee in slight flexion	1. Femur stabilized ☐	1. Heel of hand against base of patella, forearm lies along thigh 2. Palm of other hand placed on top of first hand ☐	1. Patella moved distally ☐ 2. Patellar compression against femur avoided ☐ 3. Full PROM achieved ☐ 4. Femur stabilized ☐	1. Full PROM ☐ 2. End feel ☐	1. Verbal (clear/ concise) ☐ 2. Demonstration (clear) ☐	1. Adequate support of limb/limb segment ☐ 2. Comfortable grip ☐ 3. Safe body mechanics of therapist ☐ Comments:
PATELLAR MEDIAL-LATERAL GLIDE	1. Supine 2. Roll supports knee in slight flexion	1. Femur and tibia stabilized ☐	1. Palmar aspect of thumbs positioned along lateral border of patella 2. Pads of index fingers on medial border of patella ☐	1. Patella moved medially ☐ 2. Patella moved laterally ☐ 3. Patellar compression against femur avoided ☐ 4. Full PROM achieved ☐ 5. Femur and tibia stabilized ☐	1. Full PROM ☐ 2. End feel ☐	1. Verbal (clear/ concise) ☐ 2. Demonstration (clear) ☐	1. Adequate support of limb/limb segment ☐ 2. Comfortable grip ☐ 3. Safe body mechanics of therapist ☐ Comments:
TIBIAL ROTATION	1. Sitting 2. Pad placed under distal thigh to maintain thigh in horizontal position 3. Knee flexed 90° 4. Tibia in full internal rotation	1. Femur stabilized ☐	1. Distal tibia and fibula ☐	1. Tibia externally rotated to the limit of motion ☐ 2. Full PROM achieved ☐ 3. Femur stabilized ☐	1. Full PROM ☐ 2. End feel ☐	1. Verbal (clear/concise) ☐ 2. Demonstration (clear) ☐	1. Adequate support of limb/limb segment ☐ 2. Comfortable grip ☐ 3. Safe body mechanics of therapist ☐ Comments:

Muscle	Start Position	Stabilization	End Position	Measurement of Joint Positioning Using Universal Goniometer	Recording	Instructions	Handling/Comments
HAMSTRINGS	1. Sitting grasping edge of plinth ☐ 2. Towel placed under distal thigh ☐ 3. Ankle relaxed in plantarflexion ☐ 4. Nontest leg: foot supported on stool ☐	1. Pelvis and femur stabilized ☐	1. Knee extended to limit of motion ☐ 2. Full PROM achieved ☐ 3. Pelvis and femur stabilized ☐	Knee extension 1. Axis: over the lateral epicondyle of the femur ☐ 2. Stationary arm: parallel longitudinal axis of femur, pointing toward greater trochanter ☐ 3. Movable arm: parallel longitudinal axis of fibula, pointing toward lateral malleolus ☐	1. Full PROM ☐ 2. End feel ☐	1. Verbal (clear/concise) ☐ 2. Demonstration (clear) ☐	1. Adequate support of limb/limb segment ☐ 2. Comfortable grip ☐ 3. Safe body mechanics of therapist ☐ Comments:
RECTUS FEMORIS (PRONE ONE FOOT ON FLOOR)	1. Prone ☐ 2. Hip and knee in anatomical position ☐ 3. Towel placed under distal thigh ☐ 4. Nontest leg over side of plinth, with hip flexed and foot on floor ☐	1. Pelvis and femur stabilized ☐	1. Knee flexed to limit of motion ☐ 2. Full PROM achieved ☐ 3. Pelvis and femur stabilized ☐	Knee flexion 1. Axis: over the lateral epicondyle of the femur ☐ 2. Stationary arm: parallel longitudinal axis of femur, pointing toward greater trochanter ☐ 3. Movable arm: parallel longitudinal axis of fibula, pointing toward lateral malleolus ☐	1. Full PROM ☐ 2. End feel ☐	1. Verbal (clear/concise) ☐ 2. Demonstration (clear) ☐	1. Adequate support of limb/limb segment ☐ 2. Comfortable grip ☐ 3. Safe body mechanics of therapist ☐ Comments:

(continues)

PROM Assessment and Measurement Testing: Shoulder Complex (continued)

Muscle	Start Position	Stabilization	End Position	Measurement of Joint Positioning Using Universal Goniometer	Recording	Instructions	Handling/Comments
RECTUS FEMORIS (PRONE)	1. Prone ☐ 2. Towel placed under distal thigh ☐	1. Pelvis stabilized ☐ 2. Femur stabilized ☐	1. Knee flexed to limit of motion ☐ 2. Full PROM achieved ☐ 3. Pelvis and femur stabilized ☐	Knee flexion 1. Axis: over the lateral epicondyle of the femur ☐ 2. Stationary arm: parallel longitudinal axis of femur, pointing toward greater trochanter ☐ 3. Movable arm: parallel longitudinal axis of fibula, pointing toward lateral malleolus ☐	1. Full PROM ☐ 2. End feel ☐	1. Verbal (clear/concise) ☐ 2. Demonstration (clear) ☐	1. Adequate support of limb/limb segment ☐ 2. Comfortable grip ☐ 3. Safe body mechanics of therapist ☐ Comments:
RECTUS FEMORIS (THOMAS TEST POSITION)	1. Sitting, with edge of plinth at midthigh level ☐ 2. Patient assisted into supine ☐ 3. Nontest hip held in flexion ☐ 4. Sacrum and lumbar spine flat on plinth ☐	1. Pelvis and lumbar spine stabilized ☐ 2. Anterior pelvic tilt avoided ☐	1. Leg falls toward plinth in neutral rotation ☐ 2. Hip is extended to limit of motion ☐ 3. Knee is flexed to limit of motion ☐ 4. Full PROM achieved ☐ 5. Pelvis and lumbar spine stabilized ☐ 6. Anterior pelvic tilt avoided ☐	Knee flexion 1. Axis: over the lateral epicondyle of the femur ☐ 2. Stationary arm: parallel longitudinal axis of femur, pointing toward greater trochanter ☐ 3. Movable arm parallel longitudinal axis of fibula, pointing toward lateral malleolus ☐	1. Full PROM ☐ 2. End feel ☐	1. Verbal (clear/concise) ☐ 2. Demonstration (clear) ☐	1. Adequate support of limb/limb segment ☐ 2. Comfortable grip ☐ 3. Safe body mechanics of therapist ☐ Comments:

PROM Assessment and Measurement Testing: Ankle and Foot

	STEP 1	STEP 2							
		PROM Measurement: Using A Universal Goniometer							
Movement	**PROM Assessment of End Feel**	**Start Position**	**Axis**	**Stationary Arm**	**End Position**	**Movable Arm**	**Recording**	**Instructions**	**Handling/Comments**
ANKLE DORSI-FLEXION	1. Start position ☐ 2. Stabilized ☐ 3. Therapist distal hand placement ☐ 4. Slight traction ☐ 5. End position (full PROM achieved) ☐ 6. End feel ☐	1. Supine 2. Roll under knee about 20–30° knee flexion ☐ 3. Ankle in anatomical position ☐ 4. Tibia and fibula stabilized ☐	1. Inferior to the lateral malleolus ☐	1. Parallel longitudinal axis of fibula pointing to fibular head ☐ 2. Position maintained for start position ☐ 3. Position maintained for end position ☐	1. Ankle dorsiflexed to limit of motion ☐ 2. Full PROM achieved ☐ 3. Tibia and maintained stabilized ☐	1. Parallel to sole of heel ☐ 2. Position maintained for start position ☐ 3. Position mechanics for end position ☐	1. Full PROM ☐ 2. End feel ☐	1. Verbal (clear/ concise) ☐ 2. Demonstration (clear) ☐	1. Adequate support of limb/limb segment ☐ 2. Comfortable grip ☐ 3. Safe body of therapist ☐ Comments:
ANKLE PLANTAR-FLEXION	1. Start position ☐ 2. Stabilized ☐ 3. Therapist distal hand placement ☐ 4. Slight traction ☐ 5. End position (full PROM achieved) ☐ 6. End feel ☐	1. Supine 2. Roll under knee about 20–30° knee flexion ☐ 3. Ankle in anatomical position ☐ 4. Tibia and fibula stabilized ☐	1. Inferior to the lateral malleolus ☐	1. Parallel longitudinal axis of fibula pointing to fibular head ☐ 2. Position maintained for start position ☐ 3. Position maintained for end position ☐	1. Ankle plantarflexed to limit of motion ☐ 2. Full PROM achieved ☐ 3. Tibia and fibula stabilized ☐	1. Parallel to sole of heel ☐ 2. Position maintained for start position ☐ 3. Position maintained for end position ☐	1. Full PROM ☐ 2. End feel ☐	1. Verbal (clear/ concise) ☐ 2. Demonstration (clear) ☐	1. Adequate support of limb/limb segment ☐ 2. Comfortable grip ☐ 3. Safe body mechanics of therapist ☐ Comments:
SUBTALAR INVER-SION	1. Start position ☐ 2. Stabilized ☐ 3. Therapist distal hand placement ☐ 4. Slight traction ☐ 5. End position (full PROM achieved) ☐ 6. End feel ☐	1. Prone with feet off end of plinth ☐ 2. Ankle in anatomical position ☐ 3. Tibia and fibula stabilized ☐	1. Over midline mark, superior aspect of calcaneus ☐	1. Parallel longitudinal axis of lower leg ☐ 2. Position maintained for start position ☐ 3. Position maintained for end position ☐	1. Calcaneus inverted to limit of motion ☐ 2. Full PROM achieved ☐ 3. Tibia and fibula stabilized ☐	1. Aligned with mark over midline, posterior aspect of heel pad ☐ 2. Position maintained for start position ☐ 3. Position maintained for end position ☐	1. Full PROM ☐ 2. End feel ☐	1. Verbal (clear/ concise) ☐ 2. Demonstration (clear) ☐	1. Adequate support of imb/imb segment ☐ 2. Comfortable grip ☐ 3. Safe body mechanics of therapist ☐ Comments:

(continues)

PROM Assessment and Measurement Testing: Ankle and Foot (continued)

| | STEP 1 | STEP 2 | | | | | | | |
| | | PROM Measurement: Using A Universal Goniometer | | | | | | | |
Movement	PROM Assessment of End Feel	Start Position	Axis	Stationary Arm	End Position	Movable Arm	Recording	Instructions	Handling/Comments
SUBTALAR EVERSION	1. Start position ☐ 2. Stabilized ☐ 3. Therapist distal hand placement ☐ 4. Slight traction ☐ 5. End position (full PROM achieved) ☐ 6. End feel ☐	1. Prone with feet off end of plinth ☐ 2. Ankle in anatomical position ☐ 3. Tibia and fibula stabilized ☐	1. Over midline mark, superior aspect of calcaneus ☐	1. Parallel longitudinal axis of lower leg ☐ 2. Position maintained for start position ☐ 3. Position maintained for end position ☐	1. Calcaneus everted to limit of motion ☐ 2. Full PROM achieved ☐ 3. Tibia and fibula stabilized ☐	1. Aligned with mark over midline, posterior aspect of heel pad ☐ 2. Position maintained for start position ☐ 3. Position maintained for end position ☐	1. Full PROM ☐ 2. End feel ☐	1. Verbal (clear/concise) ☐ 2. Demonstration (clear) ☐	1. Adequate support of limb/limb segment ☐ 2. Comfortable grip ☐ 3. Safe body mechanics of therapist ☐ Comments:
GREAT TOE MTP JOINT FLEXION	1. Start position ☐ 2. Stabilized ☐ 3. Therapist distal hand placement ☐ 4. Slight traction ☐ 5. End position (full PROM achieved) ☐ 6. End feel ☐	1. Supine ☐ 2. Ankle and toes in anatomical position ☐ 3. First metatarsal stabilized ☐	1. Over dorsum or over medial aspect of first MTP joint ☐	1. Parallel longitudinal axis of first metatarsal ☐ 2. Position maintained for start position ☐ 3. Position maintained for end position ☐	1. MTP joint flexed to limit of motion ☐ 2. Full PROM achieved ☐ 3. First metatarsal stabilized ☐	1. Parallel longitudinal axis of proximal phalanx of great toe ☐ 2. Position maintained for start position ☐ 3. Position maintained for end position ☐	1. Full PROM ☐ 2. End feel ☐	1. Verbal (clear/concise) ☐ 2. Demonstration (clear) ☐	1. Adequate support of limb/limb segment ☐ 2. Comfortable grip ☐ 3. Safe body mechanics of therapist ☐ Comments:
GREAT TOE MTP JOINT EXTENSION	1. Start position ☐ 2. Stabilized ☐ 3. Therapist distal hand placement ☐ 4. Slight traction ☐ 5. End position (full PROM achieved) ☐ 6. End feel ☐	1. Supine ☐ 2. Ankle and toes in anatomical position ☐ 3. First metatarsal stabilized ☐	1. Over plantar aspect or over medial aspect of first MTP joint ☐	1. Parallel longitudinal axis of first metatarsal ☐ 2. Position maintained for start position ☐ 3. Position maintained for end position ☐	1. MTP joint extended to limit of motion ☐ 2. Full PROM achieved ☐ 3. First metatarsal stabilized ☐	1. Parallel longitudinal axis of proximal phalanx of great toe ☐ 2. Position maintained for start position ☐ 3. Position maintained for end position ☐	1. Full PROM ☐ 2. End feel ☐	1. Verbal (clear/concise) ☐ 2. Demonstration (clear) ☐	1. Adequate support of limb/limb segment ☐ 2. Comfortable grip ☐ 3. Safe body mechanics of therapist ☐ Comments:

GREAT TOE MTP JOINT ABDUCTION

1. Start position ☐
2. Stabilized ☐
3. Therapist distal hand placement ☐
4. Slight traction ☐
5. End position (full PROM achieved) ☐
6. End feel ☐

- 1. Supine
- 2. Ankle and great toe in anatomical position
- 3. First metatarsal stabilized

- 1. Over dorsum of first MTP joint

1. Parallel longitudinal axis of first metatarsal ☐
2. Position maintained for start position ☐
3. Position maintained for end position ☐

1. MTP joint abducted to limit of motion ☐
2. Full PROM achieved ☐
3. First metatarsal stabilized ☐

1. Parallel longitudinal axis of proximal phalanx of great toe ☐
2. Position maintained for start position ☐
3. Position maintained for end position ☐

1. Full PROM ☐
2. End feel ☐

1. Verbal (clear/concise) ☐
2. Demonstration (clear) ☐

1. Adequate support of limb/limb segment ☐
2. Comfortable grip ☐
3. Safe body mechanics of therapist ☐

Comments:

GREAT TOE MTP JOINT ADDUCTION

1. Start position ☐
2. Stabilized ☐
3. Therapist distal hand placement ☐
4. Slight traction ☐
5. End position (full PROM achieved) ☐
6. End feel ☐

- 1. Supine
- 2. Ankle and great toe in anatomical position
- 3. First metatarsal stabilized

- 1. Over dorsum of first MTP joint

1. Parallel longitudinal axis of first metatarsal ☐
2. Position maintained for start position ☐
3. Position maintained for end position ☐

1. MTP joint adducted to limit of motion ☐
2. Full PROM achieved ☐
3. First metatarsal stabilized ☐

1. Parallel longitudinal axis of proximal phalanx of great toe ☐
2. Position maintained for start position ☐
3. Position maintained for end position ☐

1. Full PROM ☐
2. End feel ☐

1. Verbal (clear/concise) ☐
2. Demonstration (clear) ☐

1. Adequate support of limb/limb segment ☐
2. Comfortable grip ☐
3. Safe body mechanics of therapist ☐

Comments:

GREAT TOE IP JOINT FLEXION

1. Start position ☐
2. Stabilized ☐
3. Therapist distal hand placement ☐
4. Slight traction ☐
5. End position (full PROM achieved) ☐
6. End feel ☐

- 1. Supine
- 2. Ankle and great toe in anatomical position
- 3. Proximal phalanx of great toe stabilized

- 1. Over dorsal or lateral aspect of IP joint of great toe

1. Parallel longitudinal axis of proximal phalanx of great toe ☐
2. Position maintained for start position ☐
3. Position maintained for end position ☐

1. IP joint flexed to limit of motion ☐
2. Full PROM achieved ☐
3. Proximal phalanx of great toe stabilized ☐

1. Parallel longitudinal axis of distal phalanx of great toe ☐
2. Position maintained for start position ☐
3. Position maintained for end position ☐

1. Full PROM ☐
2. End feel ☐

1. Verbal (clear/concise) ☐
2. Demonstration (clear) ☐

1. Adequate support of limb/limb segment ☐
2. Comfortable grip ☐
3. Safe body mechanics of therapist ☐

Comments:

(continues)

PROM Assessment and Measurement Testing: Ankle and Foot (continued)

Movement	STEP 1 — PROM Assessment of End Feel	STEP 2 — PROM Measurement: Using A Universal Goniometer							
		Start Position	Axis	Stationary Arm	End Position	Movable Arm	Recording	Instructions	Handling/Comments
GREAT TOE IP JOINT EXTENSION	1. Start position ☐ 2. Stabilized ☐ 3. Therapist distal hand placement ☐ 4. Slight traction ☐ 5. End position (full PROM achieved) ☐ 6. End feel ☐	1. Supine ☐ 2. Ankle and great toe in anatomical position ☐ 3. Proximal phalanx of great toe stabilized ☐	1. Over plantar or lateral aspect of IP joint of great toe ☐	1. Parallel longitudinal axis of proximal phalanx of great toe ☐ 2. Position maintained for start position ☐ 3. Position maintained for end position ☐	1. IP joint extended to limit of motion ☐ 2. Full PROM achieved ☐ 3. Proximal phalanx of great toe stabilized ☐	1. Parallel longitudinal axis of distal phalanx of great toe ☐ 2. Position maintained for start position ☐ 3. Position maintained for end position ☐	1. Full PROM ☐ 2. End feel ☐	1. Verbal (clear/concise) ☐ 2. Demonstration (clear) ☐	1. Adequate support of limb/limb segment ☐ 2. Comfortable grip ☐ 3. Safe body mechanics of therapist ☐ Comments:

Muscle Length Assessment and Measurement Testing: Ankle and Foot

Muscle	Start Position	Stabilization	End Position	Measurement of Joint Position Using Universal Goniometer	Recording	Instructions	Handling/ Comments
GASTROCNEMIUS	1. Standing ☐ 2. Lower extremity in anatomical position ☐ 3. Facing a stable plinth or wall ☐	1. Foot and toes point forward and remain flat on floor ☐	1. Patient steps ahead with nontest leg ☐ 2. Patient leans forward to place hands on stable plinth or wall ☐ 3. Knee remains extended as patient leans forward ☐ 4. Ankle dorsiflexed to limit of motion ☐ 5. Foot and toes point forward and flat on floor ☐	Ankle dorsiflexion 1. Axis: inferior to the lateral malleolus ☐ 2. Stationary arm: parallel longitudinal axis of fibula pointing to head of fibula ☐ 3. Movable arm: parallel to sole of heel ☐	1. Full PROM ☐ 2. End feel ☐	1. Verbal (clear/concise) ☐ 2. Demonstration (clear) ☐	1. Adequate support of limb/limb segment ☐ 2. Comfortable grip ☐ 3. Safe body mechanics of therapist ☐ Comments:

AROM Assessment and Measurement Testing: Head, Neck, and Trunk

AROM Measurement: Using A Tape Measure or Ruler

Movement	Start Position	Stabilization	End Position	Measurement	Recording	Instructions	Comments
TMJ: OCCLUSION AND DEPRESSION OF THE MANDIBLE	1. Sitting ☐ 2. Head and neck in anatomical position, TMJ in resting position ☐	1. Patient instructed to keep head, neck and trunk in anatomical position ☐	1. Lower jaw elevated, teeth in contact ☐ 2. Mouth opened to limit of motion ☐ 3. Full AROM achieved ☐	1. Occlusion: relative position of mandibular and maxillary teeth observed ☐ 2. Depression: distance measured between edges of upper and lower central incisors ☐	1. Full AROM ☐	1. Verbal (clear/concise) ☐ 2. Demonstration (clear) ☐ 3. Substitute movement avoided ☐	
TMJ: PROTRUSION OF THE MANDIBLE	1. Sitting ☐ 2. Head and neck in anatomical position, TMJ in resting position ☐	1. Patient instructed to keep head, neck and trunk in anatomical position ☐	1. Lower jaw protruded, lower teeth beyond upper teeth ☐ 2. Full AROM achieved ☐	1. Distance measured between upper and lower central incisor teeth ☐	1. Full AROM ☐	1. Verbal (clear/concise) ☐ 2. Demonstration (clear) ☐ 3. Substitute movement avoided ☐	
TMJ: LATERAL DEVIATION OF THE MANDIBLE	1. Sitting ☐ 2. Head and neck in anatomical position, TMJ in resting position ☐	1. Patient instructed to keep head, neck and trunk in anatomical position ☐	1. Lower jaw deviated to right ☐ 2. Lower jaw deviated to left ☐ 3. Full AROM achieved ☐	1. Distance measured between two selected points that are level (e.g. space between central incisors) ☐	1. Full AROM ☐	1. Verbal (clear/concise) ☐ 2. Demonstration (clear) ☐ 3. Substitute movement avoided ☐	
NECK FLEXION	1. Sitting ☐ 2. Head and neck in anatomical position ☐	1. Patient instructed on how to stabilize shoulder girdle and avoid thoracic and lumbar spine movements ☐	1. Neck flexed to limit of motion ☐ 2. Full AROM achieved ☐	1. Distance measured between tip of chin and suprasternal notch ☐	1. Full AROM ☐	1. Verbal (clear/concise) ☐ 2. Demonstration (clear) ☐ 3. Substitute movement avoided ☐	

NECK EXTENSION	1. Sitting ☐ 2. Head and neck in anatomical position ☐	1. Patient instructed on how to stabilize shoulder girdle and avoid thoracic and lumbar spine movements ☐	1. Neck extended to limit of motion ☐ 2. Full AROM achieved ☐	1. Distance measured between tip of chin and suprasternal notch ☐	1. Full AROM ☐	1. Verbal (clear/concise) ☐ 2. Demonstration (clear) ☐ 3. Substitute movement avoided ☐
NECK LATERAL FLEXION	1. Sitting ☐ 2. Head and neck in anatomical position ☐	1. Patient instructed on how to stabilize shoulder girdle and avoid thoracic and lumbar spine movements ☐	1. Neck laterally flexed to limit of motion ☐ 2. Full AROM achieved ☐	1. Distance measured between mastoid process and acromion process ☐	1. Full AROM ☐	1. Verbal (clear/concise) ☐ 2. Demonstration (clear) ☐ 3. Substitute movement avoided ☐
NECK ROTATION	1. Sitting ☐ 2. Head and neck in anatomical position ☐	1. Patient instructed on how to stabilize shoulder girdle and avoid thoracic and lumbar spine movements ☐	1. Neck rotated to limit of motion ☐ 2. Full AROM achieved ☐	1. Distance measured between tip of chin and lateral edge of acromion process ☐	1. Full AROM ☐	1. Verbal (clear/concise) ☐ 2. Demonstration (clear) ☐ 3. Substitute movement avoided ☐
TRUNK FLEXION-THORACOLUMBAR SPINE	1. Standing, feet shoulder width apart, knees straight ☐		1. Trunk flexed to limit of motion for thoracolumbar flexion ☐ 2. Full AROM achieved ☐	1. Distance measured between C7 and S2 at start position ☐ 2. Distance measured between C7 and S2 at end position ☐	1. Full AROM ☐	1. Verbal (clear/concise) ☐ 2. Demonstration (clear) ☐ 3. Substitute movement avoided ☐

AROM Assessment and Measurement Testing: Head, Neck, and Trunk *(Continued)*

	AROM Measurement: Using A Tape Measure or Ruler					
Movement	**Start Position**	**Stabilization**	**End Position**	**Measurement**	**Recording**	**Instructions**	**Comments**
TRUNK EXTENSION-THORACOLUMBAR SPINE	1. Standing, feet shoulder width apart, knees straight ☐ 2. Hands on iliac crests and small of back ☐		1. Trunk extended to limit of motion for thoracolumbar extension ☐ 2. Full AROM achieved ☐	1. Distance measured between C7 and S2 at start position ☐ 2. Distance measured between C7 and S2 at end position ☐	1. Full AROM ☐	1. Verbal (clear/concise) ☐ 2. Demonstration (clear) ☐ 3. Substitute movement avoided ☐	
TRUNK EXTENSION-THORACOLUMBAR SPINE (Prone Press Up)	1. Prone ☐ 2. Hands positioned on plinth at shoulder level ☐	1. Strap used to stabilize pelvis ☐	1. Patient extends elbows to raise trunk and extend thoracolumbar spine to limit of motion ☐ 2. Full AROM achieved ☐	1. Distance measured between suprasternal notch and plinth ☐	1. Full AROM ☐	1. Verbal (clear/concise) ☐ 2. Demonstration (clear) ☐ 3. Substitute movement avoided ☐	
TRUNK FLEXION-LUMBAR SPINE	1. Standing, feet shoulder width apart ☐		1. Trunk flexed to limit of motion for lumbar flexion ☐ 2. Full AROM achieved ☐	1. Mark placed over spine 15 cm above spinous process of S2 at start position ☐ 2. Distance measured between 15 cm mark and S2 at end position ☐	1. Full AROM ☐	1. Verbal (clear/concise) ☐ 2. Demonstration (clear) ☐ 3. Substitute movement avoided ☐	

TRUNK EXTENSION- LUMBAR SPINE

1. Standing, feet shoulder width apart ☐
2. Hands on iliac crests and small of back ☐

1. Trunk extended to limit of motion for lumbar extension ☐
2. Full AROM achieved ☐

1. Mark placed over spine 15 cm above spinous process of S2 at start position ☐
2. Distance measured between 15 cm mark and S2 at end position ☐

1. Full AROM ☐

1. Verbal (clear/ concise) ☐
2. Demonstration (clear) ☐
3. Substitute movement avoided ☐

TRUNK LATERAL FLEXION- THORACOLUMBAR SPINE

1. Standing, feet shoulder width apart ☐

1. Trunk laterally flexed to limit of motion ☐
2. Full AROM achieved ☐

1. Distance measured between tip of third digit and floor ☐

1. Full AROM ☐

1. Verbal (clear/concise) ☐
2. Demonstration (clear) ☐
3. Substitute movement avoided ☐

TRUNK ROTATION - THORACOLUMBAR SPINE

1. Sitting feet supported ☐
2. Arms crossed in front of chest ☐
3. Patient holds end of tape measure on lateral aspect of acromion process ☐
4. Therapist holds other end of tape measure on contralateral iliac crest or upper border of greater trochanter ☐

1. Pelvis stabilized ☐

1. Trunk rotated to limit of motion ☐
2. Full AROM achieved ☐
3. Pelvis stabilized ☐

1. Distance measured between acromion process and iliac crest or greater trochanter at start position ☐
2. Distance measured between acromion process and iliac crest or greater trochanter at end position ☐

1. Full AROM ☐

1. Verbal (clear/concise) ☐
2. Demonstration (clear) ☐
3. Substitute movement avoided ☐

CHEST EXPANSION

1. Sitting ☐
2. Tape measure position around chest at level of xiphisternum ☐
3. Full expiration made ☐

1. Full inspiration made ☐

1. Chest circumference at full expiration ☐
2. Chest circumference at full inspiration ☐

1. Full AROM ☐

1. Verbal (clear/concise) ☐
2. Demonstration (clear) ☐
3. Substitute movement avoided ☐

Muscle Length Assessment and Measurement Testing: Trunk

Muscle	Start Position	Stabilization	End Position	Measurement of Joint Position Using Tape Measure	Recording	Instructions	Comments
TRUNK EXTENSORS- AND HAMSTRINGS (TOE-TOUCH TEST)	1. Standing, knees straight ☐		1. Trunk and hips flexed as patient reaches toward toes to limit of motion 2. Full AROM achieved ☐ 3. Knees maintained in extension ☐	1. Distance measured between most distant point reached by both hands and floor ☐	1. Full AROM ☐	1. Verbal (clear/ concise) ☐ 2. Demonstration (clear) ☐ 3. Substitute movement avoidedt ☐	

Answer Guides for Chapter Exercises and Questions

This appendix contains answers to the exercises and questions at the end of each chapter. In some cases, it is possible to provide concrete answers to the exercises and questions, but for some exercises and questions, there may be suitable alternate answers not identified here.

Chapter 1: Principles and Methods

1. Joint Movements

i. Flexion: Bending of a part so that the anterior surfaces come closer together; extension; sagittal plane, frontal axis.

ii. Abduction: movement away from the midline of the body or body part; adduction; frontal plane, sagittal axis.

iii. Internal rotation: turning of the anterior surface of a part toward the midline of the body; external rotation; horizontal plane, vertical/longitudinal axis.

iv. Lateral flexion: trunk or neck bending movements that occur in a lateral direction either to the right or left; lateral flexion to the opposite side; frontal plane, sagittal axis.

v. Horizontal adduction: starting with the shoulder or hip at 90° flexion or 90° abduction, movement of the arm or thigh, respectively, in either an anterior direction or toward the midline of the body; horizontal abduction; horizontal plane, vertical axis.

2. Osteokinematics and Arthrokinematics

A. *Osteokinematics* is the study of the movement of the bone in space (1). *Arthrokinematics* is the study of the movement occurring between the articular surfaces of the bones, within the joint (1).

B. *Osteokinematics:* to assess knee joint flexion PROM, the therapist stabilizes the femur and moves the tibia in a posterior direction to the limit of motion; observes, measures, and records the limited posterior movement of the tibia (i.e., limited knee flexion PROM); and considers the impact of the decreased knee flexion PROM on the patient's ADL.

C. *Arthrokinematics:* with the above knowledge, the therapist, knowing that the tibial articular surface is concave, applies the concave-convex rule: with the femur stabilized as the knee is flexed, the tibia moves in a posterior direction, and the concave tibial articular surface will glide in the same direction as the tibia moves (i.e., posterior). The therapist may conclude that the decreased posterior motion of the tibia (i.e., limited knee flexion PROM) is caused by a decreased posterior glide of the tibial articular surface. The therapist may decide that treatment is needed to restore posterior glide of the tibial articular surface to increase knee flexion PROM.

3. Contraindications and Precautions for ROM Assessment

A. AROM and PROM assessment techniques are contraindicated when muscle contraction (AROM) or motion (AROM and PROM) of the part could disrupt the healing process or result in injury or deterioration of the patient's condition.

B. The therapist would likely not perform an assessment of AROM and PROM in this case because the patient is under the influence of alcohol and may not be able to respond appropriately during the assessment.

If alcohol were not a factor, the therapist would consider the following precautions: status of fracture healing unknown; osteoporosis (general and upper extremity bone density); degree of pain experienced; and psychological state. The therapist may proceed with caution, carefully monitoring the patient's response to assessment.

4. The Rationale for the Assessment of AROM and PROM

A. Anatomical position for the knee and ankle (see Figs. 1-13 through 1-15).

ii. The hamstrings could restrict knee extension AROM because the muscles are already lengthened over the flexed hip joint in high sitting.

Alternate start position: supine as the hip is in extension, placing the hamstrings on slack at the non-test joint.

iii. Assessing Mr. Fitzgerald's AROM would provide the therapist with information about his ability to follow directions, attention span, and willingness to move; coordination; movements that cause or increase pain; ability to move the part through a full ROM; and ability to perform ADL.

iv. The therapist could not determine the reason for the decreased movement from the AROM assessment alone. The therapist must perform additional assessment techniques, such as assessment of the PROM, muscle strength, and special tests as required. Assessment of PROM will indicate if there is lack of movement at the joint; muscle strength testing will indicate if the muscle is too weak to move the limb through the PROM available at the joint. Special tests may also be necessary to determine the reason for the limited movement.

v. Mr. Fitzgerald's PROM would be assessed to determine the amount of movement possible at the joint; the quality of movement throughout the ROM; what structure(s) limit the movement by assessing the end feel; the presence or absence of pain; and whether a capsular or non-capsular pattern of movement exists.

B. Knee flexion AROM = PROM and the empty end feel with the complaint of knee pain indicates the joint cannot be moved through more than 60° flexion due to pain. Further assessment of the knee is required to determine the cause of the knee pain.

Knee extension AROM < PROM and the end feel is firm. Full extension PROM is possible at the knee joint and the end feel is normal, but the patient cannot actively move the knee into full knee extension. This is probably due to the knee extensor muscles being too weak to move the knee through the available full knee extension PROM.

Ankle dorsiflexion: the limited AROM is only slightly less than the limited PROM. The firm end feel and stretching sensation over the calf indicate that the resistance of the stretched calf muscles limits the ankle ROM.

5. Assessment and Measurement of AROM and PROM Using the Universal Goniometer

A. ii. a) You may have used some or all of the following substitute movements: trunk extension, scapular depression, shoulder flexion, wrist flexion.

b) Substitute motion can be avoided if the therapist provides appropriate instruction to the patient,

manually stabilizes the proximal joint segment (i.e., humerus in this case), and/or positions the patient to prevent unwanted movement.

c) The change in position from sitting to supine lying should have reduced the possible substitute movement, as the trunk and scapula are better stabilized.

6. Validity and Reliability: Universal Goniometer

A. *Validity* is "the degree to which an instrument measures what it is supposed to measure" (2, p. 171). *Reliability* is "the extent to which the instrument yields the same measurement on repeated uses either by the same operator (intraobserver reliability) or by different operators (interobserver reliability)" (3, p. 49).

B. Reliable joint ROM measurements are obtained by having the same therapist take the repeated measures, using a rigid standardized measurement protocol.

This involves using the same goniometer in the same clinical setting; assessing the patient at the same time of day and in a consistent manner relative to the application of treatment techniques; and using the same patient position, instructions, and accurate method of applying and reading the goniometer.

8. Using the OB "Myrin" Goniometer to Measure Joint ROM

i. The OB goniometer consists of a fluid-filled rotatable container consisting of a compass needle to measure movements in the horizontal plane, and an inclination needle to measure movements in the vertical plane. The floor of the container has a scale marked in 2° increments. The OB goniometer is attached via Velcro straps and plastic extension plates to the limb segment at a predetermined position in relation to bony landmarks, either proximal or distal to the joint being assessed.

With the patient in the start position, the fluid-filled container is rotated until the 0° arrow lines up directly underneath the needle used for the measurement. The patient moves through the ROM and the number of degrees the needle moves away from the 0° arrow on the scale is recorded as the joint ROM.

ii. The *advantages* of using the OB goniometer to measure joint ROM compared to the universal goniometer are:

It is not necessary to align the inclinometer with the joint axis.

Rotational movements using a compass inclinometer are measured with ease.

Assessment of trunk and neck ROM is done easily.

There is little change in the alignment of the goniometer throughout the ROM.

PROM is more easily assessed using the OB goniometer, as the therapist does not have to hold the goniometer and can stabilize the proximal joint segment with one hand while passively moving the distal segment with the other hand.

The *disadvantages* of using the OB goniometer compared to the universal goniometer are:

It is expensive and bulky compared to the universal goniometer.

It cannot be used to measure the small joints of the hand and foot.

Magnetic fields, other than those of Earth, will cause the compass needle to deviate and must be avoided.

References

1. MacConaill MA, Basmajian JV. *Muscles and Movements: A Basis for Human Kinesiology.* 2nd ed. New York: Robert E. Krieger; 1977.
2. Currier DP. *Elements of Research in Physical Therapy.* 3rd ed. Baltimore: Williams & Wilkins; 1990.
3. Sim J, Arnell P. Measurement validity in physical therapy research. *Phys Ther.* 1993;73:48–56.

Chapter 2: Relating Treatment to Assessment

1. *Purpose*: The therapist selects assessment or treatment based on the outcome required.

   General Procedure: The therapist employs the general procedure as follows:

   Explanation and instruction: to explain and demonstrate the assessment or treatment to the patient and obtain the patient's informed consent.

   Expose the region to be assessed or treated and drape the patient as required.

   Start position: appropriate for the assessment or treatment; ensures the patient is safe, comfortable, and adequately supported.

   Stabilization: to allow only the desired movement.

   Movement: the appropriate movement is performed.

   Assistance: provided for passive movement.

   End position is achieved.

   Substitute movement: ensure no substitute movement.

   Purpose-Specific Procedure: Purpose-specific procedure is carried out to meet the purpose of the assessment or treatment.

   Charting: For assessment, record deviations from standardized testing procedure and assessment findings. For treatment, record purpose-specific procedures used in treatment and any change in the patient's condition.

2. The purpose for which assessment and treatment are used is different. Assessment is used to assess deficiencies. Treatment is used to alleviate deficiencies.

Therefore, after employing the general procedure used for similar assessment and treatment, purpose-specific procedures are used to meet the purpose of either the assessment or the treatment used.

3. The general procedure (i.e., explanation and instruction, expose the region, start position, stabilization, movement, assistance, end position, and substitute movement) is the same. The purpose, purpose-specific procedure, and charting are different).

4. A. Active exercise

   B. Relaxed passive movement

   C. Prolonged passive stretch

5. A. Muscle length assessment

   B. Prolonged passive stretch

   C. The general procedure for the treatment is identical to the general procedure used to assess muscle length for tensor fascia latae. Therefore, the practical evaluation form for the assessment of tensor fascia latae muscle length (see Appendix E) can be used to check the correctness of the general procedure used to treat and increase the length of the tensor fascia latae. To meet the specific purpose of the treatment (i.e., to increase muscle length), the muscle would be held on stretch for a prescribed length of time.

6. A. PROM assessment

   B. Relaxed passive movement

   C. The general procedure for the treatment is identical to the general procedure used to assess PROM for hip flexion. Therefore, the practical evaluation form for the assessment of hip flexion PROM (see Appendix E) could be used to check the correctness of the general procedure used to treat and maintain the hip flexion ROM. The passive movement would then be performed according to the treatment prescription (e.g., a prescribed number of repetitions, a prescribed number of times a day).

7. A. AROM assessment

   B. Active exercise

   C. The general procedure for the treatment is identical to the general procedure used to assess AROM for elbow flexion. The general treatment procedure specific to maintaining or increasing elbow flexion AROM would be performed according to the exercise prescription (e.g., a prescribed number of repetitions, a prescribed number of times a week).

Chapter 3: Shoulder Complex

1. Palpation

A. i. Horizontal abduction and adduction; axis.

   Shoulder elevation through flexion/glenohumeral joint flexion and extension; axis (i.e., 2.5 cm inferior to the lateral aspect of the acromion process).

   ii. Shoulder elevation through flexion/glenohumeral joint flexion and extension; stationary arm.

iii. Shoulder internal and external rotation; axis.

iv. Shoulder elevation through flexion/glenohumeral joint flexion and extension; moveable arm.

Shoulder elevation through abduction/glenohumeral joint abduction/adduction; moveable arm. Horizontal abduction and adduction; moveable arm.

2. Assessment of AROM at the Shoulder Complex

A. i. The <u>shoulder complex</u> is made up of the sternoclavicular, acromioclavicular, scapulothoracic, and glenohumeral articulations.

ii. The <u>shoulder girdle</u> is made up of the sternoclavicular, acromioclavicular, and scapulothoracic articulations.

iii. The <u>shoulder joint</u> is made up of the glenohumeral joint (the shoulder joint can also be referred to as the glenohumeral joint).

B. True

C. Refer to the section in Chapter 3 titled "General Scan: Upper Extremity Active Range of Motion."

D i. Elevation, depression, protraction, retraction, medial (downward) rotation, and lateral (upward) rotation. Elevation—movement of the scapula in an upward or cranial direction. Depression—movement of the scapula in a downward or caudal direction. Protraction—movement of the scapula in a lateral direction over the thorax. Retraction—movement of the scapula in a medial direction over the thorax. Medial (downward) rotation—movement of the inferior angle of the scapula toward the midline and movement of the glenoid cavity in a downward (caudal) direction. Lateral (upward) rotation—movement of the inferior angle of the scapula away from the midline and movement of the glenoid cavity in an upward (cranial) direction. Scapular medial (downward) rotation—shoulder extension and adduction to place the hand across the small of the back.

ii. Scapular lateral (upward) rotation—shoulder elevation through flexion or abduction.

E. i. Extension: Scapular anterior tilting, scapular elevation, and shoulder abduction; with the patient in sitting, trunk flexion and ipsilateral trunk rotation may also occur.

ii. Abduction: Contralateral trunk lateral flexion, scapular elevation, and shoulder flexion.

iii. External rotation: In supine with the shoulder in 90° abduction: elbow extension, scapular depression, and shoulder adduction. In sitting with the arm at the side: scapular depression, shoulder adduction, and trunk rotation.

iv. Horizontal abduction: Scapular retraction, ipsilateral trunk rotation.

3. Assessment and Measurement of PROM at the Shoulder Complex

Scapular Elevation

i. Scapulothoracic, acromioclavicular, and sternoclavicular are the articulations where motion could be decreased.

ii. Elevation of the clavicle is associated with scapular elevation.

iii. <u>Inferior</u> glide would be decreased—because the medial end of the clavicle is a convex surface vertically, and the manubrial surface of the sternoclavicular joint is reciprocally concave. Based on the concave/convex theory of movement, a convex surface will glide in the opposite direction to the movement of the bony segment it is a part of. If the manubrium is fixed and the lateral end of the clavicle moves upward (superiorly), the articular surface of the clavicle will glide downward (inferiorly) at the sternoclavicular joint.

Shoulder Elevation Through Flexion and Through Abduction

i. Glenohumeral, scapulothoracic, acromioclavicular, sternoclavicular are the articulations that participate in shoulder elevation through flexion or abduction.

ii. Glenohumeral joint: proximal component—glenoid cavity of the scapula, concave; distal component—head of the humerus, convex. Sternoclavicular joint: medial component—lateral aspect of the manubrium sternum and the adjacent superior surface of the first costal cartilage; convex horizontally, concave vertically; lateral component—medial end of the clavicle; concave horizontally, convex vertically.

Glenohumeral Joint Abduction

i. The therapist places one hand on the superior aspect of the ipsilateral shoulder girdle (i.e., over the scapula and clavicle) to stabilize the shoulder girdle and allow isolated GH joint motion.

ii. Inferior glide of the humeral head would be decreased. The head of the humerus is convex and articulates with the concave glenoid cavity. Based on the concave/convex theory of movement, a convex surface will glide in the opposite direction to the movement of the bony segment it is a part of. If the humerus moves superiorly with glenohumeral joint abduction, the convex head of the humerus will glide inferiorly at the joint during this movement.

Shoulder Extension

The elbow should be in flexion to prevent restriction of shoulder extension due to passive insufficiency of the two-joint biceps brachii muscle (1).

Shoulder Horizontal Adduction

i. Start positions: The patient is sitting. The shoulder is in neutral rotation and in either 90° abduction or 90° flexion. The elbow is flexed and the forearm is in midposition. The start position of the shoulder should be recorded.

Shoulder horizontal abduction would also be assessed using the above start positions.

ii. Posterior glide of the humeral head would be restricted because the head of the humerus is convex and articulates with the concave glenoid cavity. Based on the concave/ convex theory of movement, a convex surface will glide in the opposite direction to the movement of the bony segment it is a part of. If the humerus moves anteriorly with glenohumeral joint horizontal adduction, the convex head of the humerus will glide posteriorly at the joint during this movement.

Shoulder Internal Rotation

i. Motion would be decreased at the glenohumeral joint.

ii. PROM would be assessed to determine end feel for shoulder internal rotation.

iii. If your partner presented with a full PROM for shoulder internal rotation and the end feel was firm, this end feel would be considered a normal end feel. However, if your partner presented with a decreased PROM and the end feel was firm, this end feel would be considered abnormal.

iv. Normal limiting factors that would create a normal firm end feel for shoulder internal rotation are tension in the posterior glenohumeral joint capsule, infraspinatus, and teres minor.

Other Questions

A. Glenohumeral joint movements of abduction, flexion, extension, horizontal abduction and adduction, internal and external rotation

B. i. The AROM may be less than the PROM because the patient may not understand the movement to be performed; may be unwilling to move through the full available ROM; may experience pain that stops the movement when performed actively; or may have muscle weakness that prevents moving the part through the full available PROM.

ii. If AROM = PROM, this may indicate a restriction in mobility at the glenohumeral joint. The cause of this restriction is determined by identifying the end feel at 30° flexion PROM. Possible causes of the restricted ROM could include pain, soft tissue (capsule, ligament, muscle) stretch, bone contacting bone, soft tissue swelling, joint effusion, spasm, or an internal derangement of the joint.

4. Muscle Length Assessment and Measurement

Pectoralis Major

i. Origin (2)—Clavicular head: anterior border of the sternal half of the clavicle; Sternal head: ipsilateral half of the anterior surface of the sternum; cartilage of the first 6 or 7 ribs; sternal end of 6th rib; aponeurosis of the external abdominal oblique. Insertion (2)—Lateral lip of the intertubercular groove of the humerus.

ii. Shoulder horizontal abduction and external rotation are the movements that would position the origin and insertion farther apart.

iii. The therapist would note a firm end feel if the pectoralis major is shortened.

iv. If the pectoralis major is shortened, shoulder horizontal abduction ROM will be restricted proportional to the decrease in muscle length. To assess this restriction, the goniometer axis is placed *on top of the acromion process*, the stationary arm is aligned *perpendicular to the trunk*, and the movable arm is aligned parallel to the *longitudinal axis of the humerus*.

Pectoralis Minor

i. Origin (2)—Outer surfaces of ribs 2 to 4 or 3 to 5 near the costal cartilages; fascia over corresponding external intercostals. Insertion (2)—Medial border and upper surface of the coracoid process of the scapula.

ii. Scapular elevation and retraction would place the muscle on stretch.

iii. If the pectoralis minor is shortened, with the patient in supine, the therapist, standing at the head of the plinth, will observe the shoulder girdle on the affected side to be resting in a protracted position away from the surface of the plinth.

5. Functional ROM at the Shoulder Complex

A. The function of the shoulder complex is to position or move the arm in space for the purpose of hand function.

B. i. It would not be possible to complete any of the activities with the glenohumeral joint fixed in anatomical position using no compensatory movement of other body parts.

ii. Combing hair—shoulder girdle elevation; neck flexion, lateral flexion, and rotation; shoulder internal and external rotation. Brushing teeth—neck flexion and rotation; shoulder internal and external rotation. Eat soup with a spoon—neck and trunk flexion/extension; shoulder internal rotation.

C. i. Extension: Pulling a window down to close it; pushing oneself up on the sides of the tub to get out of the bathtub.

ii. Elevation through flexion: Reaching to place an object on a high shelf; changing a light bulb on the ceiling.

iii. Flexion below shoulder level: Eating with a spoon or fork; drinking from a cup.

iv. External rotation: Combing the hair; manipulating the clasp of a necklace behind the neck.

v. Horizontal adduction: Washing the axilla and the skin over the scapula on the contralateral side of the body; writing on a blackboard at shoulder level.

D. i. Scapulohumeral rhythm is the coordinated movement pattern achieved through scapulothoracic and glenohumeral movement (3–6).

ii. The ratio of glenohumeral motion to scapular motion is 2:1—that is, 2° of glenohumeral motion to every degree of scapular motion (3,5,7,8).

iii. Factors affecting the rhythm are the plane of elevation, arc of elevation, amount of load on the arm, and individual differences (9).

iv. Movement occurs at the glenohumeral, sternoclavicular, acromioclavicular, scapulothoracic, and spinal joints.

v. Setting phase: 0°–60° shoulder flexion; 0°–30° shoulder abduction. The scapula remains relatively stationary, or slightly medially (downward) or laterally (upward) rotates. Most movement occurs at the glenohumeral joint.

vi. From the end of the setting phase to 170° of motion there is a predictable scapulohumeral rhythm of 2° glenohumeral joint motion for every 1° of scapular motion. Scapular motion includes lateral (upward) rotation, accompanied by secondary rotations of posterior tilting (sagittal plane) and a posterior rotation (transverse plane) (10). Full shoulder elevation through abduction depends on full external rotation of the humerus. Full shoulder elevation through flexion depends on the ability to rotate the humerus internally through range (11). The final degrees of elevation beyond 170° are achieved through contralateral trunk lateral flexion and/or trunk extension.

References

1. Gajdosik RL, Hallett JP, Slaughter LL. Passive insufficiency of two-joint shoulder muscles. *Clin Biomech*. 1994;9:377–378.
2. Standring S, ed. Gray's Anatomy: The Anatomical Basis of Clinical Practice. 39th ed. Elsevier Churchill Livingstone, London, 2005.
3. Levangie PK, Norkin CC. *Joint Structure & Function: A Comprehensive Analysis*. 3rd ed. Philadelphia: FA Davis; 2001.
4. Smith LK, Lawrence Weiss E, Lehmkuhl LD. *Brunnstrom's Clinical Kinesiology*. 5th ed. Philadelphia: FA Davis; 1996.
5. Cailliet R. *Shoulder Pain*. 3rd ed. Philadelphia: FA Davis; 1991.
6. Soderberg GL. *Kinesiology: Application to Pathological Motion*. 2nd ed. Baltimore: Williams & Wilkins; 1997.
7. Rosse C. The shoulder region and the brachial plexus. In: Rosse C, Clawson DK, eds. *The Musculoskeletal System in Health and Disease*. New York: Harper & Row; 1980.
8. Inman VT, Saunders M, Abbot LC. Observations on the function of the shoulder joint. *J Bone Joint Surg*. 1944;26:1–30.
9. Matsen FA, Lippitt SB, Sidles JA, Harryman DT. *Practical Evaluation and Management of the Shoulder*. Philadelphia: WB Saunders; 1994.
10. Peat M. The shoulder complex: a review of some aspects of functional anatomy. *Physiother Canada*. 1977;29:241–246.
11. Mallon WJ, Herring CL, Sallay PI, et al. Use of vertebral levels to measure presumed internal rotation at the shoulder: a radiologic analysis. *J Shoulder Elbow Surg*. 1996;5:299–306.

Chapter 4: Elbow and Forearm

1. Palpation

A. i. Elbow flexion/extension: Goniometer axis—lateral epicondyle of the humerus; Stationary arm—tip of the acromion process; Moveable arm—styloid process of the radius.

ii. Forearm supination/pronation: Goniometer axis—head of the third metacarpal or tip of the middle digit; Stationary arm—none (perpendicular to the floor); Moveable arm—parallel to the pencil or parallel to the tips of the four extended fingers.

2. Assessment Process

Records patient's history.

Explains rationale and component parts of assessment.

Observation.

Assessment of AROM.

Measurement of AROM, as required.

Assessment of PROM.

Measurement of PROM, as required.

Assessment and measurement of muscle length, as required.

Assessment of muscle strength.

Application of other assessment techniques, as required.

3. Assessment of AROM at the Elbow and Forearm Articulations

A. Proximal components of the elbow joint: trochlea of the humerus (convex anteroposteriorly); capitulum of the humerus (convexa).

Distal components of the elbow joint: trochlea notch of the ulna (concave); proximal aspect of the head of the radius (concave).

Superior radioulnar joint (located within the capsule of the elbow joint): radial head (convex); radial notch of the ulna (concave).

Inferior radioulnar joint: ulnar head (convex); ulnar notch of the radius (concave).

B. i. Elbow flexion: Bending of the elbow so that the anterior surface of the forearm moves toward the anterior surface of the arm. Elbow extension: Straightening of the elbow. These movements occur around a frontal axis in the sagittal plane.

ii. Forearm supination: rotation of the forearm so that the palm faces upward toward the ceiling. Forearm pronation: rotation of the forearm so that the palm faces downward toward the floor.

a) With the elbow flexed 90°, these movements occur around the axis for supination and pronation (see Fig. 4-2) (i.e., the longitudinal axis, in the frontal plane).

b) With the elbow in 0°, these movements occur in the transverse plane around a longitudinal axis. Shoulder internal rotation augments forearm pronation and shoulder external rotation augments forearm supination, with the elbow extended at 0°.

C. i. Forearm supination: ipsilateral trunk lateral flexion, shoulder adduction, and shoulder external rotation.

ii. Elbow extension: trunk flexion, shoulder extension, and scapular elevation.

iii. Elbow flexion: trunk extension, shoulder flexion, and scapular depression.

iv. Forearm pronation: contralateral trunk lateral flexion, shoulder abduction and shoulder internal rotation.

D. AROM may be less than PROM because the patient may: not understand the movement to be performed, be unwilling to move through the full available PROM, experience pain that stops the movement when performed actively, or have muscle weakness that prevents moving the part through the full available PROM.

4. Assessment and Measurement of PROM at the Elbow and Forearm

Elbow Flexion

i. A soft or firm or hard end feel are the normal end feels expected when assessing elbow flexion.

ii. True

iv. Refer to Table 4-1.

Elbow Extension/Hyperextension

i. Biceps brachii. The muscle is placed on stretch if the shoulder is in *extension*, and the forearm is *pronated*. Therefore, the therapist ensures the forearm is *supinated* and the shoulder is in *anatomical* (i.e., 0°) to avoid biceps brachii from restricting elbow extension.

ii. Posterior glide of the trochlea of the ulna and the radial head would cause decreased elbow extension PROM.

iii. The proximal aspect of the radial head and the trochlear surface of the ulna are concave surfaces. Based on the concave/convex theory of movement, a concave surface will glide in the same direction of movement as the bony segment it is a part of. The ulna and radius bone segments move in a posterior direction when the elbow is extended, therefore the concave articular surfaces with glide in a posterior direction.

Forearm Supination

i. Motion could be decreased at the superior radioulnal joint, the inferior radioulnar joint and/or the humeroradial joint in the presence of decreased forearm supination PROM.

ii. The radial head spins on the capitulum when the forearm is supinated.

iii. Anterior glide of the radial head could be limited if forearm supination ROM is decreased.

iv. The radial head is a convex surface and the radial notch of the ulna is a concave surface. Based on the concave/convex theory of movement, a convex surface will glide in the opposite direction as the bone segment of which it is a part. The radius moves posteriorly and the radial head glides anteriorly when the forearm is supinated.

v. In full supination, the radius lies <u>alongside</u> the ulna.

Forearm Pronation

ii. Normal end feels for forearm pronation are hard or firm.

iii. A hard end feel for forearm pronation is the result of contact of the radius and the ulna. A firm end feel for forearm pronation results from tension in the quadrate ligament, the dorsal radioulnar ligament of the inferior radioulnar joint, the distal tract of the interosseous membrane, supinator and biceps brachii muscles with the elbow in extension.

iv. From full supination to full pronation the radius <u>rotates</u> around the relatively <u>stationary</u> ulna.

5. Muscle Length Assessment and Measurement

Triceps

i. Origin (1): Long head: infraglenoid tubercle of the scapula; Lateral head: posterolateral surface of the humerus between the radial groove and the insertion of teres minor; lateral intermuscular septum; Medial head: posterior surface of the humerus below the radial groove between the trochlea of the humerus and the insertion of teres major; medial and lateral intermuscular septum. Insertion (1): Posteriorly on the proximal surface of the olecranon; some fibers continue distally to blend with the antebrachial fascia.

ii. Shoulder flexion and elbow flexion would place the triceps on stretch.

iii. A therapist would identify a <u>firm</u> end feel at the limit of <u>elbow flexion</u> PROM in the presence of a shortened triceps muscle.

6. Functional ROM at the Elbow and Forearm

A. i. a) In standing it would not be possible to contact parts of the body proximal to the hips, and the posterolateral aspect of the contralateral hip with the elbow fixed in 0° extension.

b) In sitting it would not be possible to contact parts of the body proximal to the mid-thigh level with the elbow fixed in 0° extension.

ii. Eating, drinking, brushing the teeth, combing or washing the hair, using the phone, dressing (i.e., doing up buttons, putting on a belt), and perineal hygiene would be impossible to perform with the elbow fixed in 0° extension.

B. i. a) If standing it would be very difficult to contact areas distal to the mid-calf.

b) If sitting it would be very difficult to contact areas distal to the mid-calf.

ii. In most cases, all personal care ADL (i.e., feeding and personal hygiene) can be performed with the elbow fixed in a position of 90° flexion (2, 3).

C. The ROM requirements for ADL are influenced by the design of the furniture used, the placement of utensils, and the patient's posture. The start and the end positions and technique used to complete the activity also affect the ROM requirements. Therefore, the ROM values provided below are a guide only.

   i. Drinking from a cup requires about 129° (4) of elbow flexion.

   ii. Holding the telephone to the ear requires about 136° to 140° (5, 6) of elbow flexion.

   iii. Tying a shoe lace requires about 16° (5) of elbow flexion.

   iv. Combing the hair on the back of the head requires about 144° (5) of elbow flexion.

   v. Reaching for a wallet in a back pocket requires about 70° (5) of elbow flexion

D. i. Forearm pronation is required to pick up a small object from a table top.

   ii. Forearm supination is required to receive change in the palm of the hand.

   iii. Forearm pronation and forearm supination are required to eat with a fork.

   iv. Forearm supination is required to reach a wallet in a back pocket.

   v. Forearm supination is required to comb the hair on the vertex of the head.

E. According to Morrey and colleagues (5), many self-care activities can be accomplished within the arc of movement from 30° to 130° elbow flexion and from 50° of pronation to 50° of supination.

References

1. Standring S, ed. Gray's Anatomy: The Anatomical Basis of Clinical Practice. 39th ed. Elsevier Churchill Livingstone, London, 2005.

2. Vasen AP, Lacey SH, Keith MW, Shaffer JW. Functional range of motion of the elbow. *J Hand Surg [Am].* 1995; 20:288–292.

3. Nagy SM, Szabo RM, Sharkey NA. Unilateral elbow arthrodesis: the preferred position. *J South Orthop Assoc.* 1999;8(2):80–85.

4. Safaee-Rad R, Shwedyk E, Quanbury AO, Cooper JE. Normal functional range of motion of upper limb joints during performance of three feeding activities. *Arch Phys Med Rehabil.* 1990;71: 505–509.

5. Morrey BF, Askew LJ, An KN, Chao EY. A biomechanical study of normal functional elbow motion. *J Bone Joint Surg [Am].* 1981;63:872–876.

6. Packer TL, Peat M, Wyss U, Sorbie C. Examining the elbow during functional activities. *Occup Ther J Res.* 1990;10: 323–333.

Chapter 5: Wrist and Hand

1. Palpation

   i. Styloid process of ulna: Wrist flexion and extension.

   ii. Distal palmar crease: Finger IP and MCP joint flexion (linear measurement of finger flexion to evaluate impairment of hand function).

   iii. Third metacarpal bone: Wrist radial and ulnar deviation; abduction of the third metacarpal; MCP joint flexion and extension of the middle digit.

   iv. First carpometacarpal joint: Thumb CM joint flexion and extension.

   v. Capitate bone: Wrist radial and ulnar deviation.

   vi. Lateral aspect of the PIP joint line: PIP joint flexion and extension.

2. Assessment Process

   i. True

   ii. False—PROM is used to determine an end feel.

   iii. True

   iv. False—AROM can also be measured using a goniometer.

3. Assessment of AROM at the Wrist and Hand Articulations

A. Make a fist: observe AROM of finger flexion, thumb flexion and adduction, and wrist extension. The hand is opened and fingers spread as far as possible: observe AROM of finger extension and abduction, thumb extension, and wrist flexion.

B. i. Radiocarpal joint—the proximal surface of the proximal row of carpal bones (i.e., the scaphoid, lunate, triquetrum) is convex and articulates with the concave surface of the distal aspect of the radius and the articular disc of the inferior radioulnar joint. Midcarpal joint—the proximal aspect of the distal row of carpal bones has a concave surface laterally (formed by the trapezoid and trapezium) and a convex surface medially (formed by the hamate and capitate). These surfaces articulate with the corresponding convex (formed by the scaphoid) and concave (formed by the scaphoid, lunate, and triquetrum) surfaces, respectively, on the distal aspect of the proximal row of carpal bones.

   ii. The CM joint of the thumb is formed by the distal surface of the trapezium, which is concave anteroposteriorly and convex mediolaterally and articulates with the corresponding reciprocal surface of the base of the first metacarpal.

   iii. The MCP joints are each formed proximally by the convex head of the metatarsal articulating with the concave base of the adjacent proximal phalanx. The IP joints are each formed by the convex head of the proximal phalanx articulating with the concave base of the adjacent distal phalanx.

C. i. Wrist extension—movement of the hand in a posterior direction so that the posterior aspect of the hand moves toward the posterior aspect of the forearm; movement occurs in a sagittal plane around a frontal axis.

   ii. Thumb abduction—the thumb moves in an anterior direction in a plane perpendicular to the palm of the hand; movement occurs in an oblique sagittal plane around an oblique frontal axis.

iii. Thumb extension at the CM joint—the thumb moves in the plane of the palm of the hand in a lateral direction away from the index finger; movement occurs in an oblique frontal plane around an oblique sagittal axis.

iv. Finger abduction—movement of the finger away from the midline of the hand (i.e., the third digit); movement occurs in the frontal plane around a sagittal axis.

v. Finger flexion at the PIP joint—bending of the finger so that the anterior aspect of the finger at the middle phalanx moves closer to the anterior aspect of the finger at the proximal phalanx; movement occurs in the sagittal plane around a frontal axis.

D. Ulnar deviation of the fingers, wrist flexion, or wrist extension are the subsitute movements that may give the appearance of a greater range of wrist ulnar deviation than is actually present.

4. Assessment and Measurement of PROM at the Wrist and Hand

Wrist Ulnar Deviation

i. Firm

ii. Refer to Table 5-1.

iv. The goniometer is positioned on the posterior aspect of the wrist joint with the axis over the capitate bone.

v. False. The movable arm of the goniometer is aligned with the longitudinal axis of the third metacarpal. Maintaining this alignment prevents motion of the third finger at the MCP joint from being incorporated into the measurement for wrist ulnar deviation ROM.

Wrist Extension

i. An anterior glide of the proximal row of carpal bones at the radiocarpal joint could be decreased if wrist extension PROM is decreases.

ii. Based on the concave/convex theory of movement, a convex surface will glide in the opposite direction to the movement of the bony segment it is a part of. Therefore, during wrist extension, as the distal end of the bones that make up the proximal row of carpal bones move in a posterior direction, the convex surfaces of the proximal ends of the proximal row of carpal bones glide in the opposite direction (i.e., anteriorly) on the fixed concave surface of the distal radius and articular disc of the inferior radioulnar joint.

iii. The goniometer alignment for wrist extension is also used to assess wrist flexion and muscle length for the long finger flexors (flexor digitorum superficialis and profundus, flexor digiti minimi, and palmaris longus) and the long finger extensors (extensor digitorum communis, extensor indicis proprius, and extensor digiti minimi.

iv. When assessing wrist extension PROM the fingers are relaxed and should be free to move into flexion to prevent stretch of the long finger flexors that could limit wrist extension PROM.

MCP Joint Extension of the Fingers and Thumb

i. In this case the end feel occurred before the full normal PROM was reached, so the firm end feel would not be considered a normal end feel. A normal end feel exists when there is a full normal PROM at the joint and the normal anatomy at the joint stops movement.

ii. A posterior glide of the base of the proximal phalanx of the thumb would be decreased with decreased thumb MCP joint extension. Based on the concave/convex theory of movement, the concave surface of the base of the proximal phalanx will glide in the same direction as the movement of the proximal phalanx it is a part of. As the thumb extends, the proximal phalanx moves in a posterior direction and the concave base of the phalanx glides in a posterior direction.

iii. Flexion, extension is the capsular pattern at the MCP joints.

iv. The wrist is positioned in slight flexion to prevent stretch of the long finger flexors from restricting MCP joint extension ROM.

Finger MCP Joint Abduction

i. Firm

ii. Refer to Table 5-2.

Thumb CM Joint

i. Carpometacarpal flexion, extension, and abduction (opposition—using the ruler on the universal goniometer to take a linear measurement)

ii. Stabilize the trapezium, wrist, and forearm.

Ring Finger PIP Flexion

i. Hard/soft/firm

ii. Refer to Table 5-2.

Thumb Opposition

i. Opposition is a sequential movement that incorporates <u>abduction, flexion,</u> and <u>adduction</u> of the first metacarpal, with simultaneous <u>rotation</u> (1).

ii. <u>First CM</u> Joint

5. Muscle Length Assessment and Measurement

Flexor Digitorum Superficialis, Flexor Digitorum Profundus, Flexor Digiti Minimi, and Palmaris Longus

i. Elbow extension; the elbow is held in this position to ensure full stretch is placed on the flexor digitorum superficialis and palmaris longus that have origins proximal to the elbow joint.

ii. If the length of the finger flexors is decreased, with the elbow extended, the forearm supinated and the fingers <u>extended</u>, wrist <u>extension</u> PROM will be restricted proportional to the decrease in muscle length. To assess this PROM restriction using a universal goniometer, the goniometer axis is placed at the <u>level of the ulnar styloid process</u>, the stationary arm is aligned parallel to the <u>longitudinal axis of the ulna</u>, and the movable arm is aligned parallel to the <u>longitudinal axis of the fifth metacarpal</u>. The therapist will note a <u>firm</u> end feel at the end of the restricted wrist PROM.

Lumbricales

i. The wrist is positioned in extension to place the flexor digitorum profundus on stretch and thus assist in stabilizing the origin of the lumbricales on the tendons of the flexor digitorum profundus.

ii. If the length of the lumbricales is decreased, with the wrist in extension and the fingers <u>flexed</u>, MCP joint <u>extension</u> PROM will be restricted proportional to the degree of muscle shortness.

Extensor Digitorum Communis, Extensor Indicis Proprius, and Extensor Digiti Minimi

i. If the length of the long finger extensors is decreased, with the elbow <u>extended</u>, forearm pronated, and fingers <u>flexed</u>, wrist <u>flexion</u> PROM will be restricted proportional to the degree of muscle shortness.

6. Functional ROM at the Wrist and Hand

A. Wrist extension and ulnar deviation (2) are the two most important wrist positions or movements for ADL.

B. For feeding activities (i.e., drinking from a cup or glass, eating using a fork or spoon, and cutting using a knife), the ROM requirements are approximately <u>3°</u> wrist flexion to <u>35°</u> wrist extension (3,4) and from <u>20°</u> ulnar deviation to <u>5°</u> of radial deviation (4).

C. The wrist: Optimizes the function of the hand to touch, grasp, or manipulate objects; positions the hand in space relative to the forearm (5); serves to transmit load between the hand and forearm (5); serves to control the length–tension relations of the extrinsic muscles of the hand.

D. The functions of the hand are: Grasp, communication, manipulation of objects, receiving of sensory information from the environment.

E. <u>CM</u> joints. In the clinical setting, it is not possible to directly measure movements at the CM joints of the second through fifth metacarpals.

F. i. Wrist flexion—hooking a bra at the back, brushing one's teeth.

ii. Wrist extension—writing, holding a glass.

iii. Wrist radial deviation—hammering, painting a wall using long brush strokes.

iv. Wrist ulnar deviation—hammering, opening a jar.

v. Finger flexion—writing, turning a doorknob to open a door

vi. Finger extension—carrying a tray over one's shoulder with the wrist in extension, using the hand to push up on a chair seat to standing;

vii. Thumb opposition—picking up the telephone receiver, threading a needle.

viii. Marked loss of wrist ROM may not significantly hinder a patient's ability to carry out ADL; however, activities of work or recreation were not included in this study.

References

1. Levangie PK, Norkin CC. *Joint Structure and Function: A Comprehensive Analysis*. 3rd ed. Philadelphia: FA Davis; 2001.
2. Ryu J, Cooney WP, Askew LJ, et al. Functional ranges of motion of the wrist joint. *J Hand Surg [Am]*. 1991;16: 409–419.
3. Brumfield RH, Champoux JA. A biomechanical study of normal functional wrist motion. *Clin Orthop*. 1984;187: 23–25.
4. Safaee-Rad R, Shwedyk E, Quanbury AO, Cooper JE. Normal functional range of motion of upper limb joints during performance of three feeding activities. *Arch Phys Med Rehabil*. 1990;71:505–509.
5. Nordin M, Frankel VH. *Basic Biomechanics of the Musculoskeletal System*. 3rd ed. Philadelphia: Lippincott Williams & Wilkins; 2001.

Chapter 6: Hip

1. Palpation

B. i. Hip flexion/extension; axis.

ii. Hip internal/external rotation; movable arm.

iii. Hip abduction/adduction; axis.

iv. Hip flexion/extension; movable arm.

v. Hip internal/external rotation; axis.

C. i. Adductor magnus

ii. Biceps femoris, semitendinosus, semimembranosus

2. Assessment of AROM at the Hip Joint

A. Acetabulum—concave shape; femoral head—convex shape.

B. i. Hip extension: movement of the thigh in a posterior direction, in a sagittal plane about a frontal axis; reciprocal movement—flexion.

ii. Hip internal rotation: movement of the anterior surface of the thigh toward the midline of the body, in a transverse plane about a vertical/longitudinal axis; reciprocal movement—external rotation.

iii. Abduction: movement of the thigh away from the midline, in the frontal plane about a sagittal axis; reciprocal movement—adduction.

C. i. See Figures 6-11 and 6-12 and accompanying text.

ii. See Figures 6-13 and 6-14 and accompanying text.

D. Lumbar spine—flexion, extension, lateral flexion, rotation

Hip—flexion, extension, abduction, adduction, internal rotation, external rotation

Knee—flexion, extension

Ankle—dorsiflexion, plantarflexion, inversion, eversion

E. The patient must have the ability to bear full weight through the lower extremities, good balance, and adequate lower extremity muscle strength to support body weight in single-leg stance.

F.   i. Hip flexion: Posterior pelvic tilt; lumbar spine flexion.

ii. Hip abduction: External rotation and flexion of the hip; hiking of the ipsilateral pelvis.

iii. Hip internal rotation: Lateral tilting of the pelvis; in sitting, shifting body weight to raise the pelvis and lift the buttocks off the sitting surface.

3. Assessment and Measurement of PROM at the Hip Joint

A. *Hip Flexion*

i.   The knee was in flexion.

ii. The knee was in flexion to place the two-joint hamstring muscles on slack at the knee so as not to limit the hip flexion ROM.

iii. The normal end feel for hip flexion is soft or firm.

iv. Refer to Table 6–1

Hip Extension

i.   The knee was in extension on the test side.

ii. The knee was in extension to place the two-joint rectus femoris muscle on slack at the knee so that the rectus femoris does not limit the hip flexion ROM.

iii. If stabilization was inadequate, anterior pelvic tilt and extension of the lumbar spine would result in erroneously large PROM values.

iv. Spin is the femoral head motion that could be decreased.

Hip Abduction

i.   The leg(s) is/are perpendicular to an imaginary line drawn between the ASISs.

ii. Inferior glide could be restricted.

iii. The femoral head is a convex articular surface, and in accordance with the concave/convex theory of joint motion, the convex surface will move in the opposite direction to the movement of the bone that moves in a superior direction. Thus, the convex articular surface moves in an inferior direction.

Hip Internal Rotation

i.   Your partner's end feel would be considered normal if your partner had full PROM and a firm end feel.

ii. The normal limiting factors that create a normal end feel are tension in the ischiofemoral ligament, the posterior joint capsule, and the external rotator muscles of the hip.

iii. Start positions are sitting, supine, sit lying, and prone.

iv. The following femoral head glides could be limited: a posterior glide with the hip in anatomical position and an inferior glide with the hip in 90° flexion.

v.   The femoral head is a convex articular surface, and in accordance with the concave/convex theory of joint motion, the convex surface will move in the - opposite direction to the movement of the bone that moves in an anterior direction with the hip in anatomical position and a superior direction with the hip in 90° flexion. Thus, the convex articular surface of the femoral head will glide in a posterior direction with the hip in anatomical position or in an inferior direction with the hip in 90° flexion.

B. Capsular; a total joint reaction at the hip joint in which the entire joint capsule is affected.

4. Muscle Length Assessment and Measurement

Hamstrings

i.   Posterior tilt position.

ii. extended beyond 20° knee flexion.

iii. The end feel is firm.

Hip Flexors

i.   Iliacus, psoas major, tensor fascia latae, sartorius, and rectus femoris are the muscles for which muscle length is being assessed.

ii. The nontest hip is held in flexion to flatten and stabilize the lumbar spine and pelvis in a neutral position and thus avoid the substitute motions of increased anterior pelvic tilt and lumbar lordosis from obscuring the presence of a hip flexion contracture.

iii. Increased lumbar lordosis can mask a hip flexion contracture.

iv. When assessing the hips flexor muscle length the hip is positioned in abduction to place the tensor fascia latae on slack.

Tensor Fascia Latae

i.   Origin (1)—anterior aspect of the outer lip of the iliac crest; the outer surface and notch below the ASIS; and the deep surface of the fascia latae. Insertion (1)—via the iliotibial tract onto the lateral aspect of the lateral condyle of the tibia. Hip adduction, hip extension, hip lateral rotation, and knee flexion are the positions that place maximal stretch on the simulated tensor fascia latae.

ii. The ober's test: trunk prone offers optimal stability of pelvis and lumbar spine.

5. Functional ROM at the Hip Joint

B. i. Riding a bicycle; sitting with the foot across the opposite thigh to tie a shoelace; in a theater stepping sideways past others to take one's seat.

ii. Sitting with one thigh across the other; making an immediate turn in standing while pivoting on one leg and continuing the turn by adducting the contralateral leg; sitting with the legs outstretched and the legs crossed at the ankles.

iii. Mounting a bicycle; squatting to the floor to pick up an object; placing one's foot out of the car to get out of the car; kicking a door closed with the lateral aspect of the foot when the knee is flexed.

iv. Examining the skin on the sole of the foot when performing foot hygiene activities; kicking a ball with the inside of the foot; sitting reaching down to tie a shoe on the floor.

C. i. The hip joint transmits forces between the ground and the pelvis to support body weight (e.g., standing; jumping) and acts as a fulcrum for the pelvis in single-leg stance (e.g., when lifting the foot up to ascend stairs). Hip movement moves the body closer to or farther from the ground (e.g., squatting to pick up an object from the ground; rising from sitting position), brings the foot closer to the body (e.g., to cut the toenails or pull on a sock), and positions the lower limb in space (e.g., moving the foot from the gas pedal to the brake; when stepping onto large stones to cross a creek).

ii. Common ADL can be accomplished in a normal manner with hip ROM of at least 20° flexion, 20° abduction, and 20° external rotation. (2)

References

1. Standring S, ed. Gray's Anatomy: The Anatomical Basis of Clinical Practice. 39th ed. Elsevier Chruchill Livingstone, London, 2005.
2. Johnston RC. Sonidt GL. Hip motion measurements for selected activities of daily living. *Clin Orthop and Related Research.* 1970;72:205–215.

Chapter 7: Knee

1. Palpation

A.

i. Knee flexion/extension
    Goniometer axis—lateral epicondyle of the femur
    Stationary arm—greater trochanter of the femur
    Moveable arm—lateral malleolus of the fibula

ii. Hamstrings or rectus femoris
    Goniometer axis—lateral epicondyle of the femur
    Stationary arm—greater trochanter of the femur
    moveable arm—lateral malleolus of the fibula

iii. True

2. Assessment Process

Records patient's history.

Explains rationale and component parts of assessment.

Observation.

Assessment of AROM.

Measurement of AROM, as required.

Assessment of PROM.

Measurement of PROM, as required.

Assessment and measurement of muscle length, as required.

Assessment of muscle strength.

Application of other assessment techniques, as required.

3. Assessment of AROM at the Knee Articulations

A. Femorotibial articulation: proximal components—convex femoral condyles; distal components—concave tibial condyles

Patellofemoral articulation: patellar surface—the surface is divided by a vertical ridge; the articular surface is flat or slightly convex mediolaterally and supero-inferiorly

Anterior surface of the femur—the surface is divided by the intercondylar groove; the articular surface is concave mediolaterally and convex superoinferiorly.

B. Femorotibial joint movement: Knee flexion—bending of the knee so that the posterior surface of the calf moves toward the posterior surface of the thigh; Knee extension—straightening of the knee in the opposite direction to flexion. These movements occur around a frontal axis in the sagittal plane. Internal tibial rotation—turning of the anterior surface of the tibia toward the midline of the body. External tibial rotation—turning of the anterior surface of the tibia away from the midline of the body. These movements occur around a longitudinal axis in the horizontal plane.

4. Assessment and Measurement of PROM at the Knee

Knee Flexion

i. A firm or soft end feel is normal.

ii. For normal limiting factors, refer to Table 7-1.

iii. If knee flexion ROM were assessed with the hip in 0° extension, the rectus femoris would be stretched at the hip and could restrict knee flexion ROM.

Knee Extension

i. If the hip were placed in flexion, the hamstrings could restrict knee extension ROM.

ii. Anterior glide would be decreased. The tibial condyles are concave surfaces. Based on the concave/convex theory of movement, a concave surface will glide in the same direction of movement as the bony segment it is a part of. When the knee is extended the tibia moves in an anterior direction; therefore, the concave articular surface of the tibia will glide in an anterior direction.

Tibial Rotation

i. Normal end feels are firm for tibial internal rotation and firm for tibial external rotation.

iii. Normal limiting factors—Tibial internal rotation: tension in the cruciate ligaments; tibial external rotation: tension in collateral ligaments (1).

Patellar Mobility

i. Patellar glides: distal glide, medial-lateral glide.

ii. Normal vertical displacement: 8 cm (2).

iii. Normal PROM: 9.6 mm medially and 5.4 mm laterally (3).

5. Muscle Length Assessment and Measurement

Rectus Femoris

i. Pelvis

iii. a) *Supine*: The patient's supine position and holding of the nontest hip in flexion stabilize the pelvis and lumbar spine. The therapist observes the anterior superior iliac spine (ASIS) to ensure there is no pelvic tilting.

b) *Prone*: Test position 1 (See Fig. 7–21): The patient's prone position (nontest leg over the side of the plinth, hip flexed, foot on floor) stabilizes the pelvis. A strap may also be placed over the buttocks to stabilize the pelvis. Test position 2 (see Fig. 7–23) The patient's prone position helps to stabilize the pelvis. A strap may also be placed over the buttocks to stabilize the pelvis. The therapist observes the pelvis to ensure there is no anterior tilting of the pelvis.

6. Functional ROM at the Knee

A. The ROM requirements for ADL are influenced by the design of the furniture used, the placement of objects, and the patient's posture. The start and the end positions and technique used to complete the activity also affect the ROM requirements. Therefore, the ROM values provided below are a guide only.

i. About 117° (4) knee flexion

ii. About 93° (4) knee flexion

iii. About 106° (4) knee flexion

iv. About 83° to 105° (5) knee flexion

v. About 86° to 107° (5) knee flexion

B. Walking requires a Rom from about 0° of knee extension as the leg advances forward to make initial contact with the ground to a maximum of about 60° of knee flexion at initial swing so that the foot clears the ground as the extremity is advanced forward (from the Rancho Los Amigos gait analysis forms, as cited in Levangie and Norkin [6]).

C. Tibial rotation occurs in ADL that require movement into full knee extension or require knee flexion from a position of full knee extension (i.e., at the beginning of knee flexion, the tibia automatically rotates internally on the femur, and at the end of knee extension the tibia automatically rotates externally), or twisting movements of the body when the foot is planted on the ground (7).

References

1. Kapandji IA. *The Physiology of the Joints.* Vol. 2. 2nd ed. New York: Churchill Livingstone; 1982.
2. Soderberg GL. *Kinesiology: Application to Pathological Motion.* 2nd ed. Baltimore: Williams & Wilkins; 1997.
3. Skalley TC, Terry GC, Teitge RA. The quantitative measurement of normal passive medial and lateral patellar motion limits. *Am J Sports Med.* 1993;21:728–732.
4. Laubenthal KN, Smidt GL, Kettelkamp DB. A quantitative analysis of knee motion during activities of daily living. *Phys Ther.* 1972;52:34–42.
5. Livingston LA, Stevenson JM, Olney SJ. Stairclimbing kinematics on stairs of differing dimensions. *Arch Phys Med Rehabil.* 1991;72:398–402.
6. Levangie PK, Norkin CC. *Joint Structure and Function. A Comprehensive Analysis.* 3rd ed. Philadelphia: FA Davis; 2001.
7. Smith LK, Weiss EL, Lehmkuhl LD. *Brunnstrom's Clinical Kinesiology.* 5th ed. Philadelphia: FA Davis; 1996.

Chapter 8: Ankle and Foot

1. Palpation

A. i. MTP joint abduction/adduction (moveable arm), MTP joint flexion/extension (moveable arm) and IP joint flexion/extensions (stationary arm)

ii. Subtalar joint inversion/eversion (axis)

iii. Ankle dorsiflexion/plantarflexion (stationary arm)

2. Assessment Process

i. True

ii. True

iii. True

iv. False-if ROM is WNL the therapist may not measure the PROM

3. Assessment of AROM at the Ankle and Foot

i. Ankle joint—dorsiflexion/plantarflexion (oblique sagittal plane/oblique frontal axis). Subtalar joint—inversion/eversion (oblique frontal plane/oblique sagittal axis). IP joints—flexion/extension (sagittal plane/frontal axis).

4. Assessment and Measurement of PROM at the Ankle and Foot

Ankle Dorsiflexion

i. Normal end feel is firm/hard.

ii. The knee is flexed about 20° to 30° to place the

gastrocnemius on slack and prevent shortness of gastrocnemius from restricting ankle dorsiflexion ROM.

iii. *Ankle joint*—The proximal concave articulating surface of the joint, commonly referred to as the ankle mortise, is formed by the medial aspect of the lateral malleolus, the distal tibia, and the lateral aspect of the medial malleolus. This concave surface is mated with the convex surface of the body of the talus.

Ankle Plantarflexion:

i. The forefoot is mobile and the hindfoot is immobile; therefore, the therapist would align the moveable arm of the goniometer with the hindfoot, more specifically parallel to the sole of the heel. This alignment will eliminate substitute forefoot movement from the measurement.

ii. During ankle plantarflexion, the convex surface of the body of the talus glides anteriorly on the fixed ankle mortise.

iii. Normal limiting factors: tension in the anterior joint capsule, anterior portion of the deltoid, anterior talofibular ligaments, and the ankle dorsiflexors; contact between the talus and the tibia. These structures create a firm or a hard end feel.

Subtalar inversion:

i. Lateral glide of the posterior facet of the calcaneus would be limited.

ii. Medial glide of the anterior and middle facets would be limited.

iii. The posterior facet of the calcaneus is a convex articular surface, and in accordance with the concave/convex theory of joint motion, the convex surface will move in the opposite direction to the movement of the bone. Therefore, when the calcaneus moves in a medial direction, the convex articular surface moves in a lateral direction on the fixed concave surface of the talus. The anterior articular surfaces of the calcaneus are concave, and in accordance with the concave/convex theory of joint motion, the concave surface will move in the same direction as the movement of the bone. Therefore, when the calcaneus moves in a medial direction, the concave articular surfaces also move in a medial direction.

Great Toe MTP Joint Extension:

i. The firm end feel would not be normal because the structures that produce the end feel restrict the PROM before the full PROM is achieved.

ii. Dorsal glide would be restricted because the articular surface of the distal end of the proximal phalanx of the great toe is concave, and in accordance with the concave/convex theory of joint motion, the concave surface will move in the same direction as the movement of the bone. The prox-

imal phalanx moves in a dorsal direction with great toe MTP joint extension; therefore, the proximal end of the proximal phalanx will also glide in a dorsal direction.

iii. The pattern of movement restriction at the MTP joint in the presence of a capsular pattern would be extension, flexion.

5. Muscle Length Assessment and Measurement

Gastrocnemius

i. *Origin* (1): Medial head: proximal and posterior aspect of the medial condyle of the femur posterior to the adductor tubercle; Lateral head: lateral and posterior aspect of the lateral condyle of the femur; lower part of the supracondylar line. *Insertion* (1): Via the Achilles tendon into the calcaneus.

ii. Knee extension and ankle dorsiflexion would place the muscle on stretch.

iii. Firm end feel would be noted if the gastrocnemius were shortened.

6. Functional ROM at the Ankle and Foot

A. 10° of ankle dorsiflexion; 20° of plantarflexion (from the Rancho Los Amigos gait analysis forms as cited in Levangie and Norkin [2])

B. i. *Ankle dorsiflexion*—descending stairs, rising from sitting, squatting to pick up an object from the floor.

ii. *Ankle plantarflexion*—reaching for a high object, depressing the accelerator of a car, ascending stairs.

iii. *Toe extension*—reaching for a high object, walking, squatting to pick up an object from the floor.

C. The ROM requirements for ADL are influenced by the design of the furniture used, the height of the step, and the patient's height. The start and the end positions and technique used to complete the activity also affect the ROM requirements. Therefore, these ROM values are a guide only.

i. Rise from sitting on a standard-height chair: 28° (3) ankle dorsiflexion.

ii. Descend a standard-height step: 21° to 36° (4) ankle dorsiflexion.

References
1. Soames RW, ed. Skeletal system. Salmons S, ed. Muscle. Gray's Anatomy. 38th ed. New York: Churchill Livingstone; 1995.
2. Levangie PK, Norkin CC. *Joint Structure & Function: A Comprehensive Analysis*. 3rd ed. Philadelphia: FA Davis; 2001.
3. Ikeda ER, Schenkman ML, Riley PO, Hodge WA. Influence of age on dynamics of rising from a chair. *Phys Ther*. 1991; 71:473–481.
4. Livingston LA, Stevenson JM, Olney SJ. Stairclimbing kinematics on stairs of differing dimensions. *Arch Phys Med Rehabil*. 1991;72:398–402.

Chapter 9: Head, Neck, and Trunk

1. Palpation

A. i. Landmarks: tip of the chin, suprasternal notch; other movements: neck extension.

ii. Landmarks: mastoid process, lateral aspect of the acromion process; other movements: none.

iii. Landmarks: spines of C7 and S2; or the suprasternal notch (with the patient in prone); other movements: thoracolumbar spine flexion (C7 and S2).

iv. Landmarks: spine of S2; point 15 cm proximal to the spine of S2; other movements: lumbar spine extension.

v. Landmarks: lateral aspect of the acromion process; the uppermost point of the iliac crest at the midaxillary line or the superior aspect of the greater trochanter; other movements: none.

B. i. Landmarks: vertex of the head, spine of T1 or spine of the scapula; other movements: neck flexion, neck lateral flexion.

ii. Landmarks: spines of C7 and S2; other movements: thoracolumbar spine flexion.

iii. Landmarks: spine of S2; point 15 cm proximal to the spine of S2; other movements: lumbar spine extension.

iv. Landmarks: spines of T1 and S2; other movements: none.

v. Landmarks: spines of T1 and T12; other movements: none.

C. It is not necessary to identify any surface anatomy locations when using the CROM to assess neck ROM.

2. Assessment and Measurement of AROM

TMJ Movements

i. Jaw movements: depression (mouth opening), occlusion (mouth closing), lateral deviation, protraction, and retraction.

ii. The proximal joint surface consists of the concave mandibular fossa, and the convex temporal articular eminence that lies anterior to the fossa. The proximal joint surface articulates with the reciprocally shaped superior surface of the articular disc that is anteroposteriorly concavoconvex. The inferior surface of the articular disc is concave and is mated with the convex condyle of the mandible to form the lower compartment of the TMJ.

iii. TMJ movements that can be measured with a rule are mandibular depression, lateral deviation, and protrusion.

iv. Functional ROM is determined for mouth opening by placing two or three flexed proximal interphalangeal joints between the upper and lower central

incisor teeth (1). The fingers represent a distance of about 35 to 50 mm (1).

Neck Extension

Neck extension ROM will be underestimated if the mouth is open during the tape measurement; therefore, the mouth should be closed when assessing neck ROM.

Neck Left Lateral Flexion

Substitute movements to be avoided: Elevation of the shoulder girdle to approximate the ear, ipsilateral trunk lateral flexion.

Neck Right Rotation

i. Start position: The patient is in supine.

ii. The inclinometer is positioned in the midline at the base of the forehead.

Thoracolumbar Spine Flexion

Thoracolumbar spine flexion can be measured using inclinometers positioned at C7 and S2.

Lumbar Spine Flexion

Lumbar spine can be measured using a tape measure and the same anatomical landmarks (i.e., spine of S2 and a point 15 cm above S2).

Thoracolumbar Spine Extension (Prone Press-up)

Factors that may result in inaccurate ROM measurements: if the upper extremities are weak, the patient may not be able to move the trunk through the full available trunk extension ROM; the pelvis being raised from the plinth during the test motion; the tape measure not being perpendicular to the plinth.

Thoracolumbar Spine Rotation

The anatomic landmarks: lateral aspect of the acromion process; the uppermost point of the iliac crest at the midaxillary line, or the superior aspect of the greater trochanter.

Thoracolumbar Spine Lateral Flexion

Substitute movements to avoid: trunk flexion, trunk extension, ipsilateral hip and knee flexion, raising the contralateral or ipsilateral foot from the floor.

3. Muscle Length Assessment and Measurement

i. False

ii. False

iii. True

4. Functional ROM at the Head, Neck and Truck

A. i. *Thoracolumbar flexion*: Squatting to pick up an object from the floor; sitting; placing dishes in a dishwasher.

ii. *Thoracolumbar extension*: Looking at or reaching for a book on a highshelf situated directly in front of you; lying prone on the elbows to read a book; throwing a ball.

iii. *Cervical spine rotation*: Looking both ways to cross the street; indicating a negative response to a question; looking behind when backing up a car.

iv. *Cervical spine lateral flexion*: Sitting and looking under the table for a dropped object; tilting the head to remove water from one's ear; moving one's head to the side when styling the hair using a blow dryer.

B. Trunk motions or movements of the feet to reposition the body are strategies that could be used to increase the field of vision.

C. i. *Sitting and tying a shoe with the foot flat on the floor*: Cervical spine extension, thoracic and lumbar spine flexion.

ii. *Combing the hair on the back of one's head*: Cervical spine rotation; may also include cervical spine extension and lateral flexion.

iii. *Brushing one's teeth*: TMJ depression (i.e., mouth opening).

iv. *Reaching for a wallet in a back pocket*: Thoracic and lumbar spine flexion and rotation.

Reference

1. Magee DJ. *Orthopedic Physical Assessment.* 4th ed. Philadelphia: Saunders; 2002.

Index

Note: Page numbers followed by *f* denote figures; those followed by *t* denote tables.